Principles of Research Design and Drug Literature Evaluation

Edited by

Rajender R. Aparasu, MPharm, PhD, FAPhA

Professor and Chair
Department of Pharmaceutical Health Outcomes and Policy
College of Pharmacy
University of Houston
Houston, Texas

John P. Bentley, RPh, PhD, FAPhA

Professor of Pharmacy Administration
Research Professor in the Research Institute of Pharmaceutical Sciences
School of Pharmacy
University of Mississippi
Oxford, Mississippi

JONES & BARTLETT
LEARNING

World Headquarters
Jones & Bartlett Learning
5 Wall Street
Burlington, MA 01803
978-443-5000
info@jblearning.com
www.jblearning.com

Jones & Bartlett Learning books and products are available through most bookstores and online booksellers. To contact Jones & Bartlett Learning directly, call 800-832-0034, fax 978-443-8000, or visit our website, www.jblearning.com.

Substantial discounts on bulk quantities of Jones & Bartlett Learning publications are available to corporations, professional associations, and other qualified organizations. For details and specific discount information, contact the special sales department at Jones & Bartlett Learning via the above contact information or send an email to specialsales@jblearning.com.

Production Credits

Executive Publisher: William Brottmiller
Executive Editor: Rhonda Dearborn
Editorial Assistant: Sean Fabery
Associate Director of Production: Julie C. Bolduc
Production Editor: Tina Chen
Marketing Manager: Grace Richards
VP, Manufacturing and Inventory Control:
  Therese Connell

Composition: diacriTech
Cover Design: Michael O'Donnell
Photo Research and Permissions Coordinator:
  Amy Rathburn
Cover Image: © Bocos Benedict/ShutterStock, Inc.
Printing and Binding: Edwards Brothers Malloy
Cover Printing: Edwards Brothers Malloy

To order this product, use ISBN: 978-1-284-03879-8

Library of Congress Cataloging-in-Publication Data
Principles of research design and drug literature evaluation/edited by Rajender R. Aparasu, John P. Bentley.
  p. ; cm.
Includes bibliographical references and index.
ISBN 978-1-4496-9130-1
I. Aparasu, Rajender R., editor of compilation. II. Bentley, John P. (John Paul), 1970- editor of compilation.
[DNLM: 1. Pharmacology. 2. Research Design. 3. Statistics as Topic. QV 20.5]
RM301.25
615.1072'4–dc23
                                        2013050973

6048

Printed in the United States of America
18 17 16 15 14   10 9 8 7 6 5 4 3 2 1

To my dear wife, Anu,
and to my lovely kids, Shravya and Saureesh
Aparasu

———————————

To my wife and partner, Sandy,
and to my teacher, mentor, and friend, Lon Larson
Bentley

CONTENTS

PREFACE

With the increasing emphasis on evidence-based practices, there is a greater need for pharmacists to understand clinical research, evaluate scientific findings, and translate evidence to support patient-care decisions. This requires a comprehensive understanding of the principles and practice of drug literature evaluation with a strong grounding in research design and statistical methods. Most available texts emphasize statistical approaches and/or scientific literature evaluation techniques. Although there may be comprehensive books in other health professions, it is challenging to find a pharmacy textbook that covers all critical research design and evaluation elements to translate evidence into practice. We decided to edit this book to provide a balanced approach to the principles of clinical research and statistics for evaluating pharmacy literature to implement evidence-based pharmacotherapy.

Most pharmacy schools offer a course in the pharmacy professional program that covers fundamentals of research design, biostatistics, and evaluation of pharmacy literature, as required by the Accreditation Council for Pharmacy Education (ACPE). Consequently, this book is divided into three sections to provide comprehensive course content to meet and exceed these curriculum standards set by the ACPE. Section 1 of the book covers principles of scientific research with an emphasis on clinical research designs ranging from randomized controlled trials to case reports. Section 2 of the book provides the foundation necessary to understand statistics and to critically evaluate results from statistical analyses reported in the medical literature with a focus on common statistical methods. Section 3 of the book covers principles of evidence-based medicine, drug literature sources and evaluation techniques, and application of evidence to patient care. There are seven chapters in each section of the book.

Chapter 1 defines basic, applied, clinical, and translational research, and describes the steps in scientific research and evidence-based medicine. Chapter 2 explains the guiding ethical principles in clinical research and discusses the regulatory framework governing clinical research. Chapter 3 provides the basics of designing clinical research, with an emphasis on common clinical research designs and methodologies. Chapter 4 discusses the design considerations associated with randomized controlled trials, including common clinical designs and analytical framework. Chapters 5 and 6 provide observational approaches for conducting clinical research. Chapter 5 describes case-control and cohort designs and includes a discussion of common biases and analytical approaches to minimize such biases. Chapter 6 provides an overview of cross-sectional studies, pre- and post-observational studies, ecological studies, and time series evaluations. Chapter 7 presents the key steps in designing a case report and case series studies along with tools to critically evaluate these designs.

Chapter 8 discusses the summarizing, organizing, and presenting functions of statistics, commonly referred to as descriptive statistics, and also introduces the different kinds of data that are collected in clinical research. Chapter 9 provides the general foundation for applying basic tools of statistical inference, focusing on the related mechanisms of estimation and hypothesis testing. Given that many studies in the drug literature involve the comparison of two or more groups, Chapter 10 discusses commonly used statistical procedures that are used to answer research questions involving group comparisons; in addition, it describes statistical methods for assessing the correlation between two variables. Chapters 11 and 12 provide an overview of regression analysis methods that can be used to account and/or adjust for variables that cannot be handled at the design stage of an experiment. Chapter 11 describes simple linear and multiple regression approaches to address a number of research problems, such as confounding and effect modification. Chapter 12 introduces logistic regression and Cox regression methods to analyze binary and time-to-event outcomes, respectively. Chapter 13 introduces the statistical principles' underlying sample size calculation. Chapter 14 presents the elements of the systematic review process and describes meta-analysis as a method to quantitatively synthesize evidence from studies identified in a systematic review.

Chapter 15 identifies the steps involved in evidence-based medicine along with the discussion of its strengths and limitations. Chapter 16 discusses the sources and use of primary, secondary, and tertiary literature to identify clinical evidence for evidence-based medicine. Chapters 17, 18, and 19 discuss approaches to assess published primary literature for patient care. Chapter 17 provides a stepwise approach to assess published literature with an emphasis on evaluating the study objectives, methods and design, statistics, results, and discussion. Chapter 18 describes the key considerations for evaluating methodological rigor in randomized controlled trials using an example. Chapter 19 describes and applies formal criteria to evaluate observational studies using an example. Chapter 20 discusses general principles of applying evidence to patient care with an emphasis on evidence from clinical trials and practice guidelines. Finally, Chapter 21 describes the general format of a journal club and examines the characteristics of an effective journal club.

This book is designed for professional pharmacy (PharmD) students. Instructors teaching principles of research and drug literature evaluation can design the professional course primarily based on this book or can supplement this book with research articles. The contents of the book can be delivered in one or two semesters. Chapters were written by expert authors specializing in pharmacy practice and research. Each chapter includes the following elements:

- *Learning Objectives* present the chapter's desired outcomes to the reader.
- *Key Terminology* helps the reader quickly identify critical new terms.
- *Review Questions* allow readers to apply what has been learned in the chapter and assess their understanding of the content.
- *Online Resources* direct students to web sites relevant to the content.

The chapters are designed to provide the knowledge base and application techniques for research design and drug literature evaluation. In addition to figures and tables, numerous pharmacy examples and case studies are provided to aid student learning. Additional readings from pharmacy journals and a drug literature evaluation project can improve the critical thinking skills of pharmacy students. The online sources and chapter references can be used to supplement the content. This book can also be an excellent resource for students in residency and fellowship training programs. In addition, this book can be beneficial to pharmacy practitioners and professionals, especially those involved in training students, residents, and fellows.

We would greatly appreciate feedback from students and faculty for future editions. All knowledge is considered as work in progress, including the contents of this book.

Rajender R. Aparasu, MPharm, PhD, FAPhA
John P. Bentley, RPh, PhD, FAPhA

INSTRUCTOR RESOURCES

Qualified instructors can receive the full suite of Instructor Resources, including the following:

- PowerPoint Presentations, featuring more than 600 slides
- Test Bank, containing more than 300 questions
- Answer Key, including answers for the end-of-chapter Review Questions

To gain access to these valuable teaching materials, contact your Health Professions Account Specialist at http://go.jblearning.com/findarep.

STUDENT RESOURCES

The Navigate Companion Website features numerous study aids and learning tools to help students get the most out of their course and prepare for class, including:

- Interactive Glossary
- Crossword Puzzles
- Interactive Flashcards
- Matching Questions
- Web Links

FOREWORD

When Drs. Aparasu and Bentley asked me to write the foreword for this book, I hesitated. It took me a long while to finally agree. I hesitated because a book's foreword is supposed to be written by someone famous who tells the readers why the authors are qualified to write the book and why the book is important. I hesitated because I could only fulfill two of the three conditions by writing the foreword to this book: the editors are eminently qualified and it is an important contribution to the library of students and practitioners. Both of the editors are seasoned, knowledgeable, and experienced with decades of direct involvement in evidence-based research. More importantly, they have convinced a veritable "who's who" of clinical trial, health services, and comparative effectiveness researchers and drug information experts to share their expertise, insights, and pearls of wisdom.

Second, why is this book important? Dr. Bentley and I served together on the editorial staff of the *Journal of the American Pharmacists Association* (*JAPhA*) for years. During our time together, we had innumerable discussions about the importance of study design and statistical methods to the appropriate interpretation and clinical application of research findings. Through these often lengthy discussions—discussions that we had more than once because they are difficult issues to resolve when interpreting a study's findings and conclusions—we came to understand the power of the statement "every study has limitations based on its design and statistical methods." It became abundantly clear to us that while these limitations are generally *listed* in a specific section designed for that purpose in most articles, the implications of those limitations are not. What does this statement mean? Let me provide an example to illustrate.

While a research article might list "confounding by severity" as a potential study limitation in an observational study, what are the implications of that bias for someone trying to use the information contained in the article in their practice? What cautions should the practitioner exercise in interpreting and adopting the researcher's conclusions into their personal practice? Should an author present the implications of various decisions a practitioner could make based on the limitations? Should the practitioner suddenly stop prescribing beta-agonist medications because a study found a greater risk of asthma-related deaths with increasing beta-agonist use? Should the practitioner deny additional use of the medication after a certain point? What are the implications of stopping or reducing the use of rescue inhalers among severely ill asthmatics? Disease severity is a potential confounder in observational studies. Severely ill patients need their rescue inhalers more frequently because their asthma is uncontrolled and, even then, they cannot all be rescued unless the underlying reason for life threatening asthma is directly addressed. This book was designed to provide and encourage practitioner's development and use of critical drug information evaluation skills through a deeper understanding of the foundational principles of study design and statistical methods. Because guidance on how a study's limited findings should *not* be used is rare, practitioners must understand and evaluate for themselves the veracity and implications of the inherently limited primary literature findings they use as sources of drug information to make evidence-based decisions together with their patients.

The editors organized the book into three supporting sections to meet their pedagogical goals and address practitioners' needs in translating research into practice. Section 1 is titled "Principles of Clinical Research." After a discussion of the scientific method and ethical considerations associated with research, Section 1 examines the strengths, weaknesses, and implications of major experimental and nonexperimental (e.g., observational) study designs. Section 2, "Statistical Principles and Data Analysis," introduces the reader to the principles of statistical methods, data analysis, and the interpretation of statistical results, including power analysis and systematic reviews. Finally, Section 3, "Principles of Drug Literature Evaluation," introduces the reader to the principles of drug literature evaluation. From the perspective of a former editor-in-chief of a pharmacy professional journal, Section 3 provides the most important applications for translating research into practice. Section 3 provides the reader with the skills needed to evaluate studies ranging from randomized controlled trials to observational studies. It facilitates the application of the information contained in these studies. Furthermore, it assists readers in their attempts to apply information from these studies, with their limitations, to support pharmacy practice and patient-care decisions—applications that are commonly lacking with simple lists of the study's limitations. Although Section 3 is the heart of the book, it cannot survive without the study design and statistical methods foundations.

Sometimes, the difference between a foreword and a book review gets blurred—even to the writer. However, one primer on writing a book foreword that I consulted stated "…in the conclusion, remind the readers why you are writing the foreword and why it matters." As health professionals, we are tasked with protecting the lives of our patients; it is our *sine qua non*. Unfortunately, as multiple examples in this book and the literature point out, published research is not without its shortcomings and failings. Therefore, as health professionals we must be able to evaluate the strengths, weaknesses, and implications of the evidence, both new and not-so-new, for ourselves. There is no such thing as the perfect study. As health professionals, we cannot simply rely on the lists and conclusions of others; we must be prepared to make decisions based on the scientific evidence for ourselves. Thanks to the editors, authors, and content of this book, you can now be more prepared than ever for translating research into practice.

L. Douglas Ried, PhD, FAPhA
Editor-in-Chief Emeritus
Journal of the American Pharmacists Association
Professor and Associate Dean for Academic Affairs
College of Pharmacy
University of Texas at Tyler
Tyler, Texas

ACKNOWLEDGEMENTS

Many individuals have contributed to the fruition of this book. The concepts and vision for this book have evolved over 18 years of teaching professional courses in research design, biostatistics, and drug literature evaluation. Feedback from pharmacy students and regular discussions with colleagues, especially Dr. Rebecca Baer at South Dakota State University (Aparasu) and Dr. Kim Adcock at the University of Mississippi (Bentley), were instrumental in developing the master plan for this book. Sincere thanks to all of the authors for patiently working with us in developing the chapter content and for contributing their expertise to this project. The feedback from the reviewers was very helpful in improving the content and formatting of the book. The insight and support of Dr. Albert Wertheimer was instrumental in undertaking this book.

We greatly appreciate Dr. Jeffrey Sherer for helping us recruit the authors for the third section of the book and overseeing the development of initial chapter outlines. Our gratitude also goes to several of our graduate students, who offered input from a student's perspective on several chapters. We also would like to thank our respective university and college/school faculty colleagues and administration teams for providing us the time and encouragement to complete this project. Finally, we are grateful to the publishing team, both past and present, at Jones & Bartlett Learning, especially Katey Birtcher, Teresa Reilly, and Sean Fabery, for their help and support. The editorial assistance of the production staff at Jones & Bartlett Learning, especially Tina Chen, is also very much appreciated.

Rajender R. Aparasu, MPharm, PhD, FAPhA
John P. Bentley, RPh, PhD, FAPhA

ABOUT THE EDITORS

Rajender R. Aparasu, MPharm, PhD, FAPhA, is a Professor and Chair of the Department of Pharmaceutical Health Outcomes and Policy at the University of Houston College of Pharmacy. He has more than 18 years of experience in teaching and research in the area of pharmaceutical practice and policy. He has taught various professional and graduate courses in colleges of pharmacy. Dr. Aparasu is a recognized educational leader and researcher in pharmaceutical practice and policy. He was instrumental in the growth of graduate programs at the University of Houston to train the next generation of pharmacy leaders. He led the creation of one of the largest MS/Residency programs in the country in collaboration with six Texas Medical Center institutions in Houston. He has served on patient safety and medication therapy management task forces.

Dr. Aparasu has received several federal and non-federal grants to address a broad array of quality of pharmaceutical care issues, especially among the elderly. He is a peer-reviewer for numerous pharmacy and medical journals and has more than 100 presentations in national/international meetings and more than 70 peer-reviewed publications. He serves on the editorial boards of several pharmacy and healthcare journals, and has been recognized as an Exceptional Peer Reviewer by several journals. Dr. Aparasu is a grant reviewer for the American Heart Association (AHA) and the Patient-Centered Outcomes Research Institute (PCORI). He is an Associate Editor of *BMC Geriatrics* and has edited a book for graduate students titled *Research Methods for Pharmaceutical Practice and Policy*. He was recognized by his peers as a 2012 Fellow of the American Pharmacists Association for his exemplary professional achievements in practice and outstanding service to the profession.

John P. Bentley, RPh, PhD, FAPhA, is a Professor of Pharmacy Administration and a Research Professor in the Research Institute of Pharmaceutical Sciences at The University of Mississippi School of Pharmacy. In the professional pharmacy curriculum, Dr. Bentley teaches elements of research design, biostatistics, epidemiology, and drug literature evaluation. At the graduate level, he teaches several applied statistics courses, including general linear models, multivariate statistics, and elective courses focusing on the application of modern longitudinal data analysis methods and principles of statistical mediation and moderation. He has conducted research projects in a variety of areas, including quality of life; medication adherence; medication use, misuse, and outcomes; pharmaceutical marketing and patient behavior; patients' evaluation of health-care providers; pharmacy practice management; tobacco use, control, and cessation among college students; and ethics and professionalism. His statistics research interests include statistical mediation analysis and longitudinal data analysis.

Dr. Bentley has worked as a member of a number of interdisciplinary research teams and has consulted with numerous researchers concerning statistical analysis. In 2009, he was named a Fellow of the American Pharmacists Association and has been recognized as a Thelma Cerniglia Distinguished Teaching Scholar at The University of Mississippi School of Pharmacy. He has served as a peer reviewer for a number of journals and as an Associate Editor for the *Journal of the American Pharmacists Association*. Dr. Bentley received his BS in pharmacy and MBA from Drake University, his MS and PhD in pharmacy administration from The University of Mississippi, and his MS and PhD in biostatistics from The University of Alabama at Birmingham (UAB).

CONTRIBUTORS

Sandra L. Alfano, PharmD, FASHP, CIP
Research Scientist, General Internal Medicine
Chair, Human Investigation Committee I and III
Co-Chair, Embryonic Stem Cell Research Oversight Committee
Yale University
New Haven, Connecticut

Bismark Baidoo, PhD
Research Associate
Department of Pharmacy Practice and Science
College of Pharmacy
The University of Arizona
Tucson, Arizona

Karen Blumenschein, PharmD
Associate Professor, Pharmacy Practice and Science Department
Associate Professor, Martin School of Public Policy and Administration
College of Pharmacy
University of Kentucky
Lexington, Kentucky

Thomas C. Dowling, PharmD, PhD, FCCP
Associate Professor and Vice Chair
Department of Pharmacy Practice and Science
School of Pharmacy
University of Maryland
Baltimore, Maryland

Joel F. Farley, PhD
Associate Professor
Division of Pharmaceutical Outcomes and Policy
Eshelman School of Pharmacy
University of North Carolina
Chapel Hill, North Carolina

McKenzie C. Ferguson, PharmD, BCPS
Assistant Professor
Department of Pharmacy Practice
Southern Illinois University Edwardsville
Edwardsville, Illinois

Lori A. Fischbach, PhD, MPH
Associate Professor
Department of Epidemiology
Fay W. Boozman College of Public Health
University of Arkansas for Medical Sciences
Little Rock, Arkansas

Daniel L. Friesner, PhD
Professor of Pharmacy Practice &
Associate Dean for Student Affairs and Faculty Development
College of Pharmacy, Nursing, and Allied Sciences
North Dakota State University
Fargo, North Dakota

Amie Goodin, MPP
Research Administrative Coordinator
Institute for Pharmaceutical Outcomes and Policy
University of Kentucky
Lexington, Kentucky

Richard A. Hansen, PhD
Gilliland Professor and Head
Department of Health Outcomes Research and Policy
Harrison School of Pharmacy
Auburn University
Auburn, Alabama

Spencer E. Harpe, PharmD, PhD, MPH
Associate Professor of Pharmacy Practice
Chicago College of Pharmacy
Midwestern University
Downers Grove, Illinois

Catherine L. Hatfield, PharmD
Clinical Associate Professor
Director, Introductory Pharmacy Practice Experiences
Department of Clinical Sciences and Administration
College of Pharmacy
University of Houston
Houston, Texas

Jill T. Johnson, PharmD, BCPS
Associate Professor
Department of Pharmacy Practice
College of Pharmacy
University of Arkansas for Medical Sciences
Little Rock, Arkansas

Rahul Khanna, PhD
Assistant Professor of Pharmacy Administration
Research Assistant Professor in the Research Institute of Pharmaceutical Sciences
School of Pharmacy
University of Mississippi
Oxford, Mississippi

Chenghui Li, PhD
Assistant Professor
Division of Pharmaceutical Evaluation and Policy
College of Pharmacy
University of Arkansas for Medical Sciences
Little Rock, Arkansas

Bradley C. Martin, PharmD, PhD
Professor and Division Head
Division of Pharmaceutical Evaluation and Policy
College of Pharmacy
University of Arkansas for Medical Sciences
Little Rock, Arkansas

Jane R. Mort, PharmD
Professor of Pharmacy Practice
Associate Dean for Academic Programs
College of Pharmacy
South Dakota State University
Brookings, South Dakota

Jeffrey T. Sherer, PharmD, MPH, BCPS
Clinical Associate Professor
Department of Clinical Sciences and Administration
College of Pharmacy
Texas Medical Center Campus
Houston, Texas

Olayinka O. Shiyanbola, PhD
Assistant Professor of Social and Administrative Sciences
School of Pharmacy
University of Wisconsin-Madison
Madison, Wisconsin

Marion K. Slack, PhD
Professor
Department of Pharmacy Practice and Science
College of Pharmacy
The University of Arizona
Tucson, Arizona

Steven M. Smith, PharmD, MPH
Assistant Professor
Departments of Pharmacotherapy & Translational Research and Community Health
Colleges of Pharmacy and Medicine
University of Florida
Gainesville, Florida

Erin M. Timpe Behnen, PharmD, BCPS
Associate Professor of Pharmacy Practice
Director, Drug Information & Wellness Center
Southern Illinois University Edwardsville
Edwardsville, Illinois

Katy E. Trinkley, PharmD
Assistant Professor, Department of Clinical Pharmacy
Skaggs School of Pharmacy and Pharmaceutical Sciences
University of Colorado
Aurora, Colorado

REVIEWERS

Joyce Addo-Atuah, PhD
Assistant Professor of Pharmacy & Health Outcomes
College of Pharmacy
Touro College
New York City, New York

Miriam A. Ansong, RPh, EMBA, PharmD
Director, Center for Global Health Education and Resources
Associate Professor of Pharmacy Practice
School of Pharmacy
Cedarville University
Cedarville, Ohio

Aleda M. H. Chen, PharmD, MS, PhD
Assistant Professor of Pharmacy Practice
School of Pharmacy
Cedarville University
Cedarville, Ohio

Chad A. Knoderer, PharmD
Associate Professor of Pharmacy Practice
College of Pharmacy and Health Sciences
Butler University
Indianapolis, Indiana

Anandi V. Law, BPharm, MS, PhD, FAACP, FAPhA
Professor and Chair
Department of Pharmacy Practice and Administration
College of Pharmacy
Western University of Health Sciences
Pomona, California

Quang A. Le, PharmD, PhD
Assistant Professor
College of Pharmacy
Western University of Health Sciences
Pomona, California

PRINCIPLES OF CLINICAL RESEARCH

THE SCIENTIFIC APPROACH TO RESEARCH AND PRACTICE

Rajender R. Aparasu, MPharm, PhD, FAPhA

CHAPTER OBJECTIVES

▸ Define basic, applied, clinical, and translational research
▸ Understand the principles of scientific inquiry
▸ Describe the steps in scientific research and evidence-based practice
▸ Discuss the scientific basis of professional education

KEY TERMINOLOGY

Abstract
Analytical research
Applied research
Basic research
Biomedical research
Clinical research
Comparative effectiveness
   research
Descriptive research
Development
Discussion section
Empiricism
Ethics

Evidence-based
   medicine
Hypothesis
Introduction section
Journal article
Method section
Objectivity
Patient-centered
   outcomes research
Pharmaceutical practice
   and policy research
Positivism
Posters

Practice-based
   research network
Primary methods
Quality
Research
Research and development
Research design
Research methodology
Research report
Results section
Secondary methods
Theory
Translational research

INTRODUCTION

Pharmacists are a vital component of healthcare delivery and biomedical systems. Medications and clinical services are integral to the myriad roles pharmacists play in the healthcare system. Pharmaceutical research and development is instrumental in the discovery of new medications and pharmaceutical formulations. There are more than 10,000 prescription products and more than 300,000 over-the-counter products in the marketplace.[1] This is mainly attributed to research and development in basic sciences such as biology, chemistry, biochemistry, and microbiology, and applied sciences such as pharmacology, pharmaceutics, and pharmacotherapy. During the past few decades, there has been significant growth of clinical pharmacy services to meet the complexities of delivering pharmaceutical care in diverse healthcare settings. Pharmacists provide a broad range of outpatient services, such as medication therapy management, immunizations, and health screenings, and inpatient services ranging from nutrition to therapeutic drug monitoring in institutional settings. High-quality research is vital to developing new medications and clinical services; it also provides the knowledge base to effectively use these products and services.

Pharmacists have an important role to play in creating and applying scientific evidence. Although pharmacists are mostly consumers of research information, they contribute immensely to the growing scientific knowledge base relevant to the pharmacy profession. Pharmacists involved in research make a vital difference by providing evidence that others can use. This knowledge is also important in academia to train the next generation of pharmacists. In recent years, practice-based innovations have created new models in delivering pharmaceutical care. With the increasing role of evidence-based paradigms, there is greater need to critically apply and evaluate research for pharmaceutical practice and policy. Both creating and applying research evidence require an understanding of the principles of research design. This chapter defines biomedical research and evolving clinical research paradigms relevant to the pharmacy practice. It discusses the principles of research design and steps involved in scientific research inquiry. Finally, the concept of evidence-based medicine is introduced to effectively translate scientific evidence to patient care.

BIOMEDICAL RESEARCH

Pharmaceuticals and pharmacists are vital for healthcare delivery. Research drives the increasing role of pharmaceuticals and pharmaceutical services in disease state management. The National Science Foundation (NSF) has defined **research** as "systematic study directed toward fuller scientific knowledge or understanding of the subject studied."[2] **Biomedical research** is a broad area that deals with research in biological and medical sciences to understand and improve the health of patients and populations. Biomedical research can be further classified as *basic* or *applied* based on the goals of the research. **Basic research** is defined as "systematic study directed toward fuller knowledge or understanding of the fundamental aspects of phenomena and of observable facts without specific applications toward processes or products in mind."[2] It is usually conducted in laboratories to provide knowledge and understanding of natural phenomena. Some areas of inquiry in basic biomedical research are biology, physiology, biochemistry, and genetics. Although scientists involved in basic research are only focused on generalized knowledge, this knowledge is critical for applied research that is product or application oriented.

Applied research is defined as "systematic study to gain [the] knowledge or understanding necessary to determine the means by which a recognized and specific need may be met."[2] It focuses on applying basic knowledge for the purpose of developing a product or an application such as a new medication, drug regimen, or service. It has practical orientation rather than the explanation focus that is inherent in basic research. It is conducted in animals and other living systems to solve a practical problem or to create a product. Some areas of inquiry in applied biomedical research are pharmacology, medicinal chemistry, and pharmaceutics. Research and development in applied biomedical research is the engine for the pharmaceutical industry.

Drug development is specifically focused on developing new drug products. **Development** is defined as "systematic application of knowledge or understanding, directed toward the production of useful materials, devices, and systems or methods."[2] **Research and development** (R&D) refers to "creative work undertaken on a systematic basis in order to increase the stock of knowledge, including knowledge of man, culture and society, and the use of this stock of knowledge to devise new applications."[2] In the pharmaceutical industry, R&D is an expensive and time-consuming process. It takes an average of 15 years for a new product to enter the market at an average cost of $1.2 billion because of complex development, testing, legal, and regulatory considerations.[3]

Clinical research plays a vital role in the drug development process because approval of a drug by the Food and Drug Administration (FDA) requires clinical trials to demonstrate the safety and efficacy of pharmaceutical products. The National Institutes of Health (NIH) has defined **clinical research** as "research that either directly involves a particular person or group of people or uses materials from humans, such as their behavior or samples of their tissue."[4] Specifically, it is "any investigation in human subjects intended to discover or verify the clinical, pharmacological, and/or other pharmacodynamic effects of an investigational product(s), and/or to identify any adverse reactions to an investigational product(s), and/or to study absorption, distribution, metabolism, and excretion of an investigational product(s) with the object of ascertaining its safety and/or efficacy."[5] Clinical research helps in understanding and applying knowledge for products or processes in prevention, diagnosis, prognosis, treatment, and cure of diseases in humans. It is conducted in laboratories, healthcare settings, and other specialized locations according to regulatory guidelines.

Clinical research includes patient-oriented research, epidemiological and behavioral research, and health services research.[4] Patient-oriented research examines the mechanisms of human diseases, effects of drug therapies and other interventions, and use of technologies and devices in humans. Epidemiological and behavioral research evaluates the distribution of and factors associated with diseases, health behavior, and health in general. Health services research evaluates the effectiveness and efficiency of treatment, interventions, and services in real-world practice. All facets of clinical research are important to improve the health of patients. Clinical research involving pharmaceuticals and pharmacy services is vital to improving the quality of pharmaceutical care.

Pharmaceutical practice and policy research is a component of health services research that deals with issues related to pharmaceuticals, pharmacist services, and pharmacy systems. It is defined as a "multidisciplinary field of scientific investigation that examines cost, access, and quality of pharmaceutical care from clinical, sociobehavioral, economic, organizational, and technological perspectives."[6] The goal of pharmaceutical practice and policy research is to increase knowledge and understanding of pharmaceuticals, pharmacist services, and pharmacy systems for individuals and populations. New areas such as pharmacoepidemiology, pharmacoeconomics, pharmaceutical outcome research, and pharmacy practice-based research are evolving and expanding the research frontiers of pharmaceutical practice and policy research. This evidence base is critical to expanding the scope and role of pharmacists and pharmacy systems.

EVOLVING RESEARCH PARADIGMS

Translational research is the new clinical research paradigm for transferring knowledge across the research and practice continuum. According to the NIH, **translational research** includes "two areas of translation: The first area is the process of applying discoveries generated during research in the laboratory, and in pre-clinical studies, to the development of trials and studies in humans. The second area of translation concerns research aimed at enhancing the adoption of best practices in the community."[7] The first area of translation is designed to improve the trajectory of research from laboratory to patient care. This is critical for diseases such as cancer and acquired immunodeficiency syndrome (AIDS) that are in need of products to cure or treat their devastating effects. The second area of translation is gaining the support of scientists, clinicians, educators, and funding agencies to rapidly adopt evidence-based patient care practices. According to the Institute of Medicine (IOM), there is a significant gap between what patients are receiving and what they should receive, leading to a quality chasm in health care.[8] Translational research and evidence-based medicine can be instrumental in bridging this quality gap.

In recent years, there is significant interest in comparative effectiveness research due to limited data comparing two therapies, interventions, or devices. The demand for comparative effectiveness data is apparent as most clinicians want such data for clinical decisions. The efficacy data derived from placebo-controlled clinical trials are designed for the drug approval process. Comparative effectiveness research is based on the concepts of evaluation of alternatives so that the research can be used to select appropriate agents from among the alternatives to optimize patient outcomes. **Comparative effectiveness research** is the "generation and synthesis of evidence that compares the benefits and harms of alternative methods to prevent, diagnose, treat, and monitor a clinical condition or to improve delivery of care."[9] The goal of comparative research is to provide information to decision makers at both the individual and population levels.

With increasing focus on patient-centered care, a new type of clinical research called **patient-centered outcomes research** (PCOR) has evolved. PCOR is designed to incorporate patients' input in the research process and to provide relevant information to providers and patients for deciding on healthcare choices. PCOR "helps people and their caregivers communicate and make informed healthcare decisions, allowing their voices to be heard in assessing the value of healthcare options."[10] For pharmaceutical products and services, the goal of PCOR is to "assess the benefits and harms of preventive, diagnostic, therapeutic, or health delivery system interventions to inform decision making, highlighting comparisons and outcomes that matter to people."[11] The incorporation of patient-relevant outcomes is a new phenomenon as traditional clinical research, until now, emphasized outcomes from the clinician's perspective. In an effort to generate evidence for patient-oriented outcomes, the federal government has created the Patient-Centered Outcomes Research Institute (PCORI), which will fund research on (1) assessment of prevention, diagnosis, and treatment options, (2) improving access and care in healthcare systems, (3) communication and dissemination research for shared decision making, (4) addressing disparities in prevention, diagnosis, or treatment effectiveness, and (5) accelerating patient-centered outcomes research and methodological research.[11]

DETERMINANTS OF SCIENTIFIC METHODOLOGY

All scientific research is bound by principles of scientific inquiry. These include empiricism, objectivity, theory, and ethical standards.[6] **Empiricism** refers to a collection of information based on human experience. It is based on the philosophy of **positivism** that states that all information derived from sensory experience is empirical evidence of science. All aspects of science should be observed and measured to be considered scientific evidence. All clinical outcomes in research are explicitly defined and measured to be considered evidence to evaluate the safety and effectiveness of medications. Measurement and quantification are vital for scientific research. **Objectivity** means there is no subjectivity or bias in any aspect of research including definition, measurement, design, and analysis. In clinical research, the measures to define effectiveness, such as blood pressure and blood glucose, are objective, and the measurement process is often blinded to minimize any kind of subjectivity. All biases in research are minimized to increase the strength of scientific evidence.

Theory provides an understanding or explanation of natural phenomena. Theories evolve over years or decades to explain natural phenomena. In pharmaceutical research, theories are often based on the pathophysiology of a disease and the pharmacology of a medication to investigate its effects. Sociobehavioral theories are often used to understand patient and provider behavior in pharmaceutical practice and policy research. Theories are also useful in developing a research hypothesis. They provide the rationale and logic for a research question and hypothesis. Research findings are used to strengthen or dispute a theory. **Ethics** provide moral societal standards for responsible research conduct. These standards are based on respect for, fairness to, and the well-being of research participants.[12] The standards are often governed by institutional review board (IRB), state, and federal regulations. To reflect all these principles in research, Kerlinger has defined scientific research as a "systematic, controlled, empirical, and critical investigation guided by theory and hypothesis about presumed relationships among such phenomena."[13]

PROCESS OF SCIENTIFIC INQUIRY

The scientific research process involves the following steps: (1) pose a research question and hypothesis, (2) develop and implement a research plan, (3) perform data collection and analysis, and (4) prepare a research report.[6] Each of these steps is critical for scientific inquiry. The research question or hypothesis dictates the research plans and data collection. Often, practical and scientific considerations necessitate overlap of these steps of the research process. The following description uses a clinical and translational research framework to explain the research steps (**Figure 1-1**).

The first step in the scientific research process is to pose a research question and hypothesis. It is important to develop a research question that needs empirical investigation. The commonly used sources for a research question are clinical practice, policy, current issue, literature, or theory. The desirable characteristics of a research question are that it is feasible, interesting, novel, ethical, and relevant (FINER).[14] Practical considerations, such as funding, expertise, environment, and access to patient care data, are also important to address the feasibility of the research. The novelty aspect of the research question can be evaluated by conducting a literature review. The goal of the research is to add something new to the existing evidence base. The ethical principles of research are governed by local IRBs and federal regulations. This requires appropriate regulatory approvals to conduct clinical research. Research relevant to the pharmacy profession should have strong implications for pharmaceutical practice and policy. Research that is not relevant will have limited value to stakeholders such as patients, providers, payers, and policy makers. These considerations will not only help develop a good research question but also ensure value for the research (**Box 1–1**).

The population, intervention, comparator, outcomes, timeline, and setting (PICOTS) framework is often used to develop a good clinical question. This framework is ideal for comparing interventions such as medications, devices, clinical services, policies, and programs. It also provides the components of a research question.[15,16] The PICOTS framework requires the research question to identify the population to be studied, the intervention to be applied, the comparator to be used, the outcomes to be evaluated, the timeline to evaluate the outcomes, and the healthcare setting of interest (**Figure 1–2**).

The population of interest can be grouped based on age, disease, or location. The intervention is usually a pharmaceutical product or service. The comparator can be an

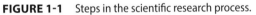

1 • Pose a research question and hypothesis

2 • Develop and implement a research plan

3 • Perform data collection and analysis

4 • Prepare a research report

FIGURE 1-1   Steps in the scientific research process.

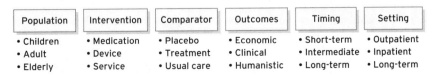

| **BOX 1-1** | **Research Question and Hypothesis** |

Question: In patients with diabetes, do clinical services by pharmacists improve short-term clinical outcomes compared with traditional care in an outpatient setting?

Hypothesis: Clinical services by pharmacists will improve short-term clinical outcomes in outpatients with diabetes compared to traditional care.

Data from Irons BK, Lenz RJ, Anderson SL, et al. *Pharmacotherapy*. 2002;22:1294–1300; and Choe HM, Mitrovich S, Dubay D, et al. *Am J Manag Care*. 2005;11:253–260.

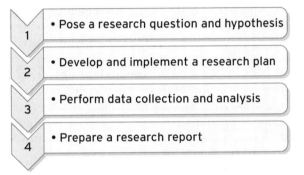

Population	Intervention	Comparator	Outcomes	Timing	Setting
• Children	• Medication	• Placebo	• Economic	• Short-term	• Outpatient
• Adult	• Device	• Treatment	• Clinical	• Intermediate	• Inpatient
• Elderly	• Service	• Usual care	• Humanistic	• Long-term	• Long-term

FIGURE 1-2   Components of a scientific research question with examples.

active medication/service or a placebo based on the goals of the research. The economic, clinical, and humanistic outcomes (ECHOs) are usually evaluated in pharmaceutical practice and policy research.[17] Costs of direct and indirect medical care are often included as economic outcomes. Clinical outcomes include morbidity and mortality measures that represent the safety and effectiveness of treatment. Humanistic outcomes include patient-reported outcomes such as health-related quality of life and functional status. The timeline for research can be short-term or long-term based on the expected effects of pharmaceutical products or services.

In addition, research can be classified as descriptive or analytical. **Descriptive research** describes or explores characteristics of a population such as prevalence of disease. **Analytical research** evaluates the relationship between two or more variables. A **hypothesis** specifies an expected relationship that is being evaluated between intervention/exposure and outcome, or two or more variables. The hypothesis is often based on existing theories. The pathophysiology of disease and pharmacology of medication provide the rationale for expected effects of pharmaceutical products. The expected relationship between clinical intervention and outcomes is usually postulated based on sociobehavioral theories. Research hypothesis is not usually specified in descriptive or exploratory research.

Developing and implementing a research plan requires a strong understanding of the principles of clinical research. Research plans include specific details of research design and methodology. Grant proposals have other requirements, such as timeline and funding details, in addition to research plans. These plans are implemented after the necessary approvals by the local IRB. **Research design** refers to the overall plan that allows researchers to gather answers to study questions and test study hypotheses.[18] The research designs can be broadly categorized into two types—experimental and observational. Experimental designs such as randomized controlled trials are the strongest study designs to test research hypotheses. The randomized designs are considered the gold standard in clinical research and are used to evaluate drug safety and efficacy. Observational research such as cohort or cross-sectional studies provides evidence of associations or relationships. The evidence from observational research is generally weaker than that from randomized controlled trials due to scientific considerations such as confounding and biases. Study design provides a structural framework for experimental or observational research.[6] Various other study designs are available to address the research question; the goal is to select the best design that can address the research question.

Research methodology provides details of data collection and measurement techniques.[6] The definitions and the measurement process of intervention and outcomes are specified in the methods. Research methods are broadly grouped as primary or secondary methods. **Primary methods** collect data specifically for research questions using techniques such as self-reported observations and biological assessments; examples include surveys and laboratory tests. These are often collected prospectively—that is, data collection begins after the study onset. **Secondary methods** involve the use of data that were collected for other purposes such as patient care or reimbursement; examples include medical charts and medical claims. These are retrospective in nature—that is, data are based on past events or existing data. Prospective methods are generally considered superior to retrospective methods because the researcher controls the data collection methods. The goal of research methods is to collect research data that are reliable (consistent) and valid (accurate). Researchers have a choice of research methods; the goal is to select the most appropriate method to collect research data (**Box 1-2**).

The research design and methodology define the data management and analysis plans. Data collected from all sources should be recorded at the patient level or other

---

BOX 1-2   Research Plan

Design:

- Choe HM et al. used randomized controlled trials to evaluate the effect of clinical services by pharmacists on glycemic control and other process measures in diabetes patients.
- Irons BK et al. used a retrospective cohort design to evaluate the clinical effectiveness of clinical services by a pharmacist in primary care for patients with diabetes.

Methods:

- Choe HM et al. prospectively collected data on glycosylated hemoglobin using a high-performance liquid chromatography machine and other secondary data were collected using chart review.
- Irons BK et al. used secondary sources like medical charts to collect data related glycosylated hemoglobin and other secondary outcomes for the study population.

BOX 1-3   Data Collection and Analysis

- Choe HM et al. analyzed data collected using Wilcoxon rank sum test and linear regression analysis. A level of $p < .05$ was set to define statistical significance.
- Irons BK et al. analyzed data collected using t-test, chi-square, analysis of variance, and Cox regression models. Two-sided tests were performed with an a priori alpha level of 0.05.

---

units of analysis to conduct appropriate statistical analyses. Data collected from surveys and laboratory tests should be gathered and coded accordingly. Similarly, data from secondary sources should be extracted and coded. Although data collection seems easy, it is often tedious and time consuming because any error can undermine the data integrity and subsequent steps in the research including statistical analyses. Statistical analysis provides the quantitative answers to the research question. It is a tool to organize, summarize, and analyze research data. Several descriptive and inferential statistics are used to analyze the data. The descriptive measures such as means, medians, and modes are often used to summarize study sample characteristics. Inferential statistics such as the t-test and analysis of variance are used to make inferences or draw conclusions based on the data collected. The appropriate statistical test is selected based on the research question, research hypothesis, research design, and methods (**Box 1-3**).

Research reports or journal articles are vital to communicate research findings to stakeholders such as patients, providers, payers, and policy makers. The **research report** or **journal article** is a detailed report that often includes the following sections: introduction, methods, results, and discussion (IMRaD).[19] It is generally peer reviewed to ensure scientific discourse and scrutiny. The **posters** are often used for a graphic/visual presentation of research in scientific conferences usually employing the IMRaD format (**Figure 1-3**).

The **abstract** is a structured summary of research to provide quick and easy-to-use information to readers. The **introduction section** of a research report or journal article includes relevant background information and covers existing literature on

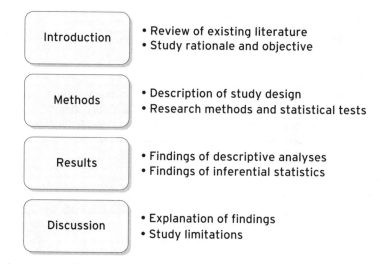

Introduction
- Review of existing literature
- Study rationale and objective

Methods
- Description of study design
- Research methods and statistical tests

Results
- Findings of descriptive analyses
- Findings of inferential statistics

Discussion
- Explanation of findings
- Study limitations

FIGURE 1-3   Components of a research report.

BOX 1-4   Key Findings and Research Report

- Choe HM et al. found a significant decrease (−2.1%) in glycosylated hemoglobin levels in the intervention group when compared to the decrease in the control group (−0.9%). Significant improvements were also seen in other process of care measures. The other results can be found in the research report.
- Irons BK et al. found no difference in glycosylated hemoglobin between the two groups. However, there was higher risk (5.19, 95% CI 2.62–10.26) of achieving the clinical goal (A1C ≤ 7%) in the study group compared to the control group. The other results can be found in the research report.

---

the subject. It provides a rationale for conducting the research. It specifies the research objective or question and research hypothesis. The **method section** includes descriptions of research design, data collection methods, and statistical tests. The **results section** describes the research findings based on the statistical analyses. The study sample is often summarized using descriptive statistics and graphs. Inferential statistics usually include confidence intervals and probability or p values. The results section provides quantitative answers to the research question. This is the most objective and unbiased section of the research report. The **discussion section** provides the interpretation and explanation of the research findings using previous research or theory. It also addresses possible limitations and future directions of the research (**Box 1-4**).

EVIDENCE-BASED MEDICINE

The goal of clinical research is to provide scientific evidence to improve the health and functioning of people. Healthcare providers, payers, and policy makers are all interested in ensuring delivery of the highest-quality patient care. **Quality** in health care refers to "the degree to which health services for individuals and populations increase the likelihood of desired health outcomes and are consistent with current professional knowledge."[20] According to the IOM, all stakeholders in health care should pursue the following six aims in the delivery of quality health care.[8] Quality health care should be (1) safe: avoid harm to patients from the healthcare delivery; (2) effective: deliver care that benefits patients; (3) patient-centered: individualize care based on patient preferences and values; (4) timely: ensure timely, needed care and avoid delays; (5) efficient: maximize the use of healthcare resources; and (6) equitable: provide care that does not vary due to personal characteristics—race or ethnicity—and minimize healthcare disparities at the individual and population levels. To achieve these aims, patients and populations should receive health care that is based on the best scientific evidence (**Figure 1-4**).

The core of **evidence-based medicine** (EBM) is to translate scientific evidence to patient care. There are several definitions of EBM. Some initially emphasize the translational aspect of evidence to practice because a "process of systematically finding, appraising, and using contemporaneous research findings as the basis for clinical decisions."[21] Others define EBM holistically as "integration of best research evidence with clinical expertise and patient values."[22] The holistic definition is the one that is most widely accepted and practiced because it not only emphasizes scientific evidence but also incorporates expertise of clinicians and patient preferences. Clinical expertise includes the knowledge, skills, and experience of practitioners to integrate evidence with patient preferences. Any care that is not patient-centered will have limited value because treatment success is dependent on individualization. This holistic approach lends equal importance to evidence (scientific), expertise (provider), and values (patient) to achieve the desired patient outcomes.

Because scientific evidence is the core of EBM, the following steps of EBM are evidence centered: (1) asking an appropriate and answerable question, (2) finding evidence, (3) appraising evidence, and (4) applying evidence to practice.[22] A simplified example is presented in **Figure 1-5**.

Each step is important to ensure that relevant evidence is obtained and combined with clinical expertise and patient values to deliver EBM. An understanding of the scientific research process and value of research evidence is critical in

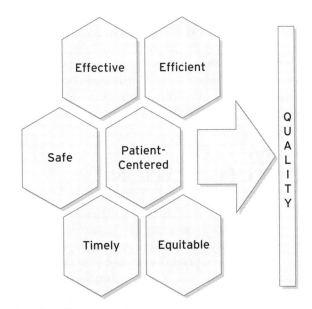

FIGURE 1-4 Six aims of quality improvements.

Data from Committee on Quality of Health Care in America. Institute of Medicine of the National Academies. *Crossing the Quality Chasm: A New Health System for the 21st Century.* Washington, DC: National Academies Press; 2001.

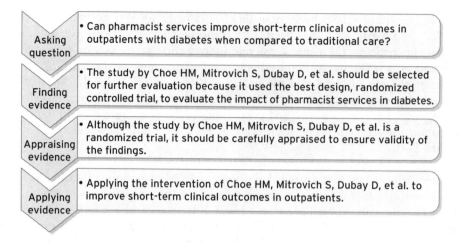

FIGURE 1-5   Example of evidence-based medicine.

Data from Choe HM, Mitrovich S, Dubay D, et al. Proactive case management of high-risk patients with type 2 diabetes mellitus by a clinical pharmacist: a randomized controlled trial. *Am J Manag Care.* 2005 Apr;11(4):253-60.

implementing EBM. If the goal of pharmaceutical practice and policy research is to develop an evidence base for pharmaceuticals, pharmacist services, and pharmacy systems, then the goal of EBM is to use the relevant scientific evidence to provide highest-quality patient care.

The research problem or question is the starting point for research. Similarly, asking the appropriate question is the starting point for providing EBM. The components of the question should include patient, intervention, comparator, and outcome (PICO). The relevant evidence is obtained after scouting for the evidence from various sources. The most relevant research is then critically appraised to ensure the validity and applicability of the evidence to patient care. This is often a time-consuming and critical process in EBM. Just because research is published in a peer-reviewed journal does not mean it is relevant or applicable to patient care.

The understanding of scientific principles is important to ensure that relevant evidence is valid and applicable. Critical appraisal of the selected research will ensure that research findings are correct (internal validity) and are applicable to the clinician's patient population (external validity). The best available and valid evidence is applied to provide patient-centered care. Medical decision making is a complex process with critical consequences; therefore, it requires "conscientious use, explicit, and judicious use of current best evidence in making decisions about the care of individual patients."[23]

SCIENTIFIC BASIS OF PROFESSIONAL EDUCATION

Scientific contributions are critical for pharmacy education and the profession. The evidence base and scientific innovations immensely contribute to the knowledge base for pharmacist training and advancement of the pharmacy profession in the healthcare system. Pharmaceutical researchers, practitioners, and educators have an important role to play to generate and translate the evidence to patient care. Pharmacist involvement is needed across the research and practice continuum, from basic research to clinical and translation research to evidence-based practice (**Figure 1-6**).

Basic and clinical researchers are vital in developing the knowledge base relevant to the pharmacy profession. Scientific breakthroughs in the basic sciences such as biology, chemistry, biochemistry, genetics, and microbiology are critical in the development of

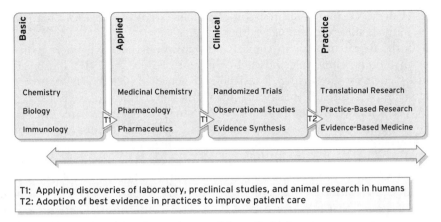

T1: Applying discoveries of laboratory, preclinical studies, and animal research in humans
T2: Adoption of best evidence in practices to improve patient care

FIGURE 1-6   Research and practice continuum of biomedical sciences.

applications in biomedical sciences. The research support by the NSF and the NIH has been instrumental in transforming the basic biomedical research landscape in the United States.[24] Pharmacists can indirectly or directly contribute to basic sciences because they have a broad understanding of basic and applied sciences relevant to pharmacy practice.

Applied scientists in pharmaceutical sciences such as medicinal chemistry, pharmaceutics, and pharmacology are instrumental in developing innovative healthcare products and services. The NIH and the pharmaceutical industry have played an important role in funding the applied biomedical sciences.[24] Foundations such as the American Cancer Society (ACS) and the American Heart Association (AHA) are also making a difference in advancing healthcare research. Pharmaceutical scientists have made immense contributions in developing and applying biomedical knowledge to products and services. Pharmacists have made enormous contributions to applied biomedical sciences and have great potential to influence the future landscape of pharmaceutical sciences. Although advanced training such as graduate degrees or fellowships is recommended to directly participate in applied research areas, pharmacists can make a difference in applied research because of their broad understanding of basic and clinical sciences.

Clinical research is the pathway to evaluate the safety and effectiveness of products and services. With increasing patient care responsibilities, the pharmacists' role in clinical research has evolved. The 1975 Millis Commission Report recognized the importance of clinical scientists who are well versed in pharmacotherapy and biomedical research and recommended the development of training programs for clinical scientists.[25] National organizations, such as the American Association of Colleges of Pharmacy (AACP) and the American College of Clinical Pharmacy (ACCP), followed up on these recommendations and developed educational and training agendas for clinical scientists.

In 2008, the ACCP Task Force report on research in the PharmD curriculum detailed research content areas and competencies. It required pharmacy students to (1) identify problems and research gaps, (2) design research to test hypotheses within the regulatory and ethical framework, (3) conduct analyses, (4) disseminate research findings, and (5) apply study findings to practice.[26] The latest curriculum standards by the Accreditation Council for Pharmacy Education (ACPE) require pharmacist education and training to incorporate (1) principles of research design and methodology, (2) regulatory and ethical principles of research, (3) methods in data management and statistical analyses, (4) principles of drug literature evaluation, and (5) practice implications of research.[27] These content areas not only emphasize the drug literature evaluation component, but also principles of research design. Sound understanding of the scientific basis of evidence creation and provision of patient care is essential for pharmacists to succeed in the highly competitive healthcare arena.

With the recent impetus in clinical and translational research, there is increased interest in training clinical scientists. In the past decade, the NIH has created the National Center for Advancing Translational Sciences (NCATS) to support clinical and translational research.[28] Specifically, the Clinical and Translational Science Awards (CTSA) program was initiated as part of NCATS to (1) develop academic infrastructure for translating biomedical research to treatments, (2) involve community practitioners and industry in translational research, and (3) train the next generation of clinical and translational researchers. Such programs are creating exciting collaborative opportunities across medicine, pharmacy, nursing, public health, and other disciplines. There are 60 academic programs in 30 states funded by the NIH as part of a CTSA consortium. Several colleges of pharmacy are part of the CTSA consortium. These programs are helping to create clinical research curriculum, training, and mentorship for pharmacy faculty and practitioners.

Practice-based research networks (PBRNs) have been instrumental in conducting clinical and translational research. A PBRN consists of a group of clinicians or practitioners involved in translational research who adopt best practices and conduct clinical research.[29] PBRNs started with primary care physicians; they now incorporate discipline-specific networks such as dentists, nurses, pharmacists, and others. These networks can be instrumental in (1) identifying problems in patient care, (2) testing effectiveness of treatments in real-world settings, and (3) evaluating patients who can benefit from treatments. PBRNs are considered the "blue highway" that links basic, clinical, and translational research.[30] The ACCP PBRN is one of the first clinical pharmacy-based research networks of clinical pharmacists in inpatient and outpatient settings. The research findings from such networks are vital for developing evidence-based practices in pharmacy.

The healthcare industry is a highly competitive marketplace with competing interests from providers, payers, and policy makers. With the increasing pressure of costs and efficiency, there is a need for providers to demonstrate value for their services based on scientific evidence. Several recent studies demonstrated the value in terms of cost, quality, and outcomes for pharmacists' services. The Ashville Project demonstrated the effect of pharmacist services for asthma on decreased costs and improved quality.[31] The Fleetwood Project showed the pharmacists' positive effect on quality and costs in long-term care.[32] A study by Chisholm-Burns et al. provided the best evidence for pharmacists' value in health care based on the data from 298 studies.[33] The meta-analyses found that pharmacist-directed patient care services have a positive effect on patient outcomes across settings and diseases. Such strong scientific evidence is vital to demonstrating pharmacists' contributions and to be recognized as healthcare providers. With increasing need for evidence for practice and policy, clinical and translational research and evidence-based practices are imperative for new models of pharmaceutical care.

SUMMARY AND CONCLUSIONS

The pharmacy profession is based on knowledge and evidence derived from scientific research. Sound understanding of the research process is critical for applying drug literature evaluation techniques for evidence-based practices. On the other hand, practice- or patient-based considerations have become paramount in research due to emerging research paradigms of clinical and translational research and patient-centered outcomes research. Pharmacists are integral to both the creation and application of evidence relevant to pharmacy practice. The goal of research is to provide evidence to improve clinical practice based on the following steps: (1) pose a research question and hypothesis, (2) develop and implement a research plan, (3) perform data collection and analysis, and (4) present a research report. Each of these steps is critical for scientific inquiry and discourse. The core of evidence-based practices is to translate evidence to patient care based on the following steps: (1) asking appropriate and answerable questions, (2) finding evidence, (3) appraising evidence, and (4) applying evidence to practice. These steps ensure that relevant evidence is obtained and combined with clinical expertise and patient values to provide EBM. New paradigms of clinical research are emerging due to payer, patient, provider, and policy considerations. Pharmacists can immensely contribute to the research and practice continuum because of their broad range of understanding of basic and applied sciences. With changes in patient care models and evolving research evidence, it is critical that pharmacists be part of the creation and application of research evidence to improve healthcare outcomes.

REVIEW QUESTIONS

1. Describe basic, applied, clinical, and translation research, using examples.
2. What are the steps in the scientific research process? Use an example.
3. What are the components of the IMRaD research report?
4. What steps are involved in evidence-based medicine? Use an example.
5. Why it is important for pharmacists to be involved in research?

ONLINE RESOURCES

Academy of Managed Care Pharmacy. Evidence-Based Medicine Training/Learning: Resources/Tools: http://amcp.org/Tertiary.aspx?id=10365

American College of Clinical Pharmacy (ACCP) Research Institute: http://www.accpri.org/

ASHP Foundation Research Resources: http://www.ashpfoundation.org/MainMenuCategories/ResearchResourceCenter/ResearchResources

University of Washington's Institute for Translational Health Sciences Clinical and Translational Sciences. Research Toolkit: http://www.researchtoolkit.org/

REFERENCES

1. Aspden P, Wolcott J, Bootman JL, Cronenwett, LR, eds. *Preventing Medication Errors: Quality Chasm Series*. Washington, DC: The National Academies Press; 2007.
2. National Science Board. Chapter 6 Glossary. In: *Science and Engineering Indicators 2008*. Volume 1, NSB 08-01; volume 2, NSB 08-01A. Arlington, VA: National Science Foundation; 2008.
3. Pharmaceutical Research and Manufacturers of America. *Pharmaceutical Industry Profile*. Washington, DC: PhRMA; April 2012.
4. Eunice Kennedy Shriver National Institute of Child Health and Human Development (NICHD). *Overview of Responsibilities for ClinicalTrials.gov: Compliance with Public Law 110-85 The Food and Drug Administration Amendments Act Title VIII Clinical Trial Databases*. In: Clinical Research Policy Guidance Document. 2010. Available at http://www.nichd.nih.gov/grants-funding/policies-strategies/policies/Documents/NICHD_ClinicalTrials_gov_Policy_final.pdf. Accessed August 29, 2013.
5. Food and Drug Administration. *ICH E6 Good Clinical Practice Consolidated Guidance*. Rockville, MD: FDA; 1996.
6. Aparasu RR. Scientific approach to pharmaceutical policy research. In: Aparasu RR, ed. *Research Methods for Pharmaceutical Practice and Policy*. Binghamton, NY: Pharmaceutical Product Press; 2010.

7. National Institutes of Health. *Institutional Clinical and Translational Science Award (U54). Research Objectives.* RFA-RM-07-007. 2006. Available at: http://grants.nih.gov/grants/guide/rfa-files/RFA-RM-07-007.html. Accessed August 29, 2013.

8. Committee on Quality of Health Care in America. Institute of Medicine of the National Academies. *Crossing the Quality Chasm: A New Health System for the 21st Century.* Washington, DC: National Academies Press; 2001.

9. Institute of Medicine. *Initial National Priorities for Comparative Effectiveness Research.* Washington, DC: National Academies Press; 2009.

10. Patient-Centered Outcomes Research Institute. *Patient-Centered Outcomes Research.* Available at: http://www.pcori.org/research-we-support/pcor/. Accessed August 29, 2013.

11. Patient-Centered Outcomes Research Institute. *National Priorities for Research and Research Agenda.* 2012. Available at: http://www.pcori.org/assets/PCORI-National-Priorities-and-Research-Agenda-2012-05-21-FINAL.pdf. Accessed August 29, 2013.

12. The National Commission for the Protection of Human Subjects of Biomedical and Behavioral Research. *The Belmont Report, Ethical Principles and Guidelines for the Protection of Human Subjects of Research.* 1979. Available at: http://www.hhs.gov/ohrp/humansubjects/guidance/belmont.htm. Accessed August 29, 2013.

13. Kerlinger FN. *Foundations of Behavioral Research.* 3rd ed. New York, NY: Holt, Rinehart and Winston; 2006.

14. Hulley SB CS. Conceiving the research question. In: Hulley SB CS, Browner WS, Grady D, Hearst N, Newman TB, eds. *Designing Clinical Research.* 2nd ed. Baltimore, MD: Williams & Wilkins; 2001:17–24.

15. Richardson WS, Wilson MC, Nishikawa J, et al. The well-built clinical question: a key to evidence-based decisions. *ACP J Club.* 1995;123(3):A12–3.

16. Velentgas P, Dreyer NA, Nourjah P, Smith SR, Torchia MM, eds. *Developing a Protocol for Observational Comparative Effectiveness Research: A User's Guide.* AHRQ Publication No. 12(13)-EHC099. Rockville, MD: Agency for Healthcare Research and Quality. 2013. www.effectivehealthcare.ahrq.gov/Methods-OCER.cfm. Accessed August 29, 2013.

17. Kozma CM, Reeder CE, Schultz RM. Economic, clinical, and humanistic outcomes: a planning model for pharmacoeconomic research. *Clin Ther.* 1993;15(6):1121–1132.

18. Polit DF, Hungler BP. *Nursing Research: Principles and Methods.* 5th ed. Philadelphia, PA: Lippincott Williams & Wilkins; 1995.

19. Pakes GE. Writing manuscripts describing clinical trials: a guide for pharmacotherapeutic researchers. *Ann Pharmacother.* 2001;35(6):770–779.

20. Institute of Medicine. *Improving Information Services for Health Services Researchers: A Report to the National Library of Medicine.* Washington, DC: National Academies Press; 1991.

21. Rosenberg W, Donald A. Evidence-based medicine: an approach to clinical problem-solving. *BMJ.* 1995;310:1122–1126.

22. Sackett DL, Strauss SE, Richardson WS, et al. *Evidence-Based Medicine: How to Practice and Teach EBM.* London, England: Churchill-Livingstone; 2000.

23. Sackett DL, et al. Evidence-based medicine: what it is and it isn't. *BMJ.* 1996;312:71–72.

24. Moses H 3rd, Martin JB. Biomedical research and health advances. *N Engl J Med.* 2011;364(6):567–571.

25. American Association of Colleges of Pharmacy. *Pharmacists for the Future: The Report of the Study Commission on Pharmacy.* Ann Arbor, MI: Health Administration Press; 1975.

26. Figg WD, Chau CH, Okita R, et al. 2008. PharmD. Pathways to biomedical research: the National Institutes of Health special conference on pharmacy research. *Pharmacotherapy.* 2008;28(7):821–833.

27. Accreditation Council for Pharmacy Education. *Accreditation Standards and Guidelines for the Professional Program in Pharmacy Leading to the Doctor of Pharmacy Degree.* Version 2.0. 2007. Available at: http://www.acpe-accredit.org/pdf/FinalS2007Guidelines2.0.pdf. Accessed August 29, 2013.

28. National Institutes of Health. National Center for Advancing Translational Sciences. Clinical and Translational Science Awards. 2012. Available at: http://www.ncats.nih.gov/files/ctsa-factsheet.pdf. Accessed August 29, 2013.

29. Agency for Health Research and Quality. Practice-Based Research Networks (PBRNs). Available at: http://pbrn.ahrq.gov/. Accessed August 29, 2013.

30. Westfall JM, Mold J, Fagnan L. Practice-based research–"blue highways" on the NIH roadmap. *JAMA.* 2007;297(4):403–406.

31. Bunting BA, Cranor CW. The Asheville Project: long-term clinical, humanistic, and economic outcomes of a community-based medication therapy management program for asthma. *J Am Pharm Assoc* (2003). 2006;46(2):133–147.

32. Lapane KL, Hughes CM, Christian JB, Daiello LA, Cameron KA, Feinberg J. Evaluation of the Fleetwood model of long-term care pharmacy. *J Am Med Dir Assoc.* 2011;12(5):355–363.

33. Chisholm-Burns MA, Kim Lee J, Spivey CA, et al. US pharmacists' effect as team members on patient care: systematic review and meta-analyses. *Med Care.* 2010;48(10):923–933.

ETHICAL CONSIDERATIONS IN CLINICAL RESEARCH

SANDRA L. ALFANO, PHARMD, CIP, FASHP

CHAPTER OBJECTIVES

▸ Explain the clinical phases of the drug approval process

▸ Understand the guiding ethical principles in clinical research

▸ Understand the regulatory framework governing clinical research, including informed consent and data confidentiality

▸ Explore key ethical challenges involved in clinical research

KEY TERMINOLOGY

Belmont Report
Beneficence
Common Rule
Conflicts of interest
Data and Safety Monitoring
    Board

Ethical principles
Human subjects research
Informed consent
Institutional review board
Justice
Phase I trials

Phase II trials
Phase III trials
Phase IV trials or post–marketing
    studies
Respect for persons
Therapeutic misconception

INTRODUCTION

Clinical research, which involves testing interventions in humans to establish their effectiveness and safety, must involve careful design and implementation to ensure the protection of the human subjects. When applied to drug development, the focus of clinical research is on establishing the efficacy and safety of the new drug. Clinical research trials are tightly controlled for both inclusion and exclusion of the participants and design of the protocol, with strict control over study procedures and interventions. It is important to recognize that the overall goal of clinical research is to develop or contribute to generalizable knowledge, which is hoped to be useful to future patients and providers. Clinical research involves actual patients with a disease; consequently, actual effects in terms of benefits and risks to these individuals also become relevant. In clinical practice, the clinician has an obligation to always act in the best interest of the patient. In clinical research, conflicts may arise as the clinician/researcher may have dual goals: to protect the patient/subject and to maintain research integrity.

A case example may help illustrate some of the conflicts that can arise.[1] In the late 1990s, researchers at the University of Pennsylvania were developing a gene transfer intervention that was intended to target the underlying pathology causing ornithine transcarbamylase (OTC) deficiency syndrome, which is a rare metabolic disorder that leads to the accumulation of ammonia in the blood. An 18-year-old man with partial OTC deficiency was recruited and consented to research. He received an infusion of the study agent and, after a short course, died. His family was distraught, claiming that they were never informed of the possibility of death from the study. A variety of disturbing facts came to light as part of the investigation of the death, including issues involving study design, consent, and conflict of interest. It was uncovered that the researcher held patents on the technology being tested, and he had founded and held significant equity in the biotech company that stood to benefit from the clinical trial. The university also held significant equity in the company. Troubling questions were raised about the researcher's conflicting interests and whether the young man had been inappropriately enrolled in the trial. In addition to the death of this young man, this tragedy has been a devastating blow to the gene transfer scientific community as a whole. This case also illustrates a conflict for the clinician (ensuring the well-being of the patient) and the researcher (striving to get research results that may lead to a future product).

In their editorial in the *American Journal of Health-System Pharmacists*, Cobaugh and Allison[2] call on pharmacists to recognize their responsibility to thoroughly understand the evidence supporting therapy choices as part of the patient care provided. This chapter provides the ethical and regulatory framework for overseeing clinical research. Specifically, it reviews the drug development process in the United States, discusses the ethical principles in human subjects research, discusses the regulatory framework in which clinical research takes place, and explores several key ethical challenges that confront those involved in the clinical research enterprise. By understanding these principles, clinicians will be better equipped to evaluate the ethical validity of research studies that may influence prescribing and drug therapy selection.

THE DRUG DEVELOPMENT PROCESS

The drug development process involves a long and expensive series of trials that are intended to lead to a commercial agent marketed for a particular indication or indications. Drug development begins with preclinical studies, which involve laboratory testing and animal testing. Suitable drug candidates identified in the laboratory are tested in animal models of the disease for pharmacologic effects, and toxicity studies are also conducted in these models. If a drug candidate is found to be promising after preclinical testing, then clinical research, which involves human testing, proceeds. See **Table 2-1** for an overview of the clinical drug testing process.

Clinical trials are conducted in phases that are sequential. **Phase I trials** involve testing a drug in humans with the intent of establishing the initial toxicity profile of the substance. The flip side of this concept is to establish the safety of the drug or, as it is sometimes phrased, show that the drug is safe for human use. Safety is a rather elusive term, however. Perhaps a more accurate term is "tolerability," which better reflects the fact that adverse effects do occur as a matter of course, but subjects (and then, eventually, patients) are able to tolerate the agent. All types of adverse effects are monitored for, reported, and compiled in the information developed about the agent. Typically, phase I trials are carried out in a cohort (group) of normal, healthy volunteers, although this is not always the case. Notably, phase I oncology trials are carried out in patients with cancer, often end-stage cancer. Phase I trials usually involve small numbers of subjects who receive the drug in a dose-escalation-by-cohort fashion. That is, the first enrollees will receive a low dose of the agent (such that the dose is not expected to have much effect) and will be monitored for toxicity. If these subjects (typically 3–6 subjects) tolerate that dose, then the next cohort of 3–6 subjects will be given a higher dose. This dose escalation and monitoring for toxicity continues until dose-limiting toxicity (DLT) is encountered. At that point, the previous dose level administered is called the maximum tolerated dose (MTD), and this is the dose that is generally recommended for the next phase of testing. The first time a drug crosses from the laboratory or animal testing into the human testing realm, the trial is referred to as a "first in human trial" (FIHT). For many drugs, there can be several phase I trials, testing different dosage forms and beginning to generate pharmacokinetic data as well.

TABLE 2-1	Clinical Drug Testing Process			
Features of Clinical Trials	**Phase I**	**Phase II**	**Phase III**	**Phase IV**
Primary Interest[a]	Toxicity (tolerability)	Preliminary efficacy and safety	Efficacy and safety	Long-term data
Target Population[b]	Healthy volunteers or subjects with the disease in question	Subjects with the disease in question	Subjects with the disease in question	Possibly subjects with other diseases
Study Design[c]	Dose escalation in cohort of patients, generally unblinded, often uncontrolled	Randomized, double-blind, placebo, or active controlled	Randomized, double-blind, placebo, or active controlled	Various depending on intent— experimental/ observational designs
Duration[d] **(subject/overall)**	About 1 month/less than a year	Months/a year or two	One to two years/ several years	Variable
Numbers Enrolled[e]	Small about 50	Medium about 100	Large 100s to 1,000s	Varies

[a] Phase I trials are intended to establish tolerability and focus primarily on toxicity. All phases, however, include reporting of toxicity data to build the profile of the drug.

[b] Phase I trials usually enroll healthy volunteers, although sometimes patients are enrolled, as in oncology phase I trials, and often in studying new drugs for Alzheimer's disease.

[c] A variety of designs can be and often are used. Placebo-controlled trials are considered strongest by the FDA.

[d] Duration is variable for each phase, but these are averages.

[e] Numbers of enrollees vary in each phase, but these are typical. Overall, it is not uncommon for a drug to be approved for marketing after having been studied in fewer than 5,000 subjects.

Once a tolerated dose is determined, a phase II trial may proceed. **Phase II trials** involve subjects with the disease in question, as these trials are designed to give initial data on efficacy and continued safety/toxicity data. This phase is also designed to collect data on pharmacokinetics, pharmacodynamics, minimum effective dose, and dose ranges that might be effective. Phase II trials are randomized trials involving fairly small numbers of subjects, about 100, and generally are short-term studies with a usual duration of months to less than a year. This phase is designed to provide preliminary evidence of efficacy and safety before large-scale trials can be conducted.

Phase III trials are designed to demonstrate efficacy in a statistically-powered sample of subjects with the disease in question. The goal of phase III trials is to generate efficacy and safety data to allow evaluation of the overall risk-to-benefit relationship of the drug. Well-done phase III trials that generate statistically significant results can be used to secure marketing approval for a given indication. Generally, phase III trials are large, enrolling hundreds or thousands of subjects, and may be long-term, extending for many months or years. The usual trial is set up as a randomized controlled trial (RCT) often involving blinding and placebo controls. Although establishing efficacy is the purpose, monitoring for safety/toxicity remains critical and will shape the eventual approval and labeling of the drug.

New drug substances for human use are under the regulatory oversight of the Food and Drug Administration (FDA), governed by the Investigational New Drug (IND) regulations in the Code of Federal Regulations (CFR) at title 21 part 312.[3] There are also regulations for biological substances at 21 CFR 600.[4] The regulations govern processes for submitting an investigational new drug application, responsibilities of sponsors and investigators, special processes for drugs intended to treat life-threatening and severely debilitating diseases, and expanded access for use of investigational drugs for treatment. All accumulating data for a particular investigational drug are compiled in an investigator's brochure, beginning with laboratory and animal data, which serves as an encyclopedia of accumulating data about the new drug. Agents that are tested in humans must be filed under an IND application with the FDA, and each protocol that is developed is submitted as part of the IND filing. When a sponsor believes data are adequate to support approval, all these data are submitted as part of a New Drug Application (NDA) for FDA approval.

Sometimes, as part of the FDA approval process, additional data collection is required by the FDA. This generally takes place as **phase IV trials or post-marketing studies** and is often intended to generate longer-term safety/toxicity data. Rarely occurring adverse effects of a drug may not have been noted during the earlier phases, but may become noticed as a new drug is prescribed to millions of patients. Collecting phase IV post-marketing safety data may help to establish the toxicity profile of the drug in a more robust fashion. At times, a phase IV trial may involve cost-effectiveness comparisons that will help in therapeutic selection among members of a drug class.

The RCT is recognized as the gold standard for conducting clinical research, as it is the strongest design to allow conclusions about causality to be drawn.[5] Randomization works to minimize bias in selection of therapeutic arm for a given subject. Strict control in the protocol procedures, and the inclusion and exclusion of subjects, serves to allow deduction about causality of the research intervention. The drug development process is a long and costly enterprise (**Figure 2-1**). According to Kaitin,[6] the average cost to bring one product to market, including failures, is $1.32 billion in 2005 dollars. For an excellent, more in-depth overview of the drug development process in the United States, consult Moore's (2003) review in *Southern Medical Journal*.[7]

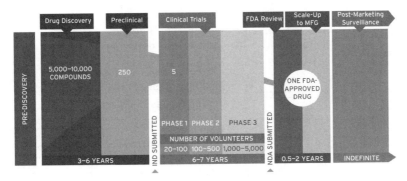

FIGURE 2-1   Research and development process in the pharmaceutical industry.
Reproduced from 2013 Profile: Biopharmaceutical Research Industry, PhRMA 2013.

DATA AND SAFETY MONITORING

It is essential that data generated during the course of a clinical trial be monitored closely, especially data related to adverse effects of the drug. Routine monitoring is a requirement because each clinical protocol must have a data and safety monitoring plan, which stipulates the responsibility for routine review, frequency of review, reporting responsibilities, and authority for modifying or stopping the study. In many large clinical trials, these responsibilities are assumed by a formal **Data and Safety Monitoring Board (DSMB)**. The DSMB reviews aggregate data that either have been unblinded or are separated by study arm to allow ongoing oversight of emerging trends in the data. Silverman[8] provides an in-depth analysis of the need for ongoing attention to ethical issues during the conduct of the clinical trial.

ETHICAL PRINCIPLES IN HUMAN SUBJECTS RESEARCH

The complex environment of clinical research and clinical drug development in particular highly depends on the participation of humans in clinical trials. However, a key fundamental concept is that participation in research is expected to be voluntary, not forced. Over the decades, there have been many examples of researchers forcing participation or deceiving participants about the true nature of the research and the risks entailed therein. During World War II, Nazi physicians performed life-threatening experiments on unwilling concentration camp detainees. Worldwide outrage over these atrocities led to development of the Nuremberg Code,[9] which emphasizes that participation in research must be *voluntary* and should never cause deliberate harm. In the United States, beginning in the 1930s, Public Health Service physicians followed the natural history of syphilis over several decades in a cohort of African-American men, who subsequently were denied antibiotic use once it was shown penicillin could be an effective treatment for syphilis. This trial became known as the Tuskegee Syphilis Study. National outrage over this reckless behavior by government-funded researchers, once exposed in 1972, led to passage of the National Research Act in 1974, which required institutions wishing to do federally-funded research to set up an institutional review board. The **institutional review board (IRB)** is charged with protecting the rights

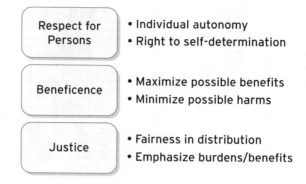

FIGURE 2-2   Ethical principles in human subjects research.

and welfare of human subjects of research, and ensuring that research is conducted in accordance with accepted ethical standards.

The National Research Act also established the National Commission for Protection of Human Subjects of Biomedical and Behavioral Research, which met over several years and, in 1979, issued a report titled "Ethical Principles and Guidelines for the Protection of Human Subjects of Research," known as the Belmont Report.[10] The **Belmont Report** articulates the fundamental **ethical principles** that must be the underpinnings of all research with human subjects: respect for persons, beneficence, and justice (**Figure 2-2**).

RESPECT FOR PERSONS

This is a concept based on Western philosophy that values individual autonomy and the individual's right to self-determination. As the Belmont Report states,

> **Respect for persons** incorporates at least two ethical convictions: first, that individuals should be treated as autonomous agents, and, second, that persons with diminished autonomy are entitled to protection.[10]

The principle of respect for persons is demonstrated through the **informed consent** process, which should be an ongoing dialogue intended to provide sufficient information so that the individual can make his/her own decision about research participation. The process involves conveying information in language that the subject can understand, assessing the comprehension of the subject, and securing voluntary agreement to participate. A written consent form is used to provide information and allow subjects to indicate agreement by signing. Consent forms must explain the purpose of the study, procedures that will be used, potential risks and benefits, economic considerations, the voluntary nature of the study and the subject's right to withdraw at any time, and an explanation of what will happen and who will pay in case the subject is injured in the study.

There is a real struggle in clinical research when developing consent documents. While their intent is to inform subjects, they often are viewed as legal documents that must contain every procedure and every risk ever possibly associated with the investigational agent. In this fashion, consent forms for investigational drug studies have become very long, very technical, and potentially overwhelming to research subjects. Ethical concerns involving the consent process focus on possibilities that subjects may not fully comprehend what is involved in the study or what risks they are willingly assuming by agreeing to participate.

In addition to those concerns inherent in clinical research with autonomous adults, it must be recognized that not every human being is capable of self-determination. Persons with diminished autonomy require special safeguards to prevent their exploitation in research. Such safeguards might involve limiting the degree of risk exposure that could be allowed, or providing for a consent monitor or advocate who would ensure the individual's welfare is protected. An example is the enrollment of adults with decisional impairment. In addition to seeking consent from the subject's legally authorized representative, limits might be placed on the acceptable levels of risk that a protocol may entail, especially if the protocol will not be of direct benefit to enrollees.

BENEFICENCE

According to the Belmont Report,

> Persons are treated in an ethical manner not only by respecting their decisions and protecting them from harm, but also by making efforts to secure their well-being. . . . In this document, **beneficence** is understood, in a stronger sense, as an obligation. Two general rules have been formulated as complementary expressions of beneficent actions in this sense: (1) do not harm and (2) maximize possible benefits and minimize possible harms.[10]

Application of this ethical principle generally takes place by doing a risk–benefit analysis, such that benefits must exceed the risks to undertake the research. Of course, such an analysis is imperfect, because research by its very nature has unknown risks and benefits. Part of the risk–benefit analysis includes deciding with imperfect knowledge when it is justifiable to seek certain benefits despite the risks involved, versus when the potential benefits are so small that the risks outweigh the benefits. It is important for each protocol that risks and benefits be monitored over time via an adequate data and safety monitoring plan. Researchers need to plan to detect and manage adverse effects as they occur and consider the need to modify or stop the research protocol. It must be recognized that research by its very nature involves risk, and indeed, subjects may be exposed to risk and may be harmed. The ethical obligation is to minimize probability of harm, while maximizing potential benefits, and to never knowingly cause (permanent) injury. Researchers are obligated to identify risks and objectively estimate their magnitude and likelihood. Both the risks and the benefits should be presented to prospective subjects in the consent form.

Several important features will influence how a protocol minimizes the risk: start with a highly competent research team and a well-designed study that incorporates procedures that have the least likelihood of harm. Build in adequate monitoring so that adverse events are quickly identified, managed, and reported. Incorporate provisions to protect privacy and confidentiality. Because clinical research, especially phase II and III trials, involves patients as research subjects, there are concerns that the research subject may suffer from the "**therapeutic misconception**."[11] That is, these research subjects may be prone to misunderstanding the risks and potential benefits associated with research participation and may have unreasonable expectations about potential individual benefits. This misunderstanding may lead to discounting of risks and overestimating personal benefits, and can be especially problematic when the treating physician is the researcher as well. Strict attention needs to be paid to accurately describing a benefit only as a potential, not a guarantee.

JUSTICE

According to the Belmont Report, there must be a sense of fairness in distributing the burdens and benefits of research. The ethic of **justice**

> . . . gives rise to moral requirements that there be fair procedures and outcomes in the selection of research subjects.[10]

Researchers have an obligation to make certain that no group inappropriately bears the burdens of research for the benefit of others. In the 1990s, this protectionist perspective underwent a paradigm shift when it was recognized that at times, clinical trials might be the best possibility of getting access to promising new drugs. An example was during the early days of the acquired immunodeficiency syndrome (AIDS) epidemic, when no drugs were yet approved to treat AIDS. Activist groups lobbied to expand access to clinical trials, not from a protection perspective, but from a perspective of fairness in distribution of potential benefits. Thus, justice requires that researchers strive to balance distribution of both the burdens and the benefits of research.

The Belmont principles remain the essential ethical principles in place to guide human research. Their application to individual research protocols involves the need to understand the principles and deal with some situations in which conflicts arise among or between them. This is the ongoing work of the IRB. It is important to note that one ethical principle does not "trump" the others. Weighing and prioritizing conflicting ethical norms is a difficult task that must involve discussion, debate, and often struggle.

REGULATORY FRAMEWORK FOR HUMAN SUBJECTS RESEARCH

In addition to the previously discussed Nuremberg Code and Belmont Report,[9,10] a number of other ethical codes exist and provide rich resources for researchers. Professional societies and special interest groups should be consulted for codes of conduct specific to specialties. In addition, several worldwide ethical guidelines exist, including the *Declaration of Helsinki*[12] and the international ethical guidelines for biomedical research issued by the Council for International Organizations of Medical Sciences (CIOMS).[13]

In the United States, the regulations for the protection of human subjects in research took shape largely after exposure of the problems associated with the Tuskegee Syphilis Study. The National Commission for the Protection of Human Subjects of Research issued the Belmont Report,[10] which provided the ethical underpinnings of human research protection regulations in the United States. These principles became codified as law in the Code of Federal Regulations (CFR) at title 45 CFR 46.[14] This set of regulations, adopted by 15 federal agencies, became known as the **Common Rule**. Notably, the FDA did not adopt these regulations wholesale, but rather, has similar regulations regarding informed consent and the IRB structure at 21 CFR 50 and 56, respectively.[15,16] The Office for Human Research Protections (OHRP)[17] provides oversight of human subjects research for the Department of Health and Human Services. The mission of the OHRP is to provide leadership in the protection of subjects involved in research by providing guidance and educational sessions for the research community. In the international setting, drug regulatory bodies have collaborated on the International Conference on Harmonisation of Technical Requirements for Registration of Pharmaceuticals for Human Use (known as ICH).[18] This is a collaboration of Europe, Japan, and the United States to achieve harmonization in regulatory approaches to oversight of the drug approval process in an efficient manner. While largely focused on drug regulatory standards, ICH also incorporates the requirement for ethical review and approval of clinical research protocols before beginning the research.

HUMAN SUBJECT RESEARCH AND INSTITUTIONAL REVIEW BOARDS

Human subjects research is defined in the Common Rule as research on:

> ...a living individual about whom an investigator (whether professional or student) conducting research obtains (1) data through intervention or interaction with the individuals or (2) identifiable private information.[14]

Although most researchers who interact or intervene with living individuals recognize that they are doing human subjects research, those who only work with identifiable private information often do not and may inadvertently fail to comply with applicable human subjects regulations. For example, conducting medical records reviews for research purposes and recording identifiable private information involves the need for review and approval of the research by the institutional review board (IRB). Although not strictly required by the regulations, most IRBs require that researchers submit proposals so that the IRB can evaluate whether the proposal involves human subject research.

IRBs are charged with protecting the rights and welfare of research subjects and ensuring sound ethical research design. By regulation, an IRB must comprise at least 5 members, at least one of whom is a scientist and one a non-scientist. In addition, there must be at least one member who is not otherwise affiliated with the institution. Membership is required to be diverse, including multiple scientific disciplines, genders, and races. The diversity of perspectives is what makes the IRB review valuable. In many IRBs for biomedical research, a pharmacist serves as a member who adds value because of his/her understanding of good research design and how to evaluate risks and benefits.

Researchers must submit information in sufficient detail in the IRB application to allow IRB review and approval. Typically, for clinical trials, this will involve submission of a detailed clinical protocol, a consent form, a sponsor's protocol, and an investigator's brochure. To approve research, an IRB must make determinations that the following criteria are met:[14]

- Risks to subjects are minimized.
- Risks to subjects are reasonable in relation to anticipated benefits to subjects, if any, and the importance of the knowledge that may reasonably be expected to result.
- Selection of subjects is equitable.
- Informed consent will be sought from each prospective subject or the subject's legally authorized representative.
- Informed consent will be appropriately documented.
- The research plan makes adequate provision for monitoring the data collected to ensure the safety of subjects.
- There are adequate provisions to protect the privacy of subjects and to maintain the confidentiality of the data.
- When some or all of the subjects are likely to be vulnerable to coercion or undue influence, additional safeguards have been included in the study to protect the rights and welfare of these subjects.

In addition to initial review and approval of protocols, IRBs are required to provide continuing review at appropriate intervals for the degree of risk associated with the protocol, but not less than once a year. If approval of a given protocol ends, all research activities must cease until reapproval is secured from the IRB. Approved research must be conducted according to the approved protocol. Any changes to the protocol must be reviewed and approved by the IRB prior to implementation, except when necessary to eliminate apparent immediate hazards to the subject(s).

In clinical drug trials, monitoring for and assessing and managing adverse events or adverse drug reactions takes a central role. All clinical drug trials must be vigilant in soliciting adverse event information from subjects and reporting these events to the sponsor, who then reports to the FDA. Only a subset of the large constellation of adverse events must be reported to the IRB: those with unanticipated problems involving risks to subjects or others.

There are various types of review that an IRB may use, including exemption determination, expedited review, or review by the full board. The Common Rule notes six exemption categories, all involving minimal risk, such as surveys/interviews, use of existing data, or specimens without identifiers. If the IRB determines the project is exempt, it does not undergo full review and may be carried out without IRB oversight. For other minimal risk protocols that do not meet one of the exemptions, it is possible that the IRB may conduct an "expedited" review, meaning it may be reviewed by the IRB chair or designee. Such protocols need to meet the full approval criteria as outlined above. For all protocols involving greater than minimal risk, review and approval by a full board must be secured before starting the research. Byerly[19] provides an in-depth review of the review types and IRB functions to help the practicing pharmacist understand these issues.

Around the turn of 21st century, institutions wishing to strengthen protections for research subjects began to form human research protection programs (HRPPs). These programs seek to create a culture of respect for, and awareness of, the rights and welfare of human research participants at the institution level while advancing scientific knowledge and facilitating the highest quality research. Such goals transcend traditional personnel and departmental jurisdictions, so the program involves integration of review and oversight functions from a number of key stakeholder groups essential to the research enterprise. In addition to protocol review and approval by IRBs, the HRPP establishes a formal process to monitor, evaluate, and continually improve the protection of human research participants. This involves oversight of research protection at the institution, as well as education of investigators and research staff about their ethical responsibility to protect research participants.

DATA CONFIDENTIALITY

Since its inception, the Common Rule required that research must include adequate provisions to protect the privacy of subjects and to maintain the confidentiality of the data (see above). Research interactions with human subjects should be conducted privately, and the data generated should be held confidentially. Because of electronic record keeping, data security measures to ensure confidentiality have increased, including use of secure servers and encryption software. In addition to the Common Rule requirements, the standards for protecting patient health information are described in the federal law known as the Health Insurance Portability and Accountability Act (HIPAA). HIPAA limits how health information can be used and disclosed to a set of activities that mainly encompass activities related to treatment, payment for treatment, and healthcare operations. Use of protected health information for research requires that the participant consent to its use through a research authorization that spells out the purpose of the research and how the data will be secured and shared.

KEY ETHICAL CHALLENGES IN CLINICAL RESEARCH

Although underlying ethical principles have been elucidated and regulations have been implemented, challenges remain in the conduct and oversight of clinical research. Some ongoing challenges involve knowing when it is appropriate to use a placebo control, how to ethically conduct phase I trials, how to avoid or manage investigator conflicts of interest in clinical research, how to differentiate research from quality improvement activities, how best to inform participants when genetic research is done, how to ensure appropriate registration of clinical trials, and dealing with myriad issues involved in clinical trials conducted in foreign countries.

Placebo use: Although the RCT, which often includes a placebo control, is considered the gold standard for clinical research, the use of a placebo control is not without ethical controversy. A placebo is generally considered an inactive or inert substance that is made to appear identical to the investigational drug being tested. According to the FDA's Robert Temple,[20] placebo-controlled trials generate the strongest efficacy data with fewest numbers of subjects. Concerns arise, however, regarding the ethics of enrolling subjects with a disease in a placebo (or no real treatment) arm. When is this justified? According to the *Declaration of Helsinki*,[12] "the benefits, risks, burdens, and effectiveness of a new intervention must be tested against those of the best current proven intervention, except in the following circumstances:"

- The use of placebo, or no treatment, is acceptable in studies where no current proven intervention exists; or
- Where, for compelling and scientifically sound methodological reasons, the use of placebo is necessary to determine the efficacy or safety of an intervention and the patients who receive placebo or no treatment will not be subject to any risk of serious or irreversible harm. Extreme care must be taken to avoid abuse of this option.

Researchers wishing to use a placebo arm must provide a justification in terms of the above factors for the IRB to consider in approval of the study.

Phase I trials: Phase I trials themselves may raise ethical concerns. If phase I trials are done in healthy volunteers, they cannot bring direct benefit to these participants. If phase I trials enroll subjects with disease (such as oncology phase I trials), then perhaps a direct benefit may result, but it is recognized that phase I trials are not designed to be of direct benefit to the participants but, rather, are designed to test safety and establish a possibly tolerable dose for future study. So why do people enroll in phase I studies?

The answer is complex and not well elucidated. Both types of subjects may enroll for altruistic reasons, in that they want to help others in the future who may suffer from debilitating disease. But as an incentive to enroll and assume the risks associated with new drug testing, healthy subjects are generally paid rather handsomely. This raises the concern that some subjects, especially those with limited means, may discount the potential risks to reap the financial reward. Conversely, patients with the disorder being studied usually are not paid and, indeed, may be subject to additional copays or other charges from a clinical trial. Although there is not much empirical data that address their reasons for participating, Glannon[21] examined this and found several motivators, such as altruism, wanting to fight as long as possible, or "therapeutic optimism" (weighing the low potential for benefit against risk when the person is facing near certain death), at play in decisions to participate in phase I trials.

Conflicts of interest: Another thorny issue at play in conducting human clinical trials involves the potential for **conflicts of interest** (COI) to affect study results. A COI is a situation in which a researcher's financial or other personal considerations may compromise, or appear to compromise, the investigator's professional judgment in conducting or reporting research. Financial interests held by those conducting research may compromise or appear to compromise the fulfillment of ethical obligations regarding the well-being of the research subjects.[22] Financial conflicts of interest, where the researcher receives large sums of money from the research sponsor, or has equity interest in a sponsor, raise the specter of concern about possible undue influence on subjects to participate in the research or bias in analysis of the data toward favorable results. Either of these behaviors will lead to concern about subject safety or concern about validity of results. Conflicts of interest are ubiquitous. The challenge is to recognize, identify, and manage them. The IRB will need to understand when a researcher's personal financial interests might have the ability to distort or affect the safety and rights of the human subjects of research or the integrity of the research, such that disclosure of the COI to research subjects or management of the conflict is necessary.

Quality improvement (QI): Another area that is often surrounded by controversy and confusion involves questions about quality improvement projects, especially in clinical settings where patients and their therapy may be involved. As QI practices have evolved to become more rigorous and controlled, they can begin to look like research studies and it becomes difficult to differentiate between the two. It is important to differentiate between human subjects research, which entails a commitment to the concept of voluntariness in participation, and QI, which explicitly is not done on a voluntary basis but rather is an operational implementation on the part of healthcare organizations.[23] Consumers as patients should have an expectation that the healthcare organization is committed to constantly improving its operations. As such, implementation of a QI project is not an optional process, but rather part of the healthcare operations. IRB review requirements are not in place for these types of projects, as they are not considered human subjects research.

Genetic research: In the age of genomics, most clinical drug research studies include a component that tests samples such as blood, saliva, cerebrospinal fluid, or tissues, such as biopsy tissues, for a variety of biomarkers or genetic makeup and mutations. Often these studies are done on leftover samples, such as samples drawn for clinical purposes, or an additional draw is added to that done for clinical reasons. These procedures generally involve minimal risk of physical harm. Instead, the primary concern is with informational risks, such as discrimination, psychological harm, or harm to family relationships if the results of the genetic testing became known to outsiders in case of a failure to keep the information secure. Another concern involves controversy over whether the results of the research testing will be shared with the participants. Because the testing involves research, which does not necessarily yield results of known validity, much research of this type does not share results with participants. However, as certain genetic mutations are becoming better associated with disease prediction, many argue that researchers and, in particular, biobanks must find a mechanism to ethically share clinically actionable information with research participants.[24]

Public registration of clinical trials: Proponents advocate the development of clinical trial registries for a variety of reasons. Originally, registries were proposed to let investigators and reviewers know about all trials, whether published or not.[25] In 2004, the International Conference of Medical Journal Editors (ICMJE) made registration of certain trials a condition of publication in an effort to encourage publication of both negative and positive trial results. More recently, there is a new FDA Amendment Act requirement for public registration of trials prior to subject enrollment, as well as a requirement to post results. The overall goals are to increase access to trials and create transparency in access to results (both positive and negative). ClinicalTrials.gov is an example of a registry, although many others exist. Although the goals of increasing public access to trials and making results available publicly may seem, on the surface, to be good, several concerns arise in how these registries perform. In 2012, Dickersin and Rennie[25] noted that ClinicalTrials.gov is coming up short in that most posted trials are not posting results. But concerns arise in simply posting results without commentary, interpretation, or context. This remains an area of interest for both researchers and the public funding the research.

Globalization of clinical research: In the 21st century, due to a burgeoning global research enterprise, there have been efforts to streamline regulatory approval in many countries. Numerous ethical concerns come into play, including whether there is adequate infrastructure for oversight/monitoring of clinical research in foreign countries; whether there are cultural differences that may make acceptance of Western ethical principles difficult; and concerns about exploitative "parachute research,"[26] where research is conducted in an ethically suspect fashion by researchers swooping into an underdeveloped country, yet once the research is concluded, the resultant pharmaceutical product is marketed in the wealthier nations and never becomes available in the locale where it was tested. IRBs are often confronted with diverse cultural practices, and it can be difficult to decide whose principles apply. There is a general recognition of the need for local review to evaluate the research project for cultural, political, and legal issues. There is also a heightened awareness about some sponsors who may use vulnerable foreign populations for risky research with little potential for future benefit.

SUMMARY AND CONCLUSIONS

Clinical research in the 21st century holds much promise for the alleviation of pain and suffering associated with many diseases. Along with such promise comes the responsibility to respect the human participants in the research and make rigorous efforts to protect their rights and well-being. This chapter provided a review of the drug approval process in the United States and the regulatory and ethical principles that guide research with human subjects. Pharmacists who are involved in the drug prescribing/selection process need to understand the clinical drug development process and the implications of ethical responsibility in the conduct of clinical research. Ethical challenges that confront the practitioner need to be considered thoughtfully as research projects are contemplated, developed, reviewed, conducted, and published.

REVIEW QUESTIONS

1. What are the fundamental ethical principles detailed in the Belmont Report and how are they implemented in clinical research?
2. In what phase of clinical trials does the evaluation of safety data take place?
3. Informed consent is a concept critical to enrollment of human subjects in clinical trials. Is there an ideal way to convey the information needed for consent?
4. Placebo controls lead to the best scientific data but may lead to ethical concerns. What are these concerns and how should they be handled?
5. What factors are necessary for an IRB to approve a protocol?

ONLINE RESOURCES

Bioethics Resources on the Web, National Institutes of Health: http://bioethics.od.nih.gov/
Collaborative Institutional Training Initiative (CITI): https://www.citiprogram.org/
Food and Drug Administration: http://www.fda.gov/
Office for Human Research Protections: http://www.hhs.gov/ohrp/
Protecting Human Subject Research Participants: http://phrp.nihtraining.com/
Yale University Human Research Protection Program: http://www.yale.edu/hrpp/

REFERENCES

1. Savulescu J. Harm, ethics committees and the gene therapy death. *J Med Ethics*. 2001;27:148–150.
2. Cobaugh DJ, Allison JJ. Understanding research principles: giving our patients the care they deserve. *Am J Health-Syst Pharm*. 2009;66:1265.
3. FDA Part 312 Investigational New Drug Application. Available at http://www.accessdata.fda.gov/scripts/cdrh/cfdocs/cfcfr/cfrsearch.cfm?cfrpart=312. Accessed October 11, 2012.
4. FDA Subchapter F-Biologics. Available at http://www.accessdata.fda.gov/scripts/cdrh/cfdocs/cfCFR/CFRSearch.cfm?CFRPart=600. Accessed October 11, 2012.
5. Hartung DM, Touchette D. Overview of clinical research design. *Am J Health-Syst Pharm*. 2009;66:398–408.
6. Kaitin KI. Deconstructing the drug development process: the new face of innovation. *Clin Pharmacol Ther*. 2010;87(3):356–361.
7. Moore SW. An overview of drug development in the United States and current challenges. *South Med J*. 2003;96(12):1244–1255.
8. Silverman H. Ethical issues during the conduct of clinical trials. *Proc Am Thorac Soc*. 2007;4:180–184.
9. Nuremberg Code. *Trials of War Criminals before the Nuremberg Military Tribunals under Control Council Law No. 10*. Washington, DC: U.S. Government Printing Office; 1949;2:181–182. Available at http://www.ushmm.org/research/doctors/Nuremberg_Code.html. Accessed October 7, 2012.
10. The National Commission for the Protection of Human Subjects of Biomedical and Behavioral Research. *The Belmont Report, Ethical Principles and Guidelines for the Protection of Human Subjects of Research, April 18, 1979*. Available at http://www.hhs.gov/ohrp/humansubjects/guidance/belmont.html. Accessed October 7, 2012.
11. Miller FG, Brody H. A critique of clinical equipoise: therapeutic misconception in the ethics of clinical trials. *The Hastings Center Report*. 2003;33(3):19–28.
12. World Medical Association. *Declaration of Helsinki: Ethical Principles for Medical Research Involving Human Subjects*. Adopted by the 18th WMA General Assembly, Helsinki, Finland, June 1964, and as revised by the 59th WMA General Assembly, Seoul, Korea, October 2008. Available at: http://www.wma.net/en/30publications/10policies/b3/index.html. Accessed October 7, 2012.
13. *International Ethical Guidelines for Biomedical Research Involving Human Subjects*, prepared by the Council for International Organizations of Medical Sciences (CIOMS) in collaboration with the World Health Organization (WHO), Geneva, Switzerland, 2002. Available at http://www.cioms.ch/. Accessed October 9, 2012.
14. Code of Federal Regulations. Title 45 Public Welfare Department of Health and Human Services; Part 46 Protection of Human Subjects; June 23, 2005. Available at http://www.hhs.gov/ohrp/humansubjects/guidance/45cfr46.html. Accessed October 7, 2012.
15. US FDA Protection of Human Subjects. Available at http://www.accessdata.fda.gov/scripts/cdrh/cfdocs/cfcfr/cfrsearch.cfm?cfrpart=50. Accessed October 12, 2012.
16. US FDA Institutional Review Boards. Available at http://www.accessdata.fda.gov/scripts/cdrh/cfdocs/cfcfr/cfrsearch.cfm?cfrpart=56. Accessed October 12, 2012.
17. Office for Human Research Protections (OHRP). Available at http://www.hhs.gov/ohrp/. Accessed October 12, 2012.
18. International Conference on Harmonisation of Technical Requirements for Registration of Pharmaceuticals for Human Use. Good Clinical Practice E6 May 1996. Available at http://www.ich.org/fileadmin/Public_Web_Site/ICH_Products/Guidelines/Efficacy/E6_R1/Step4/E6_R1__Guideline.pdf. Accessed October 9, 2012.
19. Byerly WG. Working with the institutional review board. *Am J Health-Syst Pharm*. 2009;66:176–184.
20. Temple R, Ellenberg SS. Placebo-controlled trails and active-control trials in the evaluation of new treatments. Part I: ethical and scientific issues. *Ann Intern Med*. 2000;133:455–463.

21. Glannon W. Phase I oncology trials: why the therapeutic misconception will not go away. *J Med Ethics*. 2006;32:252–255.

22. Financial Conflicts of Interest, Public Health Service, effective August 24, 2012. Available at http://grants.nih.gov/grants/policy/coi. Accessed October 10, 2012.

23. Siegel MD, Alfano SL. The ethics of quality improvement research (Editorial). *Crit Care Med*. 2009;37:791–792.

24. Wolf SM, Crock BN, Van Ness B, et al. Managing incidental findings and research results in genomic research involving biobanks and archived data sets. *Genet Med* 2012:14(4):361–384.

25. Dickersin K, Rennie D. The evolution of trial registries and their use to assess the clinical trial enterprise. *JAMA*. 2012;307:1861–1864.

26. Bastida EM, Tseng TS, McKeever C, et al. Ethics and community-based participatory research: perspectives from the field. *Health Promot Pract*. 2010;11(1):16–20.

RESEARCH DESIGN AND METHODS

RAHUL KHANNA, PHD

RAJENDER R. APARASU, MPHARM, PHD, FAPHA

CHAPTER OBJECTIVES

▸ Understand research design and methodology terminology

▸ Describe classification of research designs in clinical research

▸ Discuss common research methodologies in clinical research

▸ Explain the importance of reliability and validity in research

KEY TERMINOLOGY

Analytical studies
Biochemical methods
Biological assessments
Biophysical assessments
Case-control studies
Case report
Case series
Causality
Close-ended questions
Cohort studies
Construct validity
Content validity
Convergent validity
Criterion validity
Cross-sectional studies
Descriptive studies
Discriminant validity
Experimental designs
External validity

Face-to-face interviews
Face validity
Internal consistency
Internal validity
Inter-rater reliability
Intervention studies
Mail surveys
Microbiological methods
Observational designs
Observational technique
Obtrusive observation
Online or Internet surveys
Open-ended questions
Primary methods
Prospective cohort study
Prospective studies
Quasi-experimental
Randomized controlled
    trial

Reliability
Research design
Research methodology
Retrospective cohort
    study
Retrospective studies
Secondary methods
Self-reports
Semi-structured
    interviews
Structured (or
    standardized)
    interviews
Survey instrument
Test-retest reliability
Unobtrusive observation
Unstructured interviews
Validity

INTRODUCTION

Research design and methodology constitute the critical backbone of a sound scientific investigation. A good design increases the validity of research findings, whereas a flawed design could raise questions on the credibility of those findings. Clinical studies that are well designed provide valuable evidence to assist practitioners in making decisions that best suit the needs of the patients. When practicing evidence-based medicine (EBM), clinicians integrate their own clinical expertise with the best available clinically relevant research.[1] For a study to be considered "best available clinically relevant research," it should have a sound research design and methodology. Poorly designed studies have limited scientific value and, when incorporated into evidence-based practice, could be wasteful or sometimes harmful to patients. Consequently, an understanding of research designs and methodology is essential to evaluating and applying research evidence.

The purpose of this chapter is to introduce key issues related to clinical research design and methodology for research implementation and evaluation. The chapter describes the common terminology used for clinical research designs and methodologies. It provides a brief description of different clinical research designs using criteria such as purpose, time orientation, and investigator orientation for classification. The chapter also discusses research methodologies with an overview of primary data collection and secondary research methods. Methodological issues related to measurement, such as validity and reliability, are also discussed. The chapter concludes by describing the different data collection methods that are commonly used in clinical research.

RESEARCH DESIGN

Research design refers to the overall plan that allows researchers to gather answers to study questions and test study hypotheses.[2] The research design is the means through which researchers can answer the question under consideration. A researcher evaluates available study designs and selects the most appropriate design to answer the research question. The decision to use a particular study design hinges on the ability of that design to provide valid results. At its core, validity reflects the accuracy of study results.[3] Validity can be further distinguished into internal validity and external validity.[2] **Internal validity** reflects the extent to which clinical outcome of interest (dependent variable) in a study is caused by the treatment (independent variable). A good design increases internal validity by controlling the extraneous factors that may influence the clinical outcome of interest. Internal validity typically implies the degree of confidence a researcher has that the changes observed in the dependent variable (clinical outcome) are because of the independent variable (treatment). **External validity** refers to the extent to which the results of a study can be generalized to other settings. It reflects the degree of confidence a researcher has that the results can be replicated in other situations, settings, and populations. Both internal and external validity are essential parameters that enable researchers to judge the usefulness of a design.

CAUSALITY

Causation is one of the most commonly used terms in the scientific literature. A cause-and-effect relationship, or **causality**, exists if there is a causal relationship between the treatment (cause) and the clinical outcome (effect). No topic has received more attention in epidemiological research than the study of the causal relationship between smoking (cause) and lung cancer (effect). Given the numerous articles that have been published in scientific journals over the past few decades, it is now well known that smoking (exposure) can cause lung cancer (disease). However, for an exposure (smoking) to be considered a cause for a disease (lung cancer), there needs to be good evidence. In 1965, Sir Austin Bradford Hill listed a set of nine criteria that should be fulfilled for the relationship between two variables to be considered potentially causal.[4] As acknowledged by Hill, the fulfillment of the nine criteria does not automatically imply causation, but rather assists researchers in making decisions regarding the presence or absence of causal mechanism. The nine criteria proposed by Hill are listed in **Table 3–1**.

According to Hill, experimentation is the key requirement and strongest case for proving causality. Consequently, research designs can be broadly categorized into two types—observational and experimental. The key element that distinguishes these designs is the extent of involvement of the researcher in controlling the key independent

TABLE 3-1 Criterion for Causation Proposed by Sir Austin Bradford Hill (1965)[4]	
Criterion	**Description**
Temporality	For causation, it is essential for the cause to occur before the effect. This is a strong criterion to judge the presence or absence of causality. The fulfillment of this criterion is essential for a relationship to be termed causal. For example, an individual should be treated with medication before the occurrence of clinical outcome.
Strength	This criterion contends that the plausibility of causation increases with the strength of the relationship between two variables. For example, if the clinical outcome is significantly better among individuals treated with medication as compared to those not treated (controls), a causal relationship between treatment and outcome is likely.
Biological Gradient	Presence of a dose–response curve is an indicator of causation, wherein a linear relationship is observed between treatment and clinical outcome. Based on this criterion, causation is a plausible explanation for association between treatment and outcome if there is improvement in outcome with an increase in dose of treatment.
Consistency	This criterion determines whether the relationship between cause (independent variable) and effect (dependent variable) is observed consistently across different settings (population, time, place). If the relationship between treatment and clinical outcome is observed across different populations, time periods, and places, then causation becomes a likely explanation.
Specificity	This criterion assumes a single cause for an effect or one-to-one relationship between cause and effect. The association between treatment and clinical outcome can be explained by causation if there is only one cause for the effect.
Plausibility	For a cause to lead to an outcome there should be a biologic possibility for the relationship between the cause and the effect. In clinical research, pharmacology and disease pathology are often used to provide a biological rationale for the relationship.
Coherence	This criterion implies that the relationship between the cause and the effect should be consistent with the existing knowledge. There should not be a conflict between the causal interpretation of the relationship and the knowledge concerning the natural history and biology of the disease.
Analogy	This criterion implies that similar commonly accepted phenomenon may show causation. For example, it can be causal if the effect on medication on adverse outcome is similar to the effects seen in preclinical testing.
Experiment	The strongest case for causal mechanism is made when the researcher controls the changes in the causes (treatment) leading to changes in effect (clinical outcome). For example, causation becomes a highly plausible explanation when a randomly assigned treatment results in changes in clinical outcome.

variable (treatment) by randomization. In **observational designs**, as the name suggests, the researcher merely observes the interplay of independent variables (drug exposure) with the dependent variable (outcome of interest). The variations in exposure and outcomes are observed to evaluate their relationship or association. In **experimental designs**, the researcher controls the treatment (independent variable) that is likely to have an impact on clinical outcome (dependent variable). This is achieved in experimental studies through randomization. In addition, the other criteria, such as temporality, strength, and biological gradient, can easily be achieved in experimental studies to prove causality. Consequently, evidence from randomized controlled trials are used by the Food and Drug Administration (FDA) to establish efficacy of a drug.

RESEARCH DESIGN CLASSIFICATION

Research designs can be classified using different sets of criteria, which includes study purpose, time orientation, investigator orientation, and experimental setting (**Figure 3–1**). Although these classifications capture different dimensions of research approaches, these classifications are interlinked and sometimes overlap. As a result, a particular research design may fall under more than one category based on the approach incorporated in the study designs.

PURPOSE

The purpose of the study could be either descriptive or analytical. A researcher may decide on a particular design to just describe a phenomenon (descriptive) or provide causal interpretation of an existing phenomenon (analytical). **Descriptive studies**, as the name implies, describe or summarize information about the diseases, events, or characteristics of study subjects without making any causal inferences. Descriptive studies incorporate five important elements pertaining to a new disease or event—who, what, why, when, and where.[5] "Who" refers to the demographic characteristics, such as age and gender of study population. "What" details the case definition of the disease based on specific inclusion and exclusion criteria. With respect to the third element, "why," descriptive studies provide clues about the possible causal mechanism, which can be further studied using more advanced analytical designs. "When" pertains to the time period related to the occurrence of the disease. The last element, "where," relates to the place of occurrence of disease. Knowing the location could provide important clues to help ascertain the causation. Grimes and Schulz (2002)[5] added a sixth element, "so what," to descriptive studies. This element relates to the role played by descriptive studies in improving public health and providing information that is important in

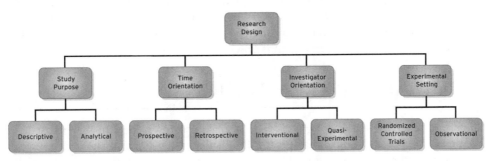

FIGURE 3-1 Research design classification.

gaining insights into the disease. For example, a descriptive study published in 1981 reported the occurrence of *Pneumocystis* pneumonia among males with a homosexual lifestyle.[6] This study was the first reported documentation of the occurrence of a disease that is now recognized as acquired immunodeficiency syndrome (AIDS), and it laid the foundation for studying the cause associated with this illness. **Analytical studies** are aimed at understanding the relationship and/or causal mechanism that may exist between two or more variables.[7] Consequently, they involve experimental or observational designs to incorporate the nine criteria proposed by Hill. These designs are often complex and resource intensive. Unlike descriptive studies, which are used to generate data for hypothesis, analytical studies are used for testing a hypothesis. The usefulness of these studies lies in their ability to test the relationship and causal pathways.

TIME ORIENTATION

Based on time orientation, research designs may be classified as prospective or retrospective. **Prospective studies** are those where the researcher collects the data after the study onset by following individuals over a period of time. The main strength of this design is to determine and define the research variables and prospectively collect relevant data to achieve the objectives. The main limitation of prospective design is that they are resource (time and cost) intensive. All experimental designs and some observational designs are prospective designs. **Retrospective studies** involve evaluation of data of past events or existing data such as medical records to achieve the research objective. In retrospective research, the event of interest has already occurred, and researchers go backward in time to determine the relationship between cause and event. The main advantage of retrospective design is that the studies are minimally resource intensive because they only involve analysis of existing data or past events. However, retrospective designs have some limitations. The researcher cannot control past events or data collection methods. Consequently, they have to rely on existing data or previous events without any say about what variables are needed and how they are defined and collected.

INVESTIGATOR ORIENTATION

Another classification criterion for research designs is based on the role played by the investigator in relation to controlling the independent variables of interest. Based on investigator orientation, research designs may be classified as intervention studies. **Intervention studies** are those where the researcher controls the treatment; this involves defining the treatment and provision of treatment randomly or non-randomly. If the intervention involves randomization, it is considered an experimental study like in a randomized controlled trial. If there is no randomization in provision of treatment, it is called **quasi-experimental** as it looks like experimental without randomization. The landmark study in pharmacy practice, the Ashville Project, was a quasi-experimental study.[8] Quasi-experimental studies are analytically similar to observational studies as the effect of non-randomized intervention is observed.

CLINICAL RESEARCH DESIGNS

There are several research designs that are available to researchers to select based on the research objectives and other practical considerations. Each of these designs has certain strengths and weaknesses. The choice of the research design and complexities of these designs often vary with the topic of research. Basic researchers often rely on experimental designs to test their research hypotheses. In clinical research, both experimental and observational designs are used to achieve research objectives. Although there are numerous study designs, the most commonly used experimental design is the randomized controlled trial (RCT). The commonly used observational designs in clinical research include cohort, case-control, cross-sectional, case series, and case reports. Each of these designs is briefly explained below.

RANDOMIZED CONTROLLED TRIALS

The **randomized controlled trial** (RCT) is an experiment that involves randomization of intervention(s) to two or more groups. The RCT is considered to be the gold standard in evaluating the safety and efficacy of an intervention.[9] There are two essential elements of RCTs.[10] The first element involves the randomization of study participants to interventional and control groups. The former represents the group in which participants are provided an intervention (also called the "experimental" or "treatment" group), while those in the latter are provided conventional or no intervention (also called the "control" group). Randomization is critical to the strength of RCTs, and is the primary reason that RCTs are the strongest research design. Because of randomization, all baseline factors are distributed evenly among the experimental and control groups, which thereby alleviates the role of systematic differences among participants in influencing study results. Thus, randomization increases internal validity of RCTs.[9] As a result, any difference observed in clinical outcomes between the two groups could be causally attributed to study intervention. The second element of RCTs is that they are always prospective; patients in the study groups are followed after the intervention to evaluate changes in the clinical outcome. Together, the two elements increase confidence among researchers in making causal inferences. The elements of RCTs that increase the internal validity of study results also contribute towards restricting their external validity (generalizability). Since RCTs are conducted in tightly controlled clinical settings, the results may not be generalizable to routine (real world) settings.

OBSERVATIONAL DESIGNS

In observational studies, as the name suggests, a researcher observes the relationship between the study variables, mainly independent (intervention or exposure) and dependent (outcome or disease), in a natural setting. Unlike experimental studies, there is no randomization of participants into experimental and control groups. Consequently, the independent variable is an exposure of interest such as medication use or an intervention. The key element in observational studies is non-randomization of the independent variable of interest. In observational studies, investigators collect data regarding exposure and outcomes using primary data techniques like interviews and surveys or use data collected previously for other purposes (secondary data) like medical charts.[11,12] Common observational studies include five types: case reports, case series, cross-sectional studies, case-control studies, and cohort studies.

   A **case report** involves a study of a single case of a new disease or manifestation, while a **case series** involves a study of multiple similar cases. Because of their simple descriptive nature, case reports (or series) are widely considered to be at the bottom of the research hierarchy and EBM. However, they serve a useful purpose by bringing attention to unusual clinical situations that otherwise may have been missed. Case reports provide clinical insights into rare events and adverse or beneficial drug effects. The information provided by case reports is instrumental in the development of new subject areas and enables the generation of a hypothesis, which can then be tested using more rigorous prospective designs.[13] Case reports are credited with the discovery of AIDS and identification of the relationship between thalidomide and birth defects.[14–16]

Cross-sectional studies examine population characteristics at a cross-section (one point) in time. Cross-sectional studies provide a snapshot of the presence of outcome and/or exposure status in the population.[17] These studies are often used to determine prevalence, that is, the proportion of individuals with a disease or outcome of interest at a given point in time.[18] As a result, they are also referred to as prevalence studies. For example, a cross-sectional design is likely to be used by a researcher who aims to assess the prevalence of rheumatoid arthritis among recipients of a state Medicaid program. The main limitation of cross-sectional studies is that they cannot be used to infer causation, since both exposure and outcome are measured at the same time. The inability to capture temporal precedence (exposure preceding outcome) makes cross-sectional designs inappropriate to study causality.

Case-control studies involve comparison of exposure status among individuals with the disease or outcome of interest (cases) and those without (controls). Cases and controls are both identified from the same source population, with the only difference being that the former experienced the outcome of interest while the latter did not. Thus, the two groups are defined by the presence or absence of outcome. Cases and controls should ideally be identical in all aspects except for the occurrence of outcome, so much so that if controls were to have the outcome, they could be classified as cases. The investigator determines the exposure history for both cases and controls going back in time (retrospectively). The likelihood ratios (rates of exposure) are statistically compared in cases and controls to evaluate the relationship between exposure and outcome. Case-control studies are the design of choice to study rare outcomes and in situations where there is a long latency period between exposure and occurrence of outcome. However, bias can creep into case-control studies if there are methodological flaws in the identification of the control group or determination of exposure status.

Cohort studies are observational studies wherein two groups, exposed and unexposed, are followed over a period of time until the development of the outcome of interest. At baseline, none of the individuals in the two groups have the outcome. The two groups are defined based on the exposure status (exposed versus unexposed) and are observed for a given time period going forward. The frequency of occurrence of the outcome in the exposed group is compared to the unexposed group. Cohort studies determine the incidence of the outcome in the exposed and unexposed groups, and therefore provide a measure of relative risk. Since exposure precedes outcomes, cohort studies are considered to be the most powerful observational design to study causation. It should be noted, though, that unlike RCTs, there is no randomization involved, and classification of individuals into exposed and unexposed groups is based on patient/provider choice. Consequently, the two groups can be different due to selection bias.

Cohort studies can be divided into two types: prospective and retrospective. In both prospective and retrospective cohort studies, exposure classification (exposed and unexposed) precedes ascertainment of outcome. In a **prospective cohort study**, the exposed and unexposed groups are classified at baseline and then followed in the future to determine the occurrence of the outcome of interest in the two groups. In a **retrospective cohort study**, a researcher uses previously collected (historical) data to identify exposure status and occurrence of the outcome in the study group. The main strength of cohort studies is their ability to ascertain temporality when examining the relationship between exposure and outcome.

RESEARCH METHODOLOGIES

Research methodology focuses on data collection and measurement techniques. Data collection is a critical step in the research process. Data collection techniques can be broadly classified into primary or secondary methods. **Primary methods** collect data specifically for the research question under consideration. Techniques such as surveys and observations are considered primary data collection methods. **Secondary methods** for data collection involve the use of data that were collected for a different purpose such as medical charts and medical claims. These data systems capture valuable data for medical and reimbursement purposes and not specifically for research. Researchers often use the available data from these data sources to investigate a research problem.

The choice of a particular data collection method is guided by several factors including the research question, population of interest, availability and feasibility of method, and cost.[19] Primary and secondary data collection methods have their advantages and limitations.[20] Primary methods enable researchers to collect data that fit the needs of the study and can be tailored in accordance with research design. However, primary data collection can be resource intensive and may require considerable cost and time. Since secondary methods employ the use of data that are already available, they are easier to conduct and less costly. The limitation of secondary data is that they may not include certain variables needed for the purposes of the study. Also, secondary data may be difficult to interpret as they may lack complete data, definition, or documentation. For example, prescriptions captured in Medicaid claims data may lack all details of medication regimen such as frequency of dosing. The decision to use a particular data collection technique is guided by three factors: reliability, validity, and practicality. The first two factors refer to the consistency and accuracy of results (discussed below), while the last factor pertains to the cost and accessibility of a data collection strategy.

RELIABILITY AND VALIDITY

The most important consideration that a researcher has to make is whether the measurement approach is reliable and valid irrespective of the approach taken for data collection. **Reliability** refers to consistency and reproducibility of results.[2,19] Results obtained from a measurement instrument should be consistent when measured repeatedly over different time periods. A commonly used metric of reliability is the **test–retest reliability**. It refers to the extent to which answers to the same instrument correlate when measured in the same sample over different time periods. For example, an electronic blood pressure monitor should give consistent blood pressure readings for the same patient over a short time period. The blood pressure measurements should consistently provide the same value for a patient at two different time periods (say, T1 and T2) that are minutes apart barring any external factor that causes substantial changes in disease state.

Another parameter to adjudicate reliability is through the assessment of **inter–rater reliability**, which refers to the extent to which results are consistent when the same measurement instrument is used by multiple raters (reproducibility). For example, the electronic blood pressure monitor will be considered reliable if it shows similar readings for the same patient when used within a few minutes by two different pharmacists. The **internal consistency** method is often used to assess the reliability of survey instruments such as the Medical Outcomes Short-Form 12 (SF-12). It involves calculating correlation coefficients of survey items or questions from the scale. A good correlation (> 0.80) between the survey questions provides evidence of reliability. Other reliability evaluation methods can also be used based on the measurement purpose.[2,19]

Validity refers to the extent to which an instrument measures what it is intended to measure. Validity reflects whether measurement is accurate. For example, it pertains to the extent to which a survey instrument like SF–12 purporting to measure quality of life actually does so. Commonly used forms of validity assessments are face validity, content validity, criterion validity, and construct validity. In **face validity**, the appearance (or face) of the instrument is used to evaluate its validity. It is the first step in evaluation and the most basic of validity assessments. A researcher can consider a survey instrument to be valid if it appears to contain questions related to quality of life. The **content validity** assesses whether the measurement contains required domains or areas to accurately measure a concept. In content validity, the researcher evaluates whether the survey instrument contains questions in specific areas, such as physical functioning, general health, and mental health, for it to be considered valid.

Construct validity refers to the extent to which an instrument measures the underlying construct that it purports to measure. The construct validity of an instrument can be further classified into criterion validity, convergent validity, and discriminant validity. **Criterion validity** refers to the ability of an instrument to correlate well with a criterion or standard. A newly developed general quality of life instrument should correlate well with a standard quality of life instrument like SF–12 to be considered valid. **Convergent validity** reflects the extent to which similar constructs correlate. Constructs that are similar in nature are expected to correlate well. For example, a new quality of life instrument should correlate well with other measures of health such as the Quality of Well-Being Scale. **Discriminant validity** reflects the extent to which an instrument purporting to measure a construct is able to differentiate it from a theoretically unrelated construct. For example, a new quality of life instrument should not correlate well with intelligence quotient (IQ) of patients because they are theoretically unrelated constructs; a low correlation is expected between the two constructs. Other evaluation methods for validity can also be used based on the research purpose.[2,19]

RESEARCH METHODS CLASSIFICATION

Research data can be collected using various techniques, which, as described earlier, can be categorized into primary and secondary methods (**Figure 3–2**). The common primary methods of data collection include self-reports, observation, and biological measurement. The three approaches differ by the level of participation by the patients (subject of investigation) and researchers in terms of gathering information. The level of participation of subjects is the highest under self-report collection techniques, and the lowest for observation techniques. The secondary data involve use of data collected for other purposes. The secondary data collected can contain self-reports, observations, and biological measures. In clinical research, the most used secondary data sources include medical charts (data collected by clinicians for patient care), medical claims (data collected by insurance for payment), national surveys (data collected by governmental agencies for policy), and research data (data collected by other researchers for different research purposes). A brief description of the three primary data collection techniques is provided below.

SELF-REPORTS

Self-reports involve data collection by direct questioning of patients. Using self-reports, data concerning patients' thoughts and perceptions, attitudes, and behaviors can

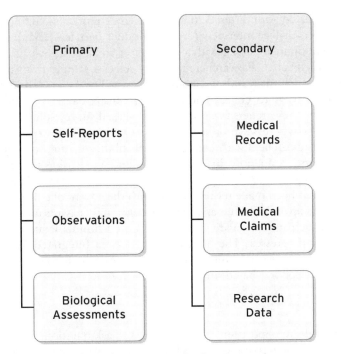

FIGURE 3-2 Data methods classification and sources for clinical research.

be collected. There are two types of self-report data collection strategies: surveys and interviews.

Surveys

A **survey instrument** includes a set of questions aimed at collecting data relevant to the purpose of the study. Questions included in the survey instrument could be either open-ended or close-ended.[2,21,22] **Open-ended questions** provide the flexibility to the patients (participants) to write responses in their own words. They lack answer choices that patients (participants) could select. An example of an open-ended question is: "What side effects of the medication are you experiencing?" Open-ended questions are intended to stimulate thoughtful responses from patients in their own words. These questions enable researchers to gather in-depth information on patient experiences and opinions. The disadvantage of open-ended questions is that they can be challenging and time consuming for patients to answer because they require patients to contemplate and provide a coherent response. Some patients may feel apprehensive about sharing their experiences and feelings in detail. The multitude of responses written could create coding challenges for the researcher. The open-ended format makes these questions unsuitable for statistical analysis. **Close-ended questions** present respondents with a specific set of response choices from which they have to choose an answer. An example of a close-ended question is: "Did you experience any side effects from the medication? [ ] Yes or [ ] No." Because these questions provide patients with options, they are easier and take less time to answer. These questions are also easy for the researchers to code and use in statistical analysis. The disadvantage of these questions is that they limit the option choices. As a result, potentially useful information may be missed if the response options do not capture the gamut of possible answers. Most research survey instruments involve close-ended questions for ease of coding and analysis.

A survey can be administered through different modes including mail, Internet, telephone, or face-to-face interview (discussed under *Interviews*). **Mail surveys** involve mailing of a questionnaire along with a cover letter and a postage-paid return envelope to selected participants.[21] Researchers typically select a sample from the list of populations of interest for time and cost considerations. The U.S. Census Bureau mostly relies on mail surveys to collect national-level census data. To conduct **online or Internet surveys**, researchers typically use web-based survey solution systems such as SurveyMonkey (www.surveymonkey.com) and Qualtrics (www.qualtrics.com). These systems provide researchers with considerable flexibility in survey design and deployment. Most course evaluations in colleges are conducted using the Internet. Surveys conducted by telephone solely depend on verbal communication. The process of telephonic surveys has been made more efficient with the advent of computer-assisted telephonic interviewing (CATI). It is an interactive system that assists interviewers in asking questions to participants. Data are entered and stored simultaneously on the computer as the interview progresses. The State and Local Area Integrated Telephone Surveys (SLAITS), like the National Immunization Survey (NIS) that collect valuable immunization data, are telephone-based surveys.

Interviews

Interviews provide an opportunity for researchers to ask questions and listen to participants' responses. **Face-to-face interviews** can be structured, semi-structured, or unstructured.[23] **Structured (or standardized) interviews** are those wherein the same set of questions is presented to all participants.[24] The set of questions and the sequence in which the questions are presented to the participants remain consistent in structured interviews.[25] Questions in structured interviews often have precoded response categories. The disadvantage of structured interviews is that they do not provide researchers with the opportunity to probe the participants on their responses. **Semi-structured interviews** include both structured and unstructured questions; they often include follow-up and/or clarifying questions.[23] **Unstructured interviews** are non-standardized and flexible, wherein the question and answer categories are not predetermined.[24] As a result, the depth and breadth of information collected from one interview to another tend to vary. The main advantage of unstructured interviews is that they help researchers in generating detailed data and provide in-depth information on a phenomenon. The disadvantage of unstructured interviews is that they could be time consuming. These interviews require highly skilled and trained interviewers who are able to control the direction of the conversation. Most of the research interviews are structured for ease of coding and analysis. The National Center for Health Statistics (NCHS) annually conducts the National Health Interview Survey (NHIS) to collect valuable healthcare data for national healthcare policy.

OBSERVATION

Another mode of data collection commonly used in clinical research is through observation of a participant's behavior. Researchers use observational techniques to gather data on participant activities, characteristics, communication, interaction, and time taken to complete a given task.[2,26] Using **observational technique**, the phenomenon of interest is watched, listened to, and recorded by the researcher.[23] Observation can be of two types: obtrusive and unobtrusive. In **obtrusive observation**, the participant is aware that he/she is being observed. The obtrusive observation method works well in situations where the researcher wants to gain insights into the participant's thought process during the performance of an activity. The disadvantage of obtrusive observation is that the participant may alter normal behavior in the presence of the observer to appear socially desirable.

In **unobtrusive observation**, the participant is unaware of the observer who may be either hidden or in disguise. Participants are less likely to alter their behaviors or activities when they are unaware that they are being observed. For example, unobtrusive observation may work well if a researcher wants to determine whether pharmacists counsel patients when filling prescription medications. In such a scenario, a researcher may put on a disguise as a pharmacy customer and observe the pharmacist–patient interaction from a distance. Both obtrusive and unobtrusive observation techniques have certain disadvantages,[27] which may limit their usefulness to only specific research settings. These techniques require highly skilled and trained observers.

BIOLOGICAL MEASURES

Biological assessments are made using biophysical, biochemical, and microbiological methods. Such clinical or laboratory tests require specialized instruments or devices such as electrocardiograms, glucometers, and microscopes. Biological assessments require skilled and knowledgeable technicians and allied healthcare professionals. These clinical tests are often conducted in laboratory settings or other specialized departments. Some consider these clinical tests to be unbiased scientific assessments because observations are made using clinical practice standards and guidelines. In recent years, there has been increasing development and marketing of devices that require minimal expertise. Some of these devices can be used by patients, such as glucometers. Biological measures are objective markers of a disease or a patient's health, and thus play a critical role in clinical research. The clinical tests are often validated before they are used in clinical practice. However, the reliability should be ascertained before they can be used for research or practice.

Biophysical assessments measure physical characteristics such as bone density, blood pressure, and forced expiratory volume. Examples of biophysical devices include x-ray, sphygmomanometer, electrocardiographs, ultrasound, and magnetic resonance imaging. **Biochemical methods** measure chemical constituents in bodily fluids such as blood or urine. Blood glucose, urine creatinine, and serum drug levels are examples of biochemical measures. These clinical tests require chemical analysis or assays using instruments such as spectroscopes and chromatography systems. **Microbiological methods** evaluate microorganisms such as bacteria or viruses in bodily fluids, such as blood or urine. These tests are based on the growth of bacterial cultures with evaluations involving microscopic examinations. In general, reliability and validity of biophysical, biochemical, and microbiological methods do not pose a problem in clinical research because these methods are based on good laboratory practices.

SUMMARY AND CONCLUSIONS

Research design and methodology represent the plan and means through which a researcher intends to collect data to address the research question. The choice of the study design and methodology are guided by several factors including the research area, availability and feasibility, and investigator expertise. Research designs can be classified based on different parameters including purpose of the study, time and investigator orientation, and experimental setting. The most common research design classifications are the experimental and observational designs. In experimental designs, a researcher randomly allocates study participants into treatment and control groups, whereas in observational designs, relationships are observed in a natural setting without any randomization. Research methodology provides the means through which data are collected. Data may be collected through primary or secondary techniques. When choosing a research methodology, researchers have to consider implications in the context of reliability and validity. Understanding the techniques of research design and methodology is important not only for researchers, but also for clinicians to evaluate the validity of research findings.

REVIEW QUESTIONS

1. What are the nine criteria of causation that were proposed by Sir Austin Bradford Hill in 1965?
2. What is the difference between prospective and retrospective study design?
3. Explain case-control and cohort study designs. How do the two designs differ?
4. Define validity and reliability using examples.
5. What are the different modes of survey administration?
6. List some biological measures and the methods used to collect the data.

ONLINE RESOURCES

e-Source: Behavioral and Social Science Research: http://www.esourceresearch.org/
Introduction to Methods for Health Service Research and Evaluation: http://ocw.jhsph.edu/index.cfm/go/viewCourse/course/HSRE/coursePage/index/

REFERENCES

1. Sackett DL, Rosenberg WM, Gray JA, Haynes RB, Richardson WS. Evidence-based medicine: what it is and what it isn't. *BMJ*. 1996;312(7023):71–72.
2. Polit DF, Hungler BP. *Nursing Research: Principles and Methods*. 5th ed. Philadelphia, PA: Lippincott Williams & Wilkins; 1995.
3. Harpe SE. Using secondary data in pharmacoepidemiology. In: Yang Y, West-Strum D. *Understanding Pharmacoepidemiology*. New York, NY: McGraw-Hill Medical; 2010:55–78.
4. Hill AB. The environment and disease: association or causation? *Proc R Soc Med*. 1965;58:295–300.
5. Grimes DA, Schulz KF. An overview of clinical research: the lay of the land. *Lancet*. 2002;359:57–61.
6. *Pneumocystis* pneumonia: Los Angeles. *Morb Mortal Wkly Rep*. 1981;30:250–252.
7. Hartung DM, Touchette D. Overview of clinical research design. *Am J Health Syst Pharm*. 2009;66(4):398–408.
8. Cranor CW, Bunting BA, Christensen DB. The Asheville Project: long-term clinical and economic outcomes of a community pharmacy diabetes care program. *J Am Pharm Assoc*. 2003;43:173–184.
9. Lu CY. Observational studies: a review of study designs, challenges and strategies to reduce confounding. *Int J Clin Pract*. 2009;63(5):691–697.
10. Roberts J, Dicenso A. Identifying the best research designs to fit the question. Part 1: quantitative designs. *Evid Based Nurs*. 1999;2(1):4–6.
11. Carlson MD, Morrison RS. Study design, precision, and validity in observational studies. *J Palliat Med*. 2009;12(1):77–82.
12. DiPietro NA. Methods in epidemiology: observational study designs. *Pharmacotherapy*. 2010;30(10):973–984.
13. Mahajan RP, Hunter JM. Case reports: should they be confined to the dustbin? *Br J Anaesth*. 2008;100:744–746.
14. McBride WG. Thalidomide and congenital abnormalities. *Lancet*. 1961;278(7216):1358.

15. Hymes KB, Cheung T, Greene JB, et al. Kaposi's sarcoma in homosexual men—a report of eight cases. *Lancet*. 1981;2(8247):598–600.

16. Lundh A, Christensen M, Jørgensen AW. International or national publication of case reports. *Dan Med Bul*. 2011;58(2):A4242.

17. Rothman KJ. *Epidemiology: An Introduction*. Oxford, England: Oxford University Press; 2002.

18. Mann CJ. Observational research methods. Research design II: cohort, cross sectional, and case-control studies. *Emerg Med J*. 2003;20:54–60.

19. Aday LA, Cornelius LJ. *Designing and Conducting Health Surveys: A Comprehensive Guide*. 3rd ed. San Francisco, CA: Jossey-Bass; 2006.

20. Hox JJ, Boeije HR. Data collection, primary versus secondary. In: Kempf-Leonard K, ed. *Encyclopedia of Social Measurement*. San Diego, CA: Academic Press; 2005:593–599.

21. Dillman DA. *Mail and Telephone Surveys: The Total Design Method*. New York, NY: John Wiley & Sons; 1978.

22. Salant P, Dillman DA. *How to Conduct Your Own Survey*. New York, NY: John Wiley & Sons; 1994.

23. Bowling A. *Research Methods in Health: Investigating Health and Health Services*. 3rd ed. Buckinghamshire, England: Open University Press; 2009.

24. Kajornboon AB. Using interviews as research instruments. *Chulalongkorn University E-Journal for Researching Teachers*. 2005;2(1). Available at: http://www.culi.chula.ac.th/e-Journal/bod/Annabel. pdf. Accessed November 11, 2012.

25. Corbetta P. *Social Research Theory, Methods and Techniques*. London, England: SAGE; 2003.

26. Schmuck R. *Practical Action Research for Change*. Arlington Heights, IL: IRI/Skylight Training and Publishing; 1997.

27. Jonassen DH, Tessmer M, Hannum WH. *Task Analysis Methods for Instructional Design*. Mahwah, NJ: Lawrence Erlbaum Associates; 1999.

4

RANDOMIZED CONTROLLED TRIALS

THOMAS C. DOWLING, PHARMD, PHD, FCCP

CHAPTER OBJECTIVES

▸ Understand the characteristics of randomized controlled trials

▸ Discuss design issues of randomized controlled trials, including sampling issues

▸ Describe common randomized controlled designs (parallel, crossover, adaptive)

▸ Explain briefly the analytical framework of randomized controlled trials

▸ Discuss the strengths and weaknesses of randomized controlled trials

KEY TERMINOLOGY

Active control
Adaptive designs
Adaptive randomization
Ascertainment bias
Attrition
Attrition bias
Bias
Blinding
Block randomization
Carryover effect
Clinical research protocol
Cluster randomization design
Crossover design
Data and safety monitoring board
Detection bias
Double-blind trial
Drug effectiveness
Drug efficacy
Effect size
Exclusion criteria

External validity
Factorial randomized trials
Hawthorne effect
Historical control
History
Inclusion criteria
Instrumentation
Intent-to-treat analysis
Interim analysis
Internal validity
Investigator bias
Maturation
Non-inferiority trials
Number needed to harm
Number needed to treat
On-treatment analysis
Open label
Parallel study design
Performance bias
Per-protocol analysis
Placebo

Power
Primary outcome
Randomization
Regression
Relative risk
Risk difference
Sample size
Selection bias
Selection bias in randomized controlled trial
Simple randomization
Single-blind trial
Stratified randomization
Study sample
Study validity
Subgroup analysis
Target population
Testing
Triple blinding
Validity
Washout period

INTRODUCTION

Randomized controlled trials provide strong evidence to support evidence-based medicine practices.[1,2] The goal of these trials is to measure a primary outcome in a highly selective group of individuals, or study participants, that are randomly assigned to receive one or more clinical interventions. In medicine, interventions may include drug therapies, prevention strategies, and medical procedures, and may occur in a variety of settings in which health care is provided, including educational research. Most randomized controlled trials are designed to determine the effect of a specific intervention on health-related outcomes, disease prevention, or progression of disease. The randomized controlled trial is widely regarded as the strongest type of study design in clinical research.

The randomized controlled trial is the most common type of trial that is used to determine the efficacy of an experimental intervention compared to a standard therapy or placebo. A key requirement in the clinical drug development cycle is the randomized controlled trial, often referred to as phase III studies or "pivotal trials" because they are used to establish the relative efficacy and safety of an investigational drug compared to a standard or control treatment group. Randomized controlled trials are required by the Food and Drug Administration (FDA) as part of a New Drug Application (NDA).[3] Adherence to very strict selection criteria, proper trial design, and minimization of bias are all critically important to establish the relative efficacy and safety of a drug. This chapter will review the most common characteristics of randomized controlled trials, including common study designs, sampling strategies, bias, and errors. The chapter will also address different ways to analyze the study data, including intention to treat and subgroup analysis.

MAXIMIZING VALIDITY

Despite having a highly qualified and dedicated research team assigned to a study, few, if any, clinical studies are designed perfectly. A study must be designed very carefully to ensure that the results obtained are valid and that the appropriate conclusions are inferred. The **validity** of a study refers to the degree to which the findings are correct. It is important to recognize the many factors that can ultimately threaten the validity and bias the study results.[4] The design and implementation are critical to maximize the validity of randomized controlled trials.

INTERNAL VALIDITY

Internal validity is the degree to which the outcome (efficacy or safety) can be explained by differences in assigned intervention (treatment). For example, a trial may set out to determine whether a new anti-hypertensive drug can reduce blood pressure in patients with hypertension. The protocol for this type of study would require very strict adherence to enrollment criteria, such that both groups (i.e., treatment vs. control) are as similar as possible before the study begins. A poorly designed study could report that a drug is effective at treating a given disease when, in fact, the patient groups were not equal or bias was introduced during the study. The process of controlling the study design factors, implemented by the scientist before conducting the study, is often referred to as the "internal validity" of the study. The best clinical trials are designed to have strong internal validity, in an effort to maximize the signal-to-noise detection. One way to strengthen internal validity in a study is to include a control group, or a group of individuals that are studied under the same experimental conditions as the treatment group. The best way to maximize internal validity is to randomly assign study participants to receive interventions so that the observed changes in the blood pressure (outcome or dependent variable) can most likely be explained by the new medication (intervention or independent variable). Some of the most important factors that may threaten the internal validity of a study include selection, history, maturation, mortality, testing, instrumentation, and statistical regression. Each of these factors is described below.

Selection

When a study involves a comparison of outcomes in a treatment group and a control group, the differences in patients' baseline characteristics (such as disease severity and demographics) in the two groups can lead to **selection bias**, and this can affect the internal validity of the study. The issue of selection bias is most problematic in retrospective trials or in observational designs because of the inability to control known and unknown baseline characteristics that influence the outcome. This is mainly attributed to lack of randomization in observational studies. In prospective randomized controlled trials, selection bias is minimized during the process of subject recruitment and the randomized phase of the trial. Furthermore, the randomization will ensure that patients in the two groups are similar with respect to known and unknown baseline characteristics.

History

Another factor that can alter the outcome of a study is related to external events that occur during the course of the study; this is referred to as **history**. Here, changes in the study outcome (dependent variable) may be attributed to these external events (such as the death of a family member or loss of a job) that occurred between study entry and evaluation time points. Thus, it may not be possible to distinguish whether or not the observed changes in outcome (blood pressure) were due to the intervention (medication) or the external events. Such external influences in the study can be minimized by the inclusion of a randomized control group in a prospective clinical trial design.

Maturation

Another way that study validity can be compromised is related to normal changes in study participants over time, often referred to as **maturation**. If there are changes that occur over the course of the study timeline, these must be accounted for at the outset of the study. Some examples of longitudinal maturation would include increase in disease severity or complexity in hypertensive patients during a study or worsening cognition over time in populations such as the elderly or those with dementia. The effect of maturation is best addressed by the use of a randomized control group, where similar changes are occurring over time in both the treatment and control groups.

Mortality/Attrition

The internal validity of a study can be compromised by the withdrawal or loss of subjects over time in the study groups, often referred to as **attrition**. This may occur due to the death of participants or dropout due to adverse events or lack of compliance to treatment regimens. This attrition poses a particular problem if it occurs to a greater extent in one group compared to another, or if it occurs in a nonrandom fashion, such as greater dropout in the treatment group due to adverse events than the control group. Attrition can also be a major contributor to bias in a study where dropout rates are significantly greater in a particular treatment group. The attrition rates have to be monitored and controlled by design or statistical analyses to minimize the effects of attrition on the internal validity of a study.

Testing

Studies that require participants to take tests or participate in their own assessment over time are susceptible to problems with internal validity due to repeated (prior) tests. Such **testing** effect for physiological or biological reasons can be "reactive" or "unreactive." A reactive effect of testing refers to situations where taking the "test" or assessment can influence subsequent tests and the outcome of the study. Studies that require self-monitoring, such as blood pressure measurements or tobacco use over time, are often considered highly reactive because the participant may alter their behaviors due to monitoring. Testing is a significant issue in psychological measurements and the testing effects are minimal in most biophysical measures. These types of threats to internal validity can be minimized by having consistent assessment methods used by unbiased investigators or research team members, or by using a randomized control group that is similarly influenced by reactive testing.

Instrumentation

Many types of studies are conducted over long periods of time and require the use of instruments to measure outcomes in the study participants over time. It is therefore possible that the changes in the instrumentation can influence the outcomes (referred to as **instrumentation**) and be attributed to the treatment or medication being studied. This may include changes in the sensitivity of the instrument, improvements in technology, and changes in the measurement techniques over time. There are significant concerns in studies involving survey instruments to evaluate symptoms or disease severity for psychiatric diseases such as depression. Consistent measurement processes in the study groups is a critical component of determining the efficacy of the study interventions.

Statistical Regression

The phenomenon of **regression** (or reversion) to the mean refers to cases where initial measurements of a variable are extremely different, either high or low, from the population mean, but then subsequent measurements are closer to the average. Such highly extreme values can often be attributed to a rare series of events that are unstable. Thus, subsequent measurements in that individual will be closer to the mean of the population of measurements, irrespective of the effects of the intervention. Sometimes this regression to the mean has been attributed to physiological processes. This occurs most often in studies that have outcomes that are susceptible to random errors. Avoiding extreme groups and using randomized control groups can minimize this internal validity problem.

External Validity

External validity indicates that the findings of a given study can be generalized to other settings or populations. For example, if a study is conducted in a small and select group of patients with hypertension who were not previously treated with medications, can the findings from this study be applied to all individuals with hypertension? The most common threats to external validity or generalizability occur in the areas of treatment interaction with subject selection, setting of the study, and historical factors.[5] Each of these factors is described below.

Interactions with Treatment and Subject Selection

This threat occurs if the effects of treatment on selected subjects differ from those of other populations. For example, this can occur if the study is conducted in military veterans who are mostly males and older adults. Clinicians often ask the following question while reading the results of a study: "Is the group of patients included in this study representative of the patients that I see in my clinic every day?" The basis for this question is whether or not the subjects selected in the clinical trial, and the results obtained in that trial, can be generalizable to other patients in different geographic regions or those with differing demographic backgrounds.

Interactions with Treatment and Pretesting

In studies involving a pretest, it is possible that the treatment will only work in those individuals who took the pretest. The process of pretesting may therefore sensitize the subjects to the treatment, and without the pretest it would be less effective or ineffective. This will make the findings not generalizable to those who were not pretested. This issue is more of a concern in studies evaluating psychological measures than studies examining biophysical measures.

Interactions with Treatment and Setting

Some clinical trials are conducted in highly specialized or artificial research settings using novel interventions and instrumentations. The results of these studies may not be extrapolated to normal settings such as rural community hospitals or outpatient clinics. For example, a university-based clinical trial in patients with hypertension (and no coexisting disease states) may have been designed to maximize internal validity, but may have low external validity because the results cannot be extrapolated to patients in a real-world setting. During controlled trials, it is also possible that subjects become more compliant to prescribed regimens or study-related procedures as a result of longitudinal learning that takes place during the trial. This is typically referred to as the **Hawthorne effect**, in which study subjects modify their behavior because of the fact that they are being studied or observed. In clinical research, subjects that are singled out for participation in clinical trials often have better outcomes than those in routine practice.[6]

Interactions with Treatment and History

It is possible that the results of a study conducted in the past may not apply today or in the future. The reason for this is that there are many factors that change in healthcare systems as time progresses, including access to care, standards of practice, and socioeconomic issues.

Multiple Treatments

The complexity of the treatment regimens or multiple treatments, as part of either the standard of care or the intervention, can have a significant effect on the results obtained. The study findings can be generalized to those with multiple treatments. Diseases often have multiple treatment approaches, where the doses and timing of a medication may be important determinants of the outcome. In such complex treatment designs, which contain a number of elements or where the study outcomes depend on factors that are outside the control of the researchers, the external validity can be challenged.

MINIMIZING BIAS

Bias can be defined as a systematic error in study design that can lead to incorrect findings. In the field of statistics, it often refers to the tendency of a measure to deviate in one direction from a true value. This type of consistent deviation from the true scenario can have disastrous effects on trial outcomes, leading to underestimation or overestimation of the true effects of the treatment. In reality, the true outcome of any medical intervention will never be known. Through employment of the experimental method, researchers try their best to measure the outcomes of a treatment and control bias in the study to yield a valid set of results from the study. However, it is never fully possible to know whether or not the results of a particular study are biased because the true results are unknown. It is important to recognize the five major types of bias that minimize the impact of these biases when designing clinical trials.[7]

INVESTIGATOR BIAS

Investigator bias refers to errors in study design, implementation, or analysis by the investigator. The research team is responsible for assessing and recording the outcomes of patients in a trial. These same investigators may also be aware of which patients are allocated to treatment and control groups, and they may unknowingly record the outcomes for patients being treated with the new drug in a more favorable way than for patients in the control group. If the study has already been completed, then the investigator may also be susceptible to **ascertainment bias**, where those responsible for analyzing or evaluating the study data are aware of which participants received the active versus control interventions. In this case, the effects of the new drug can be exaggerated if the investigators choose only those time points where the measured outcomes show the most benefit for the new drug, and ignore the data showing less impact of the new drug on the disease being treated. This type of bias can be minimized by keeping those involved in data analysis and those involved in assessing the patients during the study unaware of the treatment allocation (blinding).

SELECTION BIAS

Selection bias in randomized controlled trial refers to the preferential enrollment of specific patients into one treatment group over another.[8] During the recruitment and enrollment phases of the trial, selection bias may be introduced when allocating patients if the patients do not have equal chances to be allocated to the treatment or control arms. If patients with worse conditions are allocated to the control group, then the treatment arm may appear to be less effective, and vice versa. The most effective way to reduce selection bias is with randomization, where each subject has an equal and known chance to be enrolled in any study group. This is often accomplished using a computer algorithm to generate random numbers that are allocated to each subject.

PERFORMANCE BIAS

Performance bias refers to systematic differences in care between treatment groups, or in exposure to factors other than the intervention being studied. Once the study begins and subjects are randomized to treatment groups, performance bias can be introduced into the study if the investigators focus more attention on one group of patients compared to another. In this case, the experimental treatment group may have more intense monitoring and therefore have a greater chance of a positive outcome compared to another group that does not receive as much attention. This type of bias can be minimized by prohibiting the investigators from knowing the treatment allocations, or blinding.

ATTRITION BIAS

Attrition bias refers to differential dropout of patients in treatment and control groups. As a study is progressing, it is often observed that more subjects will drop out or become noncompliant in the treatment group that is most demanding or is associated with more side effects. Analyzing only this smaller group of patients that completed the treatment, and ignoring those who withdrew from the study, can result in attrition bias. This type of bias can be minimized by using the "intent-to-treat" analysis approach, as described in more detail later in this chapter.

DETECTION BIAS

Detection bias refers to systematic differences between groups in how outcomes are determined. It can occur when the investigator is aware of the study treatment allocation while making an assessment of the outcome in a given patient. Here, an objective assessment of the outcome cannot be made and systematic bias can lead to overestimation of the true effect of the intervention. This type of bias can be minimized by the use of non-study personnel to assess patient outcomes.

RANDOMIZATION

Randomization is the process of assigning patients to a treatment or control group randomly, or by chance alone, and is highly effective in reducing biases and confounding in a study. Biases are systematic and nonrandom deviations from the true values, whereas confounding factors influence the treatment and outcomes and, thereby, affect the study findings. In randomized trials, all study participants are given the same opportunity to be assigned to groups, thereby minimizing the biases and confounding to detect true differences in treatment groups.[4,5,7] The process of randomization can occur in several ways.

SIMPLE RANDOMIZATION

Simple randomization involves the use of a random number generator to allocate participants to study groups. This is equivalent to flipping a coin in a case of two treatment groups, where heads receives Treatment A and tails receives Treatment B. This is the simplest form of randomization, but it is also susceptible to flaws. For example, this approach can lead to unequal numbers of subjects assigned to two groups in studies with a small sample size. Having unequal numbers in each group can influence the distribution of baseline characteristics across the two groups.

BLOCK RANDOMIZATION

Block randomization refers to the process of dividing potential study subjects into a specified number of "blocks" to be randomized at the beginning of the trial, as a means of ensuring that the number of subjects in each treatment group will be equal. Here, the total number of subjects to be enrolled in the study is divided into a series of "blocks." Each block has the same number of subjects assigned from each group. If there are two treatments and one patient is assigned to each treatment, then the size of each block is 2. Once all blocks are assigned, the study will have equal numbers of subjects in each treatment group.

STRATIFIED RANDOMIZATION

Stratified randomization is the process of randomization that ensures balance of participants for predefined strata based on prognostic factors such as disease severity among the study groups. In addition to balancing the number of subjects in each treatment group, it is important to make sure that the subjects enrolled in each group have equal numbers of each stratum or level of a factor, such as age with strata of old and young patients. For example, if treatment Group A has more patients over the age of 60 than treatment Group B, the group containing older individuals may have a different response than the younger group. Thus, the trial may not be valid due to an imbalance in patient age. To achieve balance within each group, a stratified randomization process is employed. This involves stratification of patients and randomly assigning patients in each stratum. This results in groups that are balanced to account for characteristics of the study population, such as age, gender, race, and disease severity. Here, it is important that baseline measurements be taken before randomization, especially in smaller trials. In very large randomized trials, stratification is not usually required because the risk of imbalanced groups is less likely.

ADAPTIVE RANDOMIZATION

Adaptive randomization refers to the process of assigning patients to a treatment group generally based on previous success of the treatment as the trial progresses. Here, the probability of being assigned to a group changes based on the responses of the prior patients. For example, the ratio of experimental versus control may change from 1:1 to randomly assign patients to the arm in which the treatments are more favorable. In small clinical trials, prognostic factors may have a significant impact on the outcome of the study, such as age, previous treatment failures, and genetic mutations. Here, a covariate-adaptive randomization scheme may be used based on accumulating information on the distribution of covariates into the next randomization decision. These methods of adaptive randomization are not widely accepted in the scientific community, and their value has not been fully determined.[9,10]

BLINDING

Clinical trials are highly susceptible to biases that threaten the internal and external validity of the results. The best way to minimize bias related to an investigator, particularly as it relates to ascertainment, measurement, and detection bias, is by keeping those involved (patients, investigators, or monitors) in the trial unaware of the treatment allocations until the study has ended. This process is called **blinding** or masking. There are a number of ways that blinding can be applied to a clinical trial.[4,5,7]

SINGLE BLIND

In a **single-blind trial**, only one of the three categories of individuals (usually participant rather than investigator) is unaware of the intervention assignment. For example, the participant is blinded to the treatment allocation, whereas the trial investigator and assessors are aware of the intervention.

DOUBLE BLIND

In a **double-blind trial**, both the participants in the study (subjects) and those involved in the assessment (investigators and assessors) are unaware of the randomization schedule. For studies involving investigational agents, such as phase III clinical trials, at least two double-blind trials are typically required for the drug to be approved by the FDA.

TRIPLE BLIND

The most objective type of trial design is the triple-blind study. A triple-blind design is an extension of the double-blind study where patients and investigators are blinded. In **triple blinding**, an external group of individuals who are involved in monitoring the outcomes of the study are also kept unaware of the treatment allocations. For example, data may be sent to the review board in a blinded fashion as Treatment A and Treatment B. An advantage of the triple-blind study is that all individuals (patients, investigators, and monitors) involved in the allocation, evaluation, design, and monitoring are able to objectively review the study results.

OPEN LABEL

The least objective type of design is the open label study. In an **open label** study, all participants, investigators, and assessors are aware of the treatment allocation. This type of design should be avoided in studies that involve subjective assessments or outcome measurements comparing different treatments due to the potential for patient reporting and investigator bias. The open label design is usually restricted to early pharmacokinetic studies, or phase I trials, where objective information about drug exposure (such as absorption, distribution, metabolism, and excretion) and safety is learned about the investigational agent.

SAMPLE SIZE

The number of participants to be enrolled in each treatment group in a study, or **sample size**, must be determined before the study is conducted. The sample size is estimated using a series of mathematical equations based on several statistical assumptions and the difference that can be expected between the groups.[11] The goal is to determine the appropriate number of subjects that are needed to test the primary study hypothesis. The specific calculations of sample size are addressed in more detail in Chapter 13, "Sample Size and Power Analysis." Some important considerations for estimating sample size are briefly described below.

EFFECT SIZE

The **effect size** is a statistical estimation of the magnitude of effect due to treatment or association between two or more variables that is likely to occur. It can be thought of as the degree of difference between treatment groups that is clinically important—for example, a blood pressure difference of 10 mmHg. The effect size is usually estimated at the beginning of the study, and the sample size is calculated taking the effect size into consideration.

POWER

Power measures the capacity to detect a difference in the study groups if a true difference exists. The number of participants or sample size in a clinical trial has a significant impact on the ability to detect differences between groups, where a large study infers greater power to detect the true impact of the new drug or intervention than a small study. Studies with smaller numbers of subjects often suffer from low power, where a finding of "no difference in treatments" can actually be explained by having an insufficient number of subjects to show a difference, or a "false negative." Studies are typically designed to have 80% power to detect the difference in treatments equal to the "effect size" as discussed above.

RESEARCH PROTOCOL

A **clinical research protocol** is the standardized document that provides instructions to the investigators on all aspects of carrying out the study (**Table 4–1**). The protocol gives specific details on the scientific rationale, the study objectives, the hypothesis to be tested in the study, inclusion and exclusion criteria, the study design and methods, statistical information, monitoring of adverse events, and regulatory oversight. The protocol is designed so that all investigators can understand and implement the protocol in the same manner at a single site or multiple study sites. For investigational drugs, the FDA must review and approve all clinical protocols before administering the investigational

TABLE 4-1   Essential Elements of a Research Protocol
1. Introduction   a. Background/rationale
2. Clinical Study Objectives   a. Primary and secondary objectives

3. Study Design
   a. Study schematic
   b. Allocation to treatment
   c. Decision mechanism for breaking blinding

4. Subject Selection   a. Subject inclusion and exclusion criteria

5. Study Drugs
   a. Study drug compliance/adherence
   b. Withdrawal of subjects due to noncompliance
   c. Study drug supplies
      i. Formulation and packaging
      ii. Preparing and dispensing
      iii. Drug administration
   d. Storage and accountability
   e. Concomitant medications

6. Research Study Procedures
7. Safety and Effectiveness Assessments
8. Adverse Event Reporting
9. Recording/Reporting Requirement
10. Statistical Methods/Data Analysis
11. Quality Control and Quality Assurance
12. Data Handling and Record Keeping
13. Institutional Review Board Documentation
14. Study Discontinuation Criteria
15. References

agent to humans. As mandated by federal regulations, all protocols involving human subjects must also be approved by an institutional review board (IRB).[12]

SELECTING THE PARTICIPANTS

TARGET POPULATION

The **target population** is defined as the group of people with the desired clinical and demographic characteristics that will ultimately benefit from generalization of the study findings. For example, adults over 18 years of age with hypertension would be a target population for a study to evaluate the effectiveness of a new anti-hypertensive drug.

STUDY SAMPLE

The **study sample** is a more specific subset of the target population that is accessible to the investigators and that participates in the study. For example, a group of adults over 18 years of age receiving care from the University of Maryland Hypertension Clinic in Baltimore, MD, would be a study sample from the target population above.

INCLUSION/EXCLUSION CRITERIA

To control the clinical and demographic characteristics in a study sample, a set of inclusion/exclusion criteria is applied during study enrollment. Here, **inclusion criteria** relate to the specific characteristics that the investigator is most interested in studying. For example, a study may include patients with hypertension (BP > 130/80 mmHg), over the age of 60 years, and receiving an ACE inhibitor for at least 2 months to evaluate the efficacy of a new antihypertensive intervention. **Exclusion criteria** relate to factors that would confound or impair the ability to interpret the study results. For example, patients with severe kidney disease might be excluded from a study to evaluate the efficacy of a new antihypertensive agent, where drug safety may be an issue. Studies with fewer exclusion criteria are more likely to be more generalizable than those with an extensive list of exclusion criteria.

RECRUITMENT

The plan for study recruitment is an important part of the clinical protocol. The size and quality of the study sample for randomization depends on the success of the recruitment plan. The details of the recruitment strategy should be clearly described so that all personnel are able to consistently carry out the recruitment plan. The recruitment strategy is also a requirement for IRB approval, and is based on ethical principles.[13] The approach for recruiting potential subjects for a given clinical trial depends entirely on the inclusion and exclusion criteria in the protocol. For example, a randomized controlled trial to evaluate a new hypertension drug may recruit patients from an ambulatory clinic that includes a population of patients being treated for hypertension. Patients may also take an active role in seeking out clinical trials by searching the Internet. For example, the largest database of ongoing clinical trials in need of volunteers is located at ClinicalTrials .gov, which is published by the National Institutes of Health (NIH). Subjects are often recruited to participate in clinical trials by posted advertisements or use of other media outlets linked to medical research centers, ambulatory care clinics, and other hospital settings. All information and research-related data obtained by the research team about potential research subjects during the recruiting process must remain private and confidential in order to minimize the risk of revealing sensitive health information to those not approved to handle this data.

SELECTION OF CONTROL GROUP

PLACEBO CONCURRENT CONTROL

One of the most challenging aspects of designing a randomized controlled trial is the selection of a control intervention. In cases where there is no known effective therapy, an identical-appearing placebo group is most appropriate. A **placebo** consists of an inert substance (such as lactose powder) that is identical in appearance (shape and form) to the active treatment. Use of a placebo is preferred to the absence of giving a dose because it reduces the risk of bias and unblinding.

ACTIVE CONTROLS

In cases where there is a known or accepted standard of care or treatment, then participants are randomized to either the intervention or an **active control** group that is consistent with the recommended therapy. The use of active controls often occurs in hypertension trials, where it is not ethical or possible to administer an inert placebo to these patients that require treatment.

HISTORICAL (EXTERNAL) CONTROLS

In some cases, a group of participants receiving the intervention may be compared to an external group of patients that was observed at a different time (**historical control**) or in a different treatment setting. For example, a group of patients receiving the intervention (new antihypertensive combination) in an ambulatory clinic that is not related to the study site may be selected as an external control group. An advantage of this type of trial is that all participants in the study receive the intervention. Such studies involving external controls generally require larger numbers of subjects than placebo-controlled trials. A disadvantage of externally controlled studies is that participants and investigators are unblinded, and the results are susceptible to a variety of biases as described above. Generally, historical controls are not well accepted in the scientific community due to significant internal validity concerns.

NON-INFERIORITY TRIALS

The most common type of randomized controlled trial is a superiority trial, which aims to determine whether or not one treatment is better than another. In contrast, an equivalence trial aims to determine whether or not two interventions are equivalent or nearly equivalent based on a set of acceptance criteria. **Non-inferiority trials** show that the effect of a new treatment is not worse than that of an active control by some specified margin. For example, an investigator may want to know if an alternative treatment has similar clinical benefit to treat hypertension (i.e., reduce systolic blood pressure by 20 mmHg) when compared to the current standard of care. Non-inferiority trials typically have fewer patients than superiority trials and may be used when a placebo group is not ethically allowed.

STUDY DESIGN DESCRIPTION

PARALLEL

In a **parallel study design**, each subject is randomized to either to a treatment group or a placebo group only (**Figure 4-1**). All members of the group receive the treatment/placebo over the duration of the study. This is the most common design that is used for phase III comparative trials, where patients with a given disease are randomized to receive either the experimental drug or the standard therapy and followed over a specified period of time. Advantages of a parallel study include strength of the design and shorter time needed to conduct the trial. However, this type of design usually requires a large sample size when compared to crossover designs.

CROSSOVER

In a **crossover design**, each subject receives all of the interventions based on a specified sequence of events (**Figure 4-2**). For example, if two interventions are to be studied, subjects will be randomized to a treatment sequence, such as "AB" or "BA." In this case,

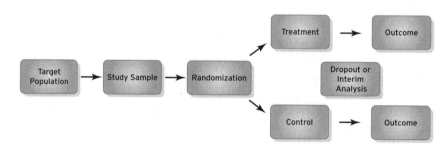

FIGURE 4-1   Parallel randomized controlled trial.

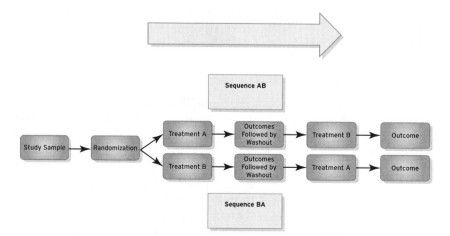

FIGURE 4-2   Crossover randomized controlled trial.

patients in the AB group receive Treatment A first, and then cross over to Treatment B after the appropriate washout period. For patients in the BA group, subjects receive Treatment B first, and then cross over to Treatment A. This type of paired design can have more statistical power with fewer subjects than a parallel design, since each subject undergoes both treatments. Disadvantages of crossover studies include the need to enroll patients with more stable disease states. They take longer to conduct due to washout periods and often have a higher dropout rate than parallel designs.

CARRYOVER AND WASHOUT

Crossover studies are susceptible to problems related to carryover and washout. **Carryover effect** refers to outcomes that remain or linger after the first treatment phase (such as Treatment A) is completed. These effects can carry over into Treatment B, which alters the baseline and subsequently alters the true treatment effect of Treatment B. The second problem relates to the **washout period**, which is the time needed for the outcomes of Treatment A to dissipate prior to beginning Treatment B. This is particularly problematic for studies involving drugs with slow elimination or long half-lives, where washout periods are typically extended over weeks or months.

FACTORIAL DESIGN

Factorial randomized trials are designed to evaluate multiple interventions in a single experiment. Factors to be studied can include multiple dose levels and multiple drug regimens. For example, in the simplest 2×2 factorial design, patients would be assigned to one of the two dose levels (i.e., 100 mg or 200 mg) and one of the two drug choices (Drug A or Drug B).

GROUP OR CLUSTER RANDOMIZATION

In a **cluster randomization design**, a specific group of subjects is selected for randomization—for example, patients enrolled in a clinic or hospital. These groups would then be randomly selected to a specific sequence of treatments or study procedures. All members of a cluster would receive the same treatment sequence.

ADAPTIVE DESIGN

One of the most state-of-the art ways to design clinical trials is using adaptive designs.[9,10] In **adaptive designs**, the conditions of a study or analysis plan are prospectively planned to be modified over time based on the results of preliminary analysis at interim time points. One potential advantage of this method over traditional designs is the ability to reduce the number of subjects to be enrolled in the active intervention group when compared to the original sample size calculation.

DESIGNING THE INTERVENTION

EFFECTIVENESS VERSUS EFFICACY

The goal of a **drug efficacy** study is to determine the effects of an intervention under tightly controlled conditions, where the study is designed to have very narrow inclusion and exclusion criteria. Most randomized controlled trials conducted during drug development (phase III) are designed to determine the efficacy of the new drug compared to placebo (or standard of care). The measures of efficacy usually include physiological measures (i.e., blood pressure, number of seizures), survival (yes/no), and quality of life (survey/questionnaire), and can be objective or subjective in nature. In contrast, **drug effectiveness** studies are designed to determine the effects of the intervention under the conditions that the drug is most often used in the clinical setting. For example, compliance to prescribed drug regimens in efficacy studies is closely monitored, whereas compliance assessment in effectiveness studies occurs in a less stringent, real-world fashion.

SAFETY

Evaluation of patient safety is an important aspect of randomized controlled trials. The measures of safety are often chosen based on the results of preclinical toxicology studies, and may include plasma and urine biochemistries (such as liver and kidney function), physical assessments and number of hospitalizations. Safety is often assessed using different dosages of the drug being investigated. Defining the relationship between the dose of the drug and the efficacy (or toxicity) requires a well-designed clinical trial. This type of trial is called a dose–response study. Addition of a placebo arm in a dose–response study is helpful to further characterize the treatment efficacy and safety of the new drug.

ADHERENCE

Lack of adherence to prescribed drug regimens can be detrimental to the success of a randomized trial. Some examples of non-adherence include taking the wrong dose at the wrong times, stopping drug therapy early, or never initiating drug therapy. The common reasons for non-adherence are low literacy, physiological factors (i.e., loss of vision or hearing), behavioral factors (i.e., social/living conditions, low motivation), inconvenience, financial factors, and perceived risk of adverse events. This ultimately leads to inaccurate dosing histories, contributes to variability in observed drug response, and confounds the assessment of dose–response. Taking accurate dose histories is an important aspect of monitoring during the clinical trial. Some strategies to improve adherence include education, counseling, and compliance aids (such as a pill box) and can be most effectively carried out by a clinical pharmacist.

STUDY MEASUREMENTS

BASELINE MEASUREMENT

It is important to accurately characterize a study population before beginning an intervention trial. This is accomplished by collecting important baseline information on all study participants in a clinical trial prior to randomization. Various types of baseline information include demographic information (age, height, weight, sex), coexisting conditions (diabetes, heart disease, hyperlipidemia), current medications, social history (alcohol, smoking history), and any other variables that may impact the outcome of interest. This baseline information is also important for subgroup analysis of the primary and secondary outcome variables. An important baseline variable may also be selected for the purpose of stratified randomization, to ensure that the potential confounding factor (such as smoking history) is evenly distributed between groups, since a balance between groups would not likely occur based on chance alone.

PROCESS MEASUREMENT

Process data are collected during the post-randomization period and provide important information on the degree of adherence to a study protocol. Examples of process variables include adherence rates, protocol deviations, attendance at study visits, and safety monitoring. Process data can also provide important insights into the degree of confounding that may be present in a study.

OUTCOME MEASUREMENT

Outcome variables are the measurements that are most likely to directly result from the study intervention. A randomized controlled trial should have only one **primary outcome** (usually efficacy), which is the main outcome of interest. It is specified before the trial begins and is usually measured objectively. The study hypothesis and sample size are developed based on the primary outcome variable. Since this primary outcome is of utmost importance, it is described in much detail in the study protocol. For example, the exact time for measuring the primary outcome may be specified, such as measuring the urine albumin concentration in the first morning urine sample using a specific urine detection assay at 30 days after beginning drug therapy.

BIOMARKERS

Intermediate markers that measure disease progression are often employed as surrogate markers in clinical trials. These biomarkers are often used as secondary outcome, or surrogate, measures. Trials that use surrogate outcomes typically enroll fewer patients than large clinical trials and occur over shorter time frames. These biomarkers are usually linked to the underlying disease process but do not directly measure disease activity. Examples of biomarkers include Cystatin-C to assess kidney function and LDL cholesterol for cardiovascular disease. Data obtained from trials using surrogate markers as primary outcome variables may be considered controversial if the biomarker is not closely linked to a clinical outcome. Health risk behaviors, such as smoking and diet, can also be considered biomarkers that are known to have an impact on an outcome such as cardiovascular disease.

SAFETY MONITORING

Monitoring the safety of each patient enrolled in a randomized controlled trial is extremely important. Adverse events are documented and reviewed by a physician investigator, along with the temporal relationship and likelihood of association with the intervention. For example, an adverse event may be classified as unlikely, possibly, probably, or definitely related to the study intervention. The appearance of serious and unexpected adverse events could lead to early discontinuation of the trial and, in the case of an FDA-regulated trial, an update to the product label. Another avenue for safety monitoring in a clinical trial is through a **data and safety monitoring board** (DSMB). The DSMB is a committee of scientists that are not associated with the conduct of the study, who evaluate adverse events at regularly scheduled intervals during the course of the study and provide feedback to the investigator and IRB regarding continuation of the study as planned.[12]

ANALYZING THE RESULTS

WHEN TO ANALYZE

Evaluation of the study endpoints usually occurs after all assessments are completed in the study sample. Some trials may have multiple measurements that were taken over a specified time frame during the study, or longitudinal assessments. Interim analysis plans are often included in protocols that allow for early escape from the intervention or when the intervention is being used for disease states with a high risk of progression (such as HIV and cancer).[14] Here, subjects are promptly removed from the study when the treatment fails, clinical conditions worsen, or one drug is shown to be highly superior to another. The decision to conduct an interim analysis is made by the external scientific review board (or DSMB) at pre-specified intervals based on statistical principles related to assumptions about the differences expected between interventions. Potential problems with interim analyses include relatively few data points, inexact inferences, and errors of interpretation. Also, interim results that are conveyed to investigators could lead to introduction of bias during the remainder of the study.

HOW TO ANALYZE

Intent-to-Treat Analysis

Attrition bias can occur when patients drop out or withdraw from a study when they are assigned to a treatment that is more demanding or associated with adverse events. By using the **intent–to-treat analysis** approach, patients are analyzed as if they completed the study in their originally assigned group. For example, if patients are allotted to a high-dose group, but then drop out or are provided a lower dose for safety/efficacy reasons, they are still analyzed as part of the high-dose group. This type of analysis gives a better indication of the effectiveness of the initial treatment.

On-Treatment (Per-Protocol) Analysis

On-treatment analysis, or **per-protocol analysis**, occurs when only those subjects who completed all aspects of the protocol are evaluated. This type of analysis is at risk of having a lower number of subjects than the total number enrolled due to protocol deviations, early withdrawals, or those lost to follow-up. This type of analysis is often used in broader sensitivity analysis, where the "per-protocol" and intent-to-treat data sets are compared to investigate any losses to internal validity. A pitfall of this type of analysis is that any exclusion of patients compromises the randomization and may lead to bias in the results.

Interim Analysis

An important ethical responsibility of investigators is to include only the minimum number of participants in a trial needed to achieve the primary objective of the study. It is possible that the initial assumptions made during the design of the study, such as the variability in treatment response or safety signals, may not hold true during the course of the study. It may, therefore, be necessary to conduct **interim analysis** to monitor study outcomes at periodic times during the course of the study.[12,14] This type of periodic monitoring or interim analysis is conducted by an independent committee or DSMB. The purpose of the DSMB is to determine whether or not the trial is meeting the primary objective and is safe to continue as planned. The DSMB reviews certain aspects of the study such as the rates of subject inclusion, rates of adverse events, outcomes based on previous experience with the drug, and statistical analysis of outcomes in the intervention and control groups. If safety concerns exist, then the DMSB committee may recommend early stopping of the trial and closure of the study.

Subgroup Analysis

Subgroup analysis is accomplished by analyzing the outcomes within categories or subgroups of participants, based on demographics or other important characteristics.[15,16] The purpose is to compare the primary outcome among subgroups of participants that completed a given study. For example, subgroups can be based on gender, ethnicity, race, or severity of disease. This approach is particularly useful in very large randomized trials, where the degree of response or nonresponse to treatment can be determined according to baseline demographics or clinical characteristics. Differences between subgroups are most appropriately assessed using statistical analysis to test for interactions between groups. Subgroups can also be arranged into those that responded to treatment (*responders*) and those that did not (*nonresponders*). A disadvantage of dividing the study participants into many subgroups is that the probability of a false positive finding increases. The subgroups can also suffer from small sample sizes, which could be insufficient to detect true differences between groups.

ANALYTICAL APPROACH

RELATIVE RISK AND RISK DIFFERENCE

When a study compares a risk of events in two or more groups, statistical tests are necessary to rule out chance variation. A detailed discussion on statistics is provided in Section 2, "Statistical Principles and Data Analysis." The simplest way to report the difference between groups involves the use of relative risk or risk difference.[17] One group may have a different rate of outcome (i.e., reduction in blood pressure) compared to another group. The **relative risk** is calculated as a ratio between risk or rate of the outcome in the treatment and control groups. This relative risk is different from the increase in risk. For example, in a clinical trial to determine whether a new blood pressure–lowering medication has a greater relative risk of a positive outcome (controlled hypertension) compared to a control group, the following 2 × 2 table is generated:

Outcome	Treatment	Control
Controlled HTN (Blood pressure < 130/80)	18 (*A*)	6 (*B*)
Uncontrolled HTN (Blood pressure > 130/80)	32 (*C*)	44 (*D*)

Here, relative risk (RR) is calculated as:

$$\text{Relative Risk} = \frac{\dfrac{A}{(A+C)}}{\dfrac{B}{(B+D)}} = \frac{\dfrac{18}{50}}{\dfrac{6}{50}} = \frac{0.36}{0.12}$$
$$= 3.00$$

The effect of a specific treatment on an event can be also calculated in terms of absolute **risk difference** (RD). This calculation is simply the difference of risk of outcomes in treatment and control groups. Here, the RD is calculated as:

$$\text{Risk Difference} = \frac{A}{(A+C)} - \frac{B}{(B+D)}$$
$$= 0.36 - 0.12 = 0.24$$

Number Needed to Treat

The effectiveness of an intervention can be assessed using a mathematical calculation called the **number needed to treat** (NNT).[17] The NNT refers to the number of patients that must receive the treatment for one patient to experience a desired outcome. It is calculated as:

$$\text{Number Needed to Treat} = \frac{1}{\text{RD}}$$

In the above hypertension example, the absolute RD was 0.24.

$$\text{Risk Difference} = 0.36 - 0.12 = 0.24$$

$$\text{Number Needed to Treat} = \frac{1}{\text{RD}} = \frac{1}{0.24} = 4.16$$

Here, the NNT is 4. This means that about one in every four patients will achieve positive blood pressure control by using the treatment instead of control. The **number needed to harm** (NNH) is calculated similarly. The NNH reflects the number of patients that must receive the treatment for one patient to experience an adverse outcome. Obviously, the NNH should be high to be considered a safe medication. Often, NNT and NNH are compared to understand the relative benefit of treatment.

STRENGTHS AND WEAKNESSES

Randomized controlled trials have an inherently strong ability to determine the unbiased efficacy of an intervention. The prospective design allows for tight control of study design, setting, and environment. Stringent pre-study and protocol specifications allow for balance of baseline variables between intervention groups, minimization of investigator and systematic bias, and a strong ability to identify causal relationships between the intervention and outcome. It is a methodologically and statistically strong research design.

However, the tenet that these trials remain the "gold standard" for evidence-based medicine has been criticized. The process of ensuring high internal validity and randomly assigning subjects to an intervention or control group can have significant limitations on generalizability. For example, the randomized trial does not provide information about which specific patients will benefit from the intervention; only that a subset of patients on average will benefit from treatment. Thus, decisions about evidence-based medicine should not be limited to only randomized controlled trials, but also include additional data obtained from phase II studies, single-case studies, epidemiological data, and phase IV post-marketing surveillance studies. Other limitations include the expense and time commitment required by investigators and participants, ethical concerns related to randomization, high dropout rates during the study, and potential Hawthorne-type longitudinal learning that limits generalizability of the results.

SUMMARY AND CONCLUSIONS

Well-designed and rigorously conducted randomized controlled trials provide critical information that can significantly impact the clinical practice of medicine. These trials can accurately determine the efficacy of a new drug or intervention using various types of randomizations and designs, active or placebo control groups, recruitment strategies, and data analysis approaches. An understanding of these clinical design issues is useful for clinicians as they take part in clinical research. It is also important to evaluate all aspects of the trial design to interpret the results of published research and consider the applicability of the study findings to practice evidence-based medicine.

REVIEW QUESTIONS

1. Describe the impact of using inclusion and exclusion criteria on the validity of a clinical trial.
2. Discuss ways to minimize attrition bias in clinical trials.
3. Briefly outline an optimal study that could be conducted to evaluate the effect of Drug X on Alzheimer's disease progression and justify your choice of design, blinding, internal/external validation, and outcome measures.
4. Compare and contrast factorial, sequential, crossover, and adaptive designs in clinical trials.

ONLINE RESOURCES

ClinicalTrials.gov: http://www.clinicaltrials.gov/
Consolidated Standards of Reporting Trials (CONSORT): http://www.consort-statement.org/home/
NIH Clinical Trials: http://www.nih.gov/health/clinicaltrials/
What Works Clearinghouse: Registry of Randomized Clinical Trials in education research: http://ies.ed.gov/ncee/wwc/references/registries/RCTSearch/RCTSearch.aspx

REFERENCES

1. Williams BA. Perils of evidence-based medicine. *Perspect Biol Med.* 2010;53(1):106–120.
2. Stolberg HO, Norman G, Trop I. Randomized controlled trials. *Am J Roentgenol.* 2004; 183(6):1539–1544.
3. Guidance for Industry. E10 Choice of Control Group and Related Issues in Clinical Trials. FDA: May 2001.
4. Appel LJ. A primer on the design, conduct, and interpretation of clinical trials. *Clin J Am Soc Nephrol.* 2006;1:1360–1367.
5. Kendall JM. Designing a research project: randomized controlled trials and their principles. *Emerg Med J.* 2003;20(2):164–168.
6. McCarney R, Warner J, Iliffe S, van Haselen R, Griffin M, Fisher P. The Hawthorne effect: a randomised, controlled trial. *BMC Med Res Methodol.* 2007;7:30.
7. Stanley K. Design of randomized controlled trials. *Circulation.* 2007;115(9):1164–1169.
8. Berger VW, Exner DV. Detecting selection bias in randomized clinical trials. *Control Clin Trials.* 1999;20(4):319–327.
9. Korn EL, Freidlin B. Outcome—adaptive randomization: is it useful? *J Clin Oncol.* 2011;29(6):771–776.
10. Guidance for Industry. Adaptive design clinical trials for drugs and biologics. FDA: February 2010.
11. Lader EW, Cannon CP, Ohman EM, et al. The clinician as investigator: participating in clinical trials in the practice setting. Appendix 1: fundamentals of study design. *Circulation.* 2004;109(21):e302–e304.

12. Silverman H. Ethical issues during the conduct of clinical trials. *Proc Am Thorac Soc.* 2007;4:80–184.

13. Belmont Report (1979). *The Belmont Report: Ethical Principles and Guidelines for the Protection of Human Subjects of Research.* Accessed December 18, 2012, from hhs.gov/ohrp/humansubjects/guidance/belmont.html.

14. Fossa SD, Skovlund E. Interim analyses in clinical trials: why do we plan them? *J Clin Oncol.* 2000;18(24):4007–4008.

15. Wang R, Lagakos SW, Ware JH, et al. Statistics in medicine—reporting of subgroup analyses in clinical trials. *N Engl J Med.* 2007;357(21):2189–2194.

16. Peduzzi P, Henderson W, Hartigan P, Lavori P. Analysis of randomized controlled trials. *Epidemiol Rev.* 2002;24(1):26–38.

17. Tripepi G, Jager KJ, Dekker FW, et al. Measures of effect: relative risks, odds ratios, risk difference, and number needed to treat. *Kidney Int.* 2007;72(7):789–791.

COHORT AND CASE-CONTROL STUDIES

LORI A. FISCHBACH, MPH, PHD

BRADLEY C. MARTIN, PHARMD, PHD

CHAPTER OBJECTIVES

▸ Describe the design characteristics of case-control and cohort designs

▸ Describe the strengths and limitations of case-control and cohort designs

▸ Identify common biases in case-control and cohort designs

▸ Calculate and interpret common measures of association used in case-control and cohort designs

KEY TERMINOLOGY

Attributable fraction in the
   exposed
Attributable risk
Attributable risk percent
Base population
Bias
Case-control
Cases
Closed cohorts
Cohort study
Concordant pair
Confounding factor
   (or confounder)
Controls
Detection bias
Diagnostic bias
Differential misclassification
Discordant pair

Effectiveness
Efficacy
Exposed group
Exposure
Exposure status
Fixed cohort
Hospital- or clinic-based
   case-control studies
Incident cases
Induction period
Information bias
Latency period
Matching
Measures of association
Measures of effect
Nested case-control
Non-differential misclassification
Odds ratio

Open cohort
Population-based case-control
Prevalent cases
Prevented fraction in the
   exposed
Primary data
Prospective cohort studies
Recall bias
Retrospective cohort studies
Rate ratio
Risk difference
Risk ratio
Secondary data
Selection bias
Temporal ambiguity
Unexposed group

INTRODUCTION

Observational epidemiologic studies such as the cohort and case-control designs are used to inform patients, clinicians, and policy makers on a wide variety of topics, including the effects of drugs and the influence of different pharmacy services on a range of outcomes in humans. Though there are more challenges in establishing causal inferences with observational studies compared to randomized controlled trials (RCTs), these studies are the only ethical way to gain insights on the effects of exposures known to have harmful effects that would be of interest to clinicians. For example, the effect of exposure to tobacco smoke, illicit drug use, or a nutrient-poor diet on disease risk cannot be examined using RCTs because it would be unethical to purposefully expose persons to these types of conditions that pose harmful effects while having virtually no health benefits. The only ethical way to enumerate the effect of these exposures on disease risk in humans is by carefully conducting observational studies.

Although RCTs are considered the "gold standard" to estimate the effect of an exposure (or treatment) on a disease outcome in humans, they are still subject to bias and other limitations. RCTs often have limited generalizability; they are primarily designed to assess **efficacy,** the effect of a treatment in ideal settings on disease outcomes, rather than **effectiveness,** the effect of the treatment in typical clinical settings on disease outcomes. Most often, clinical trials are not adequately powered to estimate the effects of treatment on rare clinical endpoints and side effects (or adverse events). For example, a cohort study detected an elevated risk of cardiac death associated with azithromycin that was undetected in clinical trials.[1] RCTs also often do not follow study subjects long enough to estimate the effect of treatments on clinical endpoints that take a long time to develop.[2] Further, if patients in clinical trials do not adhere to (or comply with) their randomly assigned treatments, then the intention-to-treat analyses that are commonly used can produce biased estimates of effect.[2]

There is a growing emphasis on observational epidemiologic designs to answer important clinical questions where there are knowledge gaps in the comparative effectiveness framework.[3] For example, a comparative effectiveness cohort study provided evidence that a newer and more expensive radiation therapy (intensity-modulated radiation therapy) was more effective than traditional radiation therapy in prostate cancer patients to prevent recurrent cancer and with fewer side effects.[4] These designs can also be used to identify new uses of existing therapies that can be confirmed by clinical trials. By using observational epidemiologic designs, safety and effectiveness can be ascertained by using data sources that represent typical care. This chapter describes two prominent and often used observational epidemiologic designs, the cohort study and the case-control study, and discusses the design, analysis, and interpretation of the results that use these approaches.

COHORT STUDIES

GENERAL DESIGN FRAMEWORK

A **cohort study** typically consists of subjects at risk for a disease(s) whose exposure status, such as aspirin use, is assessed at baseline, and who are followed up over time to detect incident (new cases of) disease, such as cardiovascular disease. The term "**exposure**" or "**exposure status**" is typically used to describe an innate trait, or contact, experience, intake, etc. with a potential risk or protective factor whose effect on the outcome is being examined in the study. **Figure 5-1** provides an illustration of a cohort study comparing two groups: one exposed to a treatment of interest and another that is unexposed.

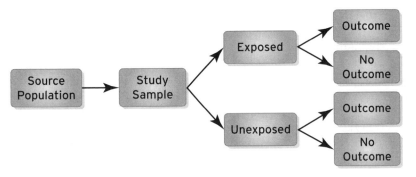

FIGURE 5-1   Diagram of a typical cohort study.

Cohort studies can be used to assess the influence of biomarkers or risk factors such as Apolipoprotein E (ApoE) e4 alleles or body mass index on the occurrence of a disease. It can also compare the effect of two or more treatments (e.g., clopidogrel compared to aspirin) on clinical outcomes. The latter parallels a clinical trial where treatment groups are formed based on whether or not they received a certain treatment versus another treatment and then are followed forward in time (or followed up) to compare the frequency of outcome(s) between the treatment groups. Unlike a clinical trial, however, the investigator does not randomly allocate or assign subjects to treatment groups, but rather observes and compares the outcome(s) between two or more groups that happened to be exposed to the treatment(s) of interest.

TYPES OF COHORT DESIGNS

Cohort studies may be considered retrospective or prospective depending on whether the subjects' current exposure and/or outcome status is being measured while the study is being conducted (prospective) or whether the subjects' past exposure and/or outcome status is being used (retrospective). **Prospective cohort studies** typically rely on actively recruiting and screening subjects, assessing baseline exposures and risk factors, and subsequently assessing the development of outcomes over a follow-up period at regular intervals. Prospective cohort studies may recruit subjects participating in surveys, from healthcare facilities, or from other sources. **Retrospective cohort studies**, sometimes referred to as historical cohort studies, use the same general framework as the prospective cohort study, but previous exposures and disease outcomes are typically measured using stored biological samples or existing records. Cohort studies using past exposure to measure the exposure of interest are followed for the incidence of the outcome after exposed members of the cohort are exposed. These studies commonly take advantage of existing data such as administrative claims data, medical records, or patient registries.

Well-designed prospective cohort studies have several advantages over retrospective cohort studies, which may include (1) tailoring the study measures specific to the research question(s), (2) purposefully capturing data on important risk factors (exposures, outcomes, confounders, etc.), (3) using reliable and validated techniques to assess exposure and outcome measures, and (4) measuring the exposure before the disease occurs, which can lead to more valid and reliable research findings. On the other hand, prospective cohort studies incur the expense of actively recruiting subjects and may take considerable time to complete, particularly for studying outcomes that take a long time to develop. Retrospective cohort studies have the advantage of being able to quickly produce study results, but can only be used to investigate exposures that have previously existed in the population (e.g., treatments that have been on the market for a sufficiently long time to observe the effect of the treatment(s) on the outcome(s)). Retrospective cohort studies are also limited because errors in the measurement of important factors (e.g., exposures, outcomes, confounders, etc.) may exist in some retrospective data sources.

Cohort studies may include closed or open cohorts. **Closed cohorts**, such as birth cohorts, start with a set group of individuals who are followed forward in time to determine if they develop the disease outcome. When this follow-up time is fixed for all individuals in the cohort, the closed cohort is called a **fixed cohort**. **Open cohorts**, for example, a cohort of persons with commercial insurance, permit persons to come in and drop out of the cohort over time and contribute variable follow-up time for the duration they are in the cohort.

EXPOSURE EVALUATION

Typically, a cohort study is initiated by a cross-sectional study to determine the baseline exposure status and to exclude subjects who are not at risk for the disease. There are important considerations to make when measuring this exposure status; the validity (accuracy) and the reliability (reproducibility) of the measure. In its simplest form, the exposure status can have two levels: those who are observed to have the exposure at baseline (the **exposed group**), and those who are observed to not have the exposure (the **unexposed group**). For example, for a cohort study examining the effect of azithromycin use on heart disease, those who were already identified as having heart disease in a baseline cross-sectional study would be excluded. The remaining subjects who take azithromycin would form the exposed group, and those who do not take azithromycin would form the unexposed group. Both groups would then be followed over time to assess differences in the development of heart disease.

Exposure status is not always classified as simply exposed or unexposed; it may also be classified by different levels (e.g., different types, dosing, or durations of therapeutic drugs) or types of exposures, and different dosing or duration of exposure to explore how the intensity of exposure influences outcome. For example, in a study examining the effect of calcium supplementation on postmenopausal bone fractures, the exposure over a year could be defined by the level or frequency of calcium supplementation intake per year; where *once a day*, *once a month*, *once a year*, and *never* would correspond to values of 365, 12, 1, and 0 times per year, respectively.

Sometimes the exposed and unexposed groups are chosen separately. In those instances, it is important that the unexposed group is similar to the exposed group with respect to important predictors of disease incidence independent of the exposure (i.e., so they have the same background risk for the outcome as the exposed group).

OUTCOME EVALUATION

A central goal of epidemiology is to identify causes (or exposures) that can explain outcomes such as disease occurrence, which are referred to as the "outcome" or "disease." The Economic, Clinical, and Humanistic Outcomes (ECHO) model classifies health outcomes into economic, clinical, and humanistic categories.[5] Economic outcomes include direct costs (e.g., costs from hospitalization), indirect costs (e.g., lost wages due to hospitalization), and intangible consequences of exposures such as treatments (e.g., pain and suffering). Clinical outcomes include measures of morbidity, mortality, or a positive health outcome such as the resolution of a disease. Humanistic outcomes include measures from a patient perspective such as functional status, quality of life, and satisfaction.[5] Cohort studies can examine the effect of an exposure on more than one outcome. For example, death, diseases, quality of life, and adverse effects of treatment can all be outcomes within a single cohort study.

ANALYTIC FRAMEWORK FOR COHORT STUDIES

The most basic presentation of a cohort study with two groups (exposed and unexposed) in a fixed cohort with cumulative incidence data begins with a 2×2 table to estimate the effect of the exposure (e.g., protease inhibitors) on the outcome (e.g., death) (**Table 5-1**).

The risk or incidence of the outcome—in this example, the risk of death—for exposed persons is:

$$R(\text{exposed}) = \frac{A}{(A + B)}$$

The risk of death for unexposed persons is:

$$R(\text{unexposed}) = \frac{C}{(C + D)}$$

These risks represent the risk of the outcome (death) over a fixed time period for subjects who were followed to detect the development of the outcome. If all subjects were followed for one year, these risks represent the annual death rates for the exposed and unexposed, but the fixed follow-up time in a cohort study may also be shorter or longer than a year.

Measures of Effect from Cohort Studies

The relative **measures of association** such as risk ratios and rate ratios are used to estimate the effect of an exposure on a disease outcome (**measures of effect** such as causal risk ratios and causal rate ratios, respectively). **Risk ratios** and **rate ratios**, which are also called relative risks, compare the risk or rate of the outcome in the exposed group relative to that in the unexposed. The null value where the exposure is not associated with the outcome is reflected by a value of 1.0. Unbiased risk ratios greater than 1 correspond to the exposure increasing the risk for the outcome (the exposure being associated with an increased likelihood of the outcome or being a "risk factor" for the outcome), and an unbiased risk ratio less than 1 would correspond to the exposure decreasing the risk for the outcome (the exposure being associated with a decreased likelihood of the outcome). For a fixed cohort, the formula for the unadjusted risk ratio (RR) is simply the risk or incidence of the outcome in the exposed group divided by the risk or incidence of the outcome in the unexposed group:

$$\text{Risk Ratio} = \frac{R(\text{exposed})}{R(\text{unexposed})} = \frac{\dfrac{A}{(A + B)}}{\dfrac{C}{(C + D)}}$$

TABLE 5-1	Cohort Control 2×2 Table		
	Outcome (e.g., dead)	**No Outcome (e.g., alive)**	**Total**
Exposed (e.g., protease inhibitors)	A	B	$A + B$
Unexposed	C	D	$C + D$
Total	$A + C$	$B + D$	$A + B + C + D$

If the risks are measured as incidence rates in an open cohort where person-time of follow-up varies, then a rate ratio can be calculated to estimate the relative effect of exposure on the outcome. The rate ratio would be interpreted similarly to the risk ratio with the null value corresponding to 1.0, where the rate would be the same in both exposure groups. In an open cohort, the follow-up time varies from person to person, and the sum of all the time that the subjects are followed before they develop the outcome or leave the study is called the person-time of follow-up. The following is the formula for the unadjusted rate ratio:

$$\text{Rate Ratio} = \frac{\text{Rate of outcome exposed}}{\text{Rate of outcome unexposed}} = \frac{\dfrac{A}{\text{Person-time in the exposed group}}}{\dfrac{C}{\text{Person-time in the unexposed group}}}$$

The risk ratio or rate ratio provides an estimate of the effect of the exposure on disease in relative or proportional terms, but one could also consider an estimate of the effect measure in absolute terms. A factor or exposure may have a strong relative effect on an outcome as indicated by having a large risk ratio, but if the outcome is rare, the absolute risk associated with the exposure may be fairly small. The **risk difference** (RD), which is also called the **attributable risk**, is the difference in risk for the outcome between an exposed and an unexposed group and is calculated as follows:

$$\text{Risk Difference} = R\left(\text{exposed}\right) - R\left(\text{unexposed}\right) = \frac{A}{\left(A+B\right)} - \frac{C}{\left(C+D\right)}$$

Another measure of effect, one that provides an indicator for the public health impact of a risk factor, is the **attributable fraction in the exposed** (AFE), which expresses the risk difference relative to the risk in the exposed group. The AFE is expressed as a percentage of the incidence of disease in the exposed group due to the exposure, which is sometimes referred to as the **attributable risk percent** (ARP). For an exposure that causes disease, this measure of impact indicates the proportion of risk in the exposed group that would not have occurred in the exposed group if they were not exposed. The higher the ARP, the greater burden the exposure contributes to the risk of the outcome in the exposed group, whereas ARPs that approach 0 indicate that almost none of the disease in the exposed group is attributable to the exposure. Similarly, an ARP that approaches 1 would indicate that nearly all the disease in the exposed group is attributed to the exposure. The ARP is calculated as a percentage as follows:

$$\text{ARP} = \frac{R\left(\text{exposed}\right) - R\left(\text{unexposed}\right)}{R\left(\text{exposed}\right)} \times 100 = \frac{\dfrac{A}{\left(A+B\right)} - \dfrac{C}{\left(C+D\right)}}{\dfrac{A}{\left(A+B\right)}} \times 100$$

For an exposure that is protective for a disease outcome, the proportion of potential cases in the exposed group which were prevented by being exposed can be measured; this is called the **prevented fraction in the exposed** (PFE). When expressed as a percentage, the PFE can be interpreted as the percentage of potential cases in the exposed group that were prevented by being exposed. The PFE can be calculated as follows:

$$\text{PFE} = 1 - \text{Risk Ratio} = 1 - \frac{\dfrac{A}{\left(A+B\right)}}{\dfrac{C}{\left(C+D\right)}}$$

TABLE 5-2 Cohort 2 × 2 Table[6]			
	Any Influenza	**No Influenza**	**Total**
Fully Vaccinated	$A = 7$	$B = 147$	154
Unvaccinated	$C = 61$	$D = 395$	456
Total	68	542	610

Using a cohort study that assessed the effectiveness of inactivated influenza vaccine in children less than three years of age, the risk ratio (RR) and risk difference (RD) were calculated.[6] **Table 5-2** shows how these are calculated when the follow-up time is fixed, where all children were followed for 3 months from January to April 2008.

$$\text{Risk Ratio} = \frac{\dfrac{A}{(A+B)}}{\dfrac{C}{(C+D)}} = \frac{\dfrac{7}{154}}{\dfrac{61}{456}} = 0.34$$

$$\text{Risk Difference} = \frac{A}{(A+B)} - \frac{C}{(C+D)} = \frac{7}{154} - \frac{61}{456} = -0.088$$

$$\text{PFE} = 1 - 0.34 = 0.66$$

The risk ratio = 0.34 corresponds to the estimate that children who were vaccinated were 34% (about one-third) as likely to develop influenza from January to April 2008, compared to unvaccinated children. The RD = −0.088 corresponds to the estimate that the risk of influenza among vaccinated children was approximately 9% less than it was for unvaccinated children (4.5% versus 13.4%) from January to April 2008. In other words, for every 100 children that were vaccinated, 9 fewer cases of flu were observed compared to 100 children who were not vaccinated in this 3-month period. Because the exposure (vaccination) in this case is protective for the outcome (influenza), the PFE instead of the AFE is estimated. The PFE of 0.66 suggests that 66% of potential cases of influenza in the vaccinated group were prevented by being vaccinated.

If the above study was conducted in an open cohort with children with various follow-up times, the results could look like those in **Table 5-3**. In this example, the sum of the follow-up times for the 154 vaccinated children was 208 person-months (which corresponds to a mean follow-up time = 2 months), and for the 456 unvaccinated children it was 684 months (mean follow-up time = 1.5 months).

$$\text{Rate Ratio} = \frac{\dfrac{A}{\text{Person-time in exposed}}}{\dfrac{C}{\text{Person-time in unexposed}}} = \frac{\dfrac{7}{208}}{\dfrac{61}{684}} = 0.38$$

$$\text{Risk Difference} = \frac{A}{\text{Person-time in exposed}} - \frac{C}{\text{Person-time in unexposed}}$$

$$= \frac{7}{208} - \frac{61}{684} = -0.056$$

TABLE 5-3 Open Cohort Table[6]		
	Any Influenza	**Person-Time (PT in Months)**
Fully Vaccinated	$A = 7$	208 = PT in exposed
Unvaccinated	$C = 61$	684 = PT in unexposed
Total	68	892

The analyses described thus far provide unadjusted estimates of the effect of an exposure on an outcome. Because of the observational nature of cohort studies, there is almost always a chance that exposed and unexposed groups may differ by risk factors for the outcome (described later in the chapter), which could distort (or confound) the true association between the exposure and the outcome. For example, vaccinated young children may be more likely to attend a daycare center where the chances of getting influenza would be more likely. In this case, failure to account for or control for being in day care (a confounder) may understate the true effect that the vaccine has on the incidence of influenza in this population. A **confounding factor (or confounder)** is associated with both the exposure (e.g., treatment) and the outcome. The issue of confounding and other biases is covered more extensively at the end of the chapter.

CASE-CONTROL STUDIES

GENERAL DESIGN FRAMEWORK

As the terms "case" and "control" imply, a **case-control** study design seeks to compare the frequency of exposure among subjects or **cases** that experience an outcome event, most commonly a disease, and **controls** who do not have the outcome event or disease. One of the distinguishing features of this type of design is that the investigator starts by selecting subjects on the basis of the outcome event. Typically, the investigator then compares the observed level of exposure in the cases and controls to estimate the effect the exposure has on the event or disease. The outcome is always defined by the case definition, and one or more exposures can be compared between cases and controls. Thus, by definition, cases are those that have already developed some outcome, such as gastric cancer, and past exposures, such as non-steroidal anti-inflammatory drug (NSAID) use, are usually measured. Most case-control studies are inherently retrospective where the outcome and exposure have occurred prior to the initiation of the investigation. **Figure 5-2** provides a diagram of a case-control study that estimates the effect of two different exposures on the disease outcome. Once cases and controls are assembled, the researcher can also collect data on a wide range of exposures, and estimate their effect on the outcome. One cannot, however, explore alternative outcomes or case definitions without adding an additional case group.

SELECTION OF CASES AND CONTROLS

Typically, cases are identified by searching existing records where events would be recorded from some source population. The source population is defined based on the sampling procedures and the eligibility criteria; for example, residing in a geographic area, having benefits with a particular insurer, or seeking care at a health facility. The records searched might include claims data, disease registries, or inpatient or outpatient medical records where

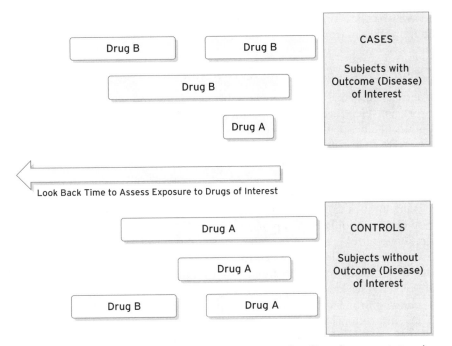

FIGURE 5-2 Diagram of a typical case-control study assessing the effect of exposure to two drugs.

disease events are routinely recorded. Cases may include newly diagnosed cases (**incident cases**) or persons with existing disease (**prevalent cases**). When feasible, incident cases are usually preferred because an association between an exposure and a prevalent disease could reflect the exposure's association with the duration of the disease and not with disease occurrence. Ideally, the case definition should be based on the best measure of the disease outcome or a less expensive measure(s) with a high sensitivity and high specificity.

A sample of controls, or those without the event or disease, should then be selected to estimate the exposure distribution in the base population. The **base population** is the population at risk for the outcome who, if they were to have the disease or event, would be selected to be a case in the study. For example, suppose a researcher is interested in examining the effect of NSAIDs on gastric cancer. Suppose a case–control design was used and cases with gastric cancer were selected from those who had undergone an upper endoscopy at a medical center in the United States, the source population. Controls should then be selected to represent the distribution of the exposure in the base population. Controls should not be selected to represent the exposure distribution in the source population if it differs from the base population. Also, controls should not be selected to represent those who do not experience the outcome or disease in the base population. Returning to the gastric cancer case–control example, because patients who undergo an upper endoscopy may have other disease conditions that are associated with NSAIDs (e.g., peptic ulcer disease), randomly selecting controls from this endoscopy center source population would likely not represent the exposure in the base population and, therefore, would likely introduce selection bias. In this example, the base population may not be identifiable unless it is known who would get an upper endoscopy at this particular medical center, if they had gastric cancer. Suppose that the cases were chosen from all gastric cancer patients in the Kaiser Permanente Southern California insurance system. If it is known that most people with this insurance will seek care within the Kaiser Permanente Southern California system and that people without this insurance will not seek care within this system, then the base population can be defined as Kaiser Permanente Southern California insurance holders, and controls can be randomly selected from these insurance holders.

TYPES OF CASE-CONTROL DESIGNS

Case-control studies may have an identifiable base population or cases and controls can come from non-identifiable base populations. A case-control study that identifies cases and controls in a defined base population is called a **population-based case-control** study. A **nested case-control** study is a type of population-based case-control study where the study is nested within a cohort study. Typically, all the incident cases from the cohort form the case group, while controls are randomly selected from (1) all subjects (case-based sampling), (2) subjects without the disease at the time the case was identified (density sampling), or (3) subjects who do not develop the disease over the entire follow-up period of risk (cumulative sampling).

Random control selection from the base population can be made in population-based case-control studies without introducing selection bias. However, base populations are often not definable. In **hospital- or clinic-based case-control studies**, cases are typically selected from people with the relevant disease of interest at a hospital or clinic, and controls are selected from people without the disease at the same institution. These institutional-based studies usually do not have an identifiable base population. In these studies, the controls, by virtue of being patients in a hospital or clinic, are ill and their illnesses may be related to the exposure status and, therefore, can lead to selection bias. Selection bias is discussed in more detailed at the end of this chapter.

DEFINING EXPOSURE TIME WINDOWS

Exposure status for cases and controls is often assessed by conducting a patient or caregiver survey or interview; searching medical, occupational, or other records; collecting biological samples; or linking by geographic residence to assess environmental exposures. Measuring and categorizing the appropriate time frame during which the exposure could affect the outcome, or the time at risk for the outcome, is important in order to obtain a valid measure of the exposure. The time at risk for the outcome can be assessed by evaluating *a priori* information regarding the clinical and pathophysiologic relation between the exposure and the outcome. This includes the **latency period,** the time period between the start of the disease and detection of the disease, and the **induction period,** the time between when the person is exposed and the disease is initiated.

The most basic approach to measuring exposure in cases and controls is to construct a binary measure of exposed and unexposed. This binary measure of exposure can take on several definitions including *currently exposed* (exposed on or immediately prior to the index case definition), *ever exposed* (exposed at any time previously in the look back time window), and *formerly exposed* (not currently exposed but exposed at some prior time period). In addition to defining exposure according to these time windows, exposure can be measured or categorized based on the intensity of exposure considering the duration and dose of exposure.

ANALYTIC FRAMEWORK FOR CASE-CONTROL STUDIES

The starting point for an analysis of an unmatched case-control study is to construct a 2 × 2 table that describes the exposure status for cases and controls as depicted in **Table 5-4**. The cells represent the numbers of cases and controls that are exposed and unexposed. Because the number of controls selected is chosen by the investigator, one cannot calculate the prevalence or incidence of disease from these data alone.

The primary analysis is based on comparing the odds of exposure for cases and controls, or the **odds ratio** (OR). The odds of exposure is a ratio of the number of people with exposure to those without exposure. The odds ratio is calculated by taking the odds of exposure among the cases and dividing that by the odds of exposure among the controls. If the odds of exposure for the cases is higher than the odds of exposure for the controls and the OR is an unbiased estimate for the association between the exposure and the outcome, then that exposure is positively associated with the outcome or a risk factor for the outcome (OR > 1); conversely, if the odds of exposure for the cases is lower than the odds of exposure for the controls and the OR is an unbiased estimate of the association between the exposure and the outcome, then that factor is negatively associated with the outcome or is protective for the outcome (OR < 1).

$$\text{Odds of being exposed among the cases} = \frac{\dfrac{A}{(A+C)}}{\dfrac{C}{(A+C)}} = \frac{A}{C}$$

$$\text{Odds of being exposed among the controls} = \frac{\dfrac{B}{(B+D)}}{\dfrac{D}{(B+D)}} = \frac{B}{D}$$

$$\text{Odds Ratio} = \frac{\text{Odds of being exposed among cases}}{\text{Odds of being exposed among controls}} = \frac{\dfrac{A}{C}}{\dfrac{B}{D}} = \frac{A \times D}{B \times C}$$

In a case-control study that explored the association between statins (HMG CoA reductase inhibitors) and prostate cancer, the following data were collected:[7]

Using the data from the 2 × 2 **Table 5–5**, the following unadjusted measures can be calculated:

$$\text{Odds of being exposed among the cases} = \frac{34}{66} = 0.52$$

$$\text{Odds of being exposed among the controls} = \frac{99}{103} = 0.96$$

$$\text{Odds Ratio} = \frac{0.52}{0.96} = \frac{34 \times 103}{66 \times 99} = 0.54$$

TABLE 5-4 Unmatched Case-Control 2 × 2 Table

	Case	Control
Exposed	A	B
Unexposed	C	D
Total	A + C	B + D

TABLE 5-5 Statin Exposure among Cases and Controls[7]

	Prostate Cancer	Control
Statin Exposed	A = 34	B = 99
Unexposed	C = 66	D = 103
Total	100	202

In this study, the OR suggests that statin use was inversely associated with prostate cancer where the odds of statin use among prostate cancer cases is approximately half the odds of statin use among controls. The authors also explored the effect of duration and cumulative dose and adjusted for a range of potential dietary and pharmacologic confounders and consistently found that statins and higher levels of statin exposure were inversely associated with prostate cancer.[7]

CONFOUNDER ADJUSTMENT

Confounding may occur in any study design including a case-control design. One approach to more efficiently control for confounding in the analysis is to match or restrict the selection of the controls based on characteristics of the cases that are likely to confound the relation between the exposure and the disease. **Matching** is a process of making the cases and controls similar (or balanced) with regard to this confounding factor so that there will be enough information in the analysis to adequately control for the factor. For example, in a study examining the effect of a new topical ointment on pressure ulcer healing in a nursing home population, each control (without pressure ulcer healing) could be selected so that the location of the pressure ulcer matched the location of the pressure ulcer for a certain case (whose pressure ulcer had healed). In matching a control to every case, there would be enough data to control for confounding by location on the body more efficiently in the analysis. Without matching, there may not be enough information on pressure ulcers from certain locations to control for location in the analysis. Case-control studies that use matching cannot estimate the influence of the matched factor on the outcome. So in the pressure ulcer example, the influence of the location on pressure ulcer healing could not be assessed.

If a case-control study uses matching, the analysis should account for the matched dependent sampling of controls. If the case-control study uses one-to-one matching, the unit of analysis becomes the matched case-control pair. **Table 5-6** displays a framework for analyzing one-to-one matched pairs, which is quite different than the framework for unmatched studies. To calculate the OR, each case-control pair is placed into one of four categories: two **concordant pair** categories where the exposure status was the same for both cases and controls and two **discordant pair** categories where the exposure status for the case was different than for the matched control. The OR can be estimated by dividing the number of pairs where the case was exposed and the control was not by the number of pairs where the case was unexposed and the control was exposed.

Using a multivariable technique, such as logistic regression or, in the case where there are matched sets, conditional logistic regression, will often be required to control for multiple confounders simultaneously. The logistic model can be used to estimate an odds ratio while controlling for confounders. In its basic form, the crude odds ratio can be obtained by exponentiation of the logit coefficient of a binary exposure variable in a model that

TABLE 5-6   One-to-One Matched Case-Control Paired Analysis

	Control Exposed	Control Unexposed	Total
Case Exposed	W	X	W + X
Case Unexposed	Y	Z	Y + Z
Total	W + Y	X + Z	W + X + Y + Z

W = Exposed Concordant Pair
X = Case Exposed, Control Unexposed Discordant Pair
Y = Case Unexposed, Control Exposed Discordant Pair
Z = Unexposed Concordant Pair
Odds Ratio = X / Y

contains only the exposure variable as an independent variable and the binary disease status (case versus control) as the dependent variable. The adjusted odds ratio is obtained the same way except that it is obtained from the exponentiated exposure coefficient from a model that includes a set of confounders. Selection bias, exposure misclassification, misclassification of cases and controls, and temporal ambiguity are additional biases that could prevent the odds ratio from being a valid measure of the effect of an exposure on a disease outcome.

ADVANTAGES AND DISADVANTAGES OF COHORT AND CASE-CONTROL DESIGNS

There is no one universally superior approach that should be used to assess the effect of an exposure on an outcome as the choice of the epidemiologic design will be influenced by the availability of data, the frequency and course of the disease being studied, how frequently persons are exposed, and the time and budgetary resources available to conduct the study, among other factors (**Table 5-7**). Cohort studies can be designed to assess the effect of exposures that do not frequently occur by intentionally sampling those persons that are exposed to those factors. Cohort studies, unlike case-control studies, also have the advantage of providing data to directly estimate measures such as risks, incidence rates, risk ratios, rate ratios, and risk differences. One drawback of cohort studies is that exceptionally large cohort studies followed for many years are required to estimate the effect of an exposure on rare disease outcomes or when it takes a long time for the exposure to cause a detectable disease. Because the case-control approach does not require following individuals forward in time, it is particularly well suited to study disease outcomes that are rare or take a particularly long time to develop. A case-control study design allows these studies to be conducted relatively quickly at significantly lower cost compared to cohort studies and, in particular, prospective cohort studies that usually include regular longitudinal assessments. However, case-control studies are typically more prone to biases.

TABLE 5-7 Advantages of Cohort and Case-Control Studies	
Advantages of Cohort Studies	**Advantages of Case-Control Studies**
Directly estimate rates, risks, rate ratios, risk ratios, and risk differences	Typically quicker and less expensive to conduct
Study rare exposures	Study rare outcomes
Study multiple outcomes	Study outcomes with long latency/induction periods
Less prone to recall biases	Study multiple exposures
More opportunity to validate study measures, if prospective	Usually require fewer subjects
Less risk of selection bias and temporal ambiguity	

DATA SOURCES FOR CASE-CONTROL AND COHORT STUDIES

Primary data obtained directly from subjects for the purpose of the study and **secondary data** obtained from existing records or data sources can be used for either cohort or case-control studies. The type of data must be considered in assessing the validity of either study, particularly as it relates to the measurement of exposures, outcomes, or variables used to control for confounding. Primary data has the advantage of being able to precisely tailor the study measures to the specific study objectives, and can include behavioral and social measures that can often confound exposure–outcome associations and are rarely available in secondary data sources. Primary data can permit collecting information on exposures not commonly recorded in secondary data such as the use of over-the-counter or illicit drugs.

Secondary data sources such as medical records or administrative claims data can be used without any direct involvement of the subject, which may greatly speed the investigation but are limited in scope to the measures that were routinely collected from the data source. Because secondary data from administrative claims data typically do not directly involve the subject or their caregivers, the estimates of the effect of an exposure on a disease may be less likely to be biased due to the fallibility of subject recall being different by disease outcome, but these estimates can be subject to measurement errors due to coding and other inaccuracies, particularly for outcomes that require additional information not included in the existing database. Studies should clearly define study measures and offer some rationale for choosing and defining study measures (e.g., the exposure, the disease outcome, confounders), including estimates of the validity of the measures, particularly for measures defining outcomes and exposures that were not collected for research purposes.

BIASES AND APPROACHES FOR MINIMIZING BIASES IN EPIDEMIOLOGIC STUDIES

A central goal in epidemiology is to identify causes that can explain outcomes such as disease occurrence. Since it is not possible to observe disease occurrence in the same population during the same time frame with and without the exposure (no person can be exposed and unexposed at the same time), we estimate the risk of disease in subjects with versus without exposure. In RCTs, randomization of study subjects to treatment groups can help make the unexposed group "comparable" to the exposed group when the sample size is large enough; thus the study population receiving treatment becomes similar to the population not receiving treatment with respect to the risk of disease occurrence in the absence of the exposure. Since observational designs do not involve randomization, it is important to control confounders that may distort the study findings.

In case-control and cohort studies, measures of association, such as risk ratios, rate ratios, risk differences, and odds ratios, are used to estimate measures of effect (causal risk ratios, causal rate ratios, and causal risk differences). To do this, causal inferences are made. Causal inferences can only be made if the findings are not explained by systematic errors in the measures of association—in other words, if the measures of association provide a valid (or unbiased) estimate of the effect of the exposure on the disease outcome. Different studies, even different RCTs, can show substantial differences in causal interpretability due to differences in validity.

Bias occurs when the estimate of the effect of the exposure on disease does not represent the true effect of the exposure on the disease outcome. A valid estimate of effect represents, aside from random error, the true effect that the exposure has on the disease in the base population. A valid estimate of the effect refers to one that is internally valid, or unbiased. This differs from an externally valid estimate, which is one that is internally valid and can be generalizable to a population outside of the study population. Biases can be classified into 3 non-mutually exclusive types: (1) confounding, (2) selection bias, and (3) information bias.

Confounding can occur in any type of study design. The example used earlier in this chapter identified that attending a daycare center (confounder) could distort or bias the estimate of the effect of a vaccine (exposure) on influenza (outcome). For a factor to be a confounder, it needs to be (1) associated with the exposure (e.g., attending day care is associated with being vaccinated); (2) a risk factor for the outcome in the unexposed group in the base population (e.g., children attending day care are more likely to experience influenza); and (3) not in the same causal pathway whereby the exposure affects the outcome (e.g., being vaccinated does not cause someone to be in day care, and then subsequently experience influenza).

Confounding can occur in a variety of situations, including (1) when an association between two variables (the exposure and disease) is due to a common cause of the exposure and the disease or (2) as a result of selection bias, such as from matching on a factor that is not a risk factor for the disease, but is associated with the exposure in a case-control study. Confounding should ideally be assessed using *a priori* knowledge of the relation between all potential confounders, the exposure, and the disease simultaneously.[8] Confounding can occur when the effect of treatment is mixed with one or more factors that distort the true treatment–outcome relation.

Approaches to control for confounding include restricting the inclusion criteria (e.g., only including children that do not attend day care), stratifying the analyses (e.g., estimating separate measures of association—risk ratios, rate ratios, odds ratios, etc.— for those that attend day care and those that do not), or most commonly by estimating measures of association utilizing a multivariate statistical model (e.g., logistic regression, Cox Proportional Hazards models) to adjust for the influence of the confounding variables. The multivariate approach is the most common because it can adjust the estimates of treatment effect for multiple confounding factors simultaneously.

Selection bias occurs when there is error in the estimate of effect due to procedures used to select subjects, or factors that influence study participation or follow-up. In cohort studies, selection bias occurs when risk for the disease outcome affects study participation differently for those exposed and unexposed. In case-control studies, selection bias occurs when (1) the exposure or factors related to the exposure affect selection of subjects differently for cases and controls, or (2) when the controls do not represent the exposure distribution in the base population, or (3) when the exposure distribution among the cases does not reflect the exposure distribution of cases in the source population.

In cohort studies, selection bias is less likely to occur than in case-control studies because selection of subjects into the cohort usually occurs before the disease occurs. Most cohort studies start with a base population consisting of exposed and unexposed subjects at risk for the outcome, and therefore, selection bias is minimized. One type of selection bias that occurs in a cohort study is selective loss to follow-up. This type of bias occurs when a lack of study participation due to loss to follow-up, non-participation, or non–response is associated with the disease (or outcome) differently for the exposure groups in a cohort study. For example, **Table 5-8** shows the results of a 1-year cohort

TABLE 5-8 Illustration of Selective Loss to Follow-Up in a 1-Year Prospective Cohort Study to Examine the Effect of a Diet Drug on Weight Loss

Hypothetical Results: No Loss to Follow-Up				Observed Results: Loss to Follow-Up			
True Causal RR = 3.3				Estimated RR = 3.0			
	Weight Loss	No Weight Loss			Weight Loss	No Weight Loss	
Diet Drug	100	400	500	Diet Drug	95	355	450
No Diet Drug	30	470	500	No Diet Drug	25	325	350
	130	870	1,000		120	680	800

study examining the effect of a diet drug on long-term weight loss, with 500 participants who were on the diet drug and 500 who were not. On the left side of the table is the hypothetical true causal risk ratio represented by a 2 × 2 table with an RR = 3.3. On the right side of the table, 10% of participants taking the diet drug and 30% not taking the diet drug were lost to follow-up, and this loss was lower for those who lost weight versus those who did not lose weight, resulting in an RR = 3.0. In this case, selection bias occurred because the outcome (weight loss) influenced study participation differently for those who were on the diet drug versus those who were not taking the diet drug.

As discussed previously, the control group in a case–control study should be selected to represent the exposure distribution of those who would be cases if they were diseased (i.e., the base population). The potential for selection bias can be reduced when cases and controls are selected from an identifiable base population, such as from population-based case-control studies and nested case-control studies. In other case-control studies, selection bias often occurs. For example, a basic case-control study investigated the use of vitamin C supplementation and prostate cancer (**Table 5–9**). The true distribution of prostate cancer and vitamin C supplementation and the causal risk ratio in the base population are depicted on the left side of the table, while vitamin C supplementation for the 80 cases and 80 controls is depicted on the right side of the table. Cases were selected from a prostate cancer screening program with recruitment at health fairs in Dallas, Texas, while controls were selected randomly from unscreened men in Dallas. Men who attended the health fairs and were screened were more likely to take vitamin C supplements than controls, so cases were more likely to take vitamin C than controls. Selection bias occurred because the controls did not represent the distribution of vitamin C use in the base population. Participation in the health fairs and then the screening program was associated with the exposure (vitamin C), and it influenced study participation differently for the cases versus controls.

Selection bias could also occur when the selection of cases seeking care at hospitals or clinics is affected by referral patterns, which also could be influenced by the exposure status of the cases. **Detection bias** occurs when the exposure affects the detection of the disease (or outcome). In case-control studies, detection bias is a type of selection bias since the exposure affects the detection of and the selection of cases, and it can occur even when the disease is correctly classified. Likewise, diagnostic bias and reporting bias, biases that result when the exposure affects the diagnosis or reporting of the disease (or outcome), are types of selection bias in case-control studies. With **diagnostic bias**, the exposure affects the diagnosis and hence the selection of cases in a case–control study.

In cohort studies and clinical trials, detection, diagnostic, and reporting biases are information biases. **Information bias** occurs when errors in the measurement or collection of data biases the estimate of effect. One type of information bias is misclassification bias. There are two types of misclassification biases: differential and non-differential.

TABLE 5-9	Illustration of Selection Bias in a Hypothetical Case-Control Study Examining the Effect of Vitamin C Supplementation and Prostate Cancer						
True Causal RR in Base Population: 1.0				OR = 2.3			
	Prostate Cancer	No Prostate Cancer				Prostate Cancer	No Prostate Cancer
Vitamin C	30	2,970	3,000		Vitamin C	40	24
No Vitamin C	70	6,930	7,000		No Vitamin C	40	56
	100	9,900	10,000			80	80

Differential misclassification of the disease occurs when the accurate measurement of the disease depends on the exposure and results in a biased estimate of effect. In cohort studies and clinical trials, differential misclassification typically results from detecting, diagnosing, or reporting the disease differently for the exposed and unexposed groups. Differential misclassification of the disease can be minimized in cohort studies by using the same methods to measure the disease in the exposed and unexposed groups. Likewise, differential misclassification of the exposure occurs when the accurate measurement of the exposure depends on the disease. **Recall bias** is a type of differential misclassification that commonly occurs in case-control studies. Recall bias often occurs when cases are more likely to recall the true level of a previous exposure compared to controls. In case-control studies, differential misclassification of the exposure can be minimized using the same methods to measure exposure data from the cases and the controls. As previously mentioned, the use of administrative claims data may reduce the occurrence of biases such as recall bias.

Non-differential misclassification[9] is a bias that occurs when the misclassification of the disease is the same for all categories of the exposure or the misclassification of the exposure is the same for all categories of the disease. Secondary data sources can be more prone to non-differential misclassification bias. Non-differential bias usually leads to bias toward showing no effect of the exposure on the outcome. This is not a serious concern when the estimated effect is still strong even in the presence of non-differential misclassification, but can be a serious concern when true causal effects are not detected due to this bias.

Temporal ambiguity, occurs when it is not clear whether the exposure affects the disease or the disease affects the exposure. In other words, it is not clear if the exposure preceded the outcome. Temporal ambiguity is not usually seen in cohort studies since the exposure is usually measured before the disease occurs. However, temporal ambiguity is common in most case-control studies that are not nested within cohort studies.

SUMMARY AND CONCLUSIONS

Well-conducted observational epidemiologic studies can provide clinicians with valuable insights about the effects of drugs, behavioral factors, practice settings, and other factors on the occurrence of disease or other outcomes. These types of studies will not replace evidence that can be obtained from well-conducted RCTs, but are critical in filling the evidence gaps when it is not ethical or feasible to conduct an RCT. There is no one universally superior design as the design will be influenced by the nature of the outcome or disease that is being studied, the exposures, and the resources available to support the study. Cohort studies mirror the clinical trial in that they start with groups exposed and unexposed and follow them forward in time to detect differences in outcomes of interest; however, assignment to exposure groups (e.g., drug groups) is not randomized, nor are all cohort studies prospective. Case-control studies are conducted by selecting cases (those with the outcome or disease of interest), identifying a set of controls without the outcome or disease of interest, and looking back in time to identify differences in exposure levels. Due to the observational nature of research using case-control or cohort study designs, researchers conducting or using this type of evidence need to be aware of the potential biases that might affect the validity of each study's findings before drawing conclusions. Common biases that can influence the validity of an epidemiologic study are selection biases—particularly for case-control studies, confounding, and information bias resulting from errors in the measurement of the study exposures and the study outcomes—and temporal ambiguity.

REVIEW QUESTIONS

1. A case-control study was conducted to examine the effect of silicone breast implants on connective tissue disease. One hundred cases were randomly selected from female patients from a large consortium of medical clinics with connective tissue disease, and controls were randomly selected from female patients without connective tissue disease in the same clinic consortium. Exposure to silicone breast implants was determined from both medical records and a questionnaire that all cases and controls were asked to fill out. If physicians at the clinics believed that there was an association between breast implants and connective tissue disease, then they may have been more likely to find and diagnose connective tissue disease in women with breast implants. The left side of the following table illustrates what the true distribution of the exposure was in the base population in a 2 × 2 format, along with the true causal risk ratio showing that the silicone breast implants did not increase the incidence of connective tissue disease (RR = 1.0). The right side of this table corresponds to data in a 2 × 2 format from the above-described case-control study.
   a) Which measure of association should be used to estimate the effect of silicone breast implants on connective tissue disease?
   b) Calculate the measure of association from 1(a).
   c) Interpret the measure of association from 1(b).
   d) Do you think that the measure of association calculated in 1(b) is a valid estimate of the causal risk ratio?
   e) What is an alternative explanation for the interpretation given in 1(c)?

True Causal RR = 1.0

	Connective Tissue Disease	No Connective Tissue Disease			Connective Tissue Disease	No Connective Tissue Disease
Silicone Breast Implants	10	4,990	5,000	Silicone Breast Implants	50	5
No Silicone Breast Implants	190	94,810	95,000	No Silicone Breast Implants	50	95
	200	99,800	100,000		100	100

2. Gulf War veterans have reported a variety of illnesses during and after their deployment to the Persian Gulf. Suppose we suspect that these veterans were exposed to potentially carcinogenic chemicals, which have not been identified. Therefore, a retrospective cohort study was conducted to examine the effect of deployment to the Persian Gulf in 1990–1991 on cancer incidence. The exposed group consisted of all U.S. military personnel veterans who were deployed to the Persian Gulf in 1990–1991 and were still alive at the end of the Gulf War. The unexposed group was selected in 2010 from surviving U.S. military veterans who were in the military sometime between 1990 and 1991, but were stationed in locations other than the Persian Gulf during that time period. Cancer incidence for both groups was determined from physician examinations conducted routinely from 2010–2013 and medical records from the 1990s–2010. The study reported that the rate of cancer among those deployed to the Persian Gulf in 1990–1991 was approximately 20% more likely than among those in the unexposed group. What is an alternative explanation for these findings?

3. A prospective cohort study is conducted to examine the effect of estrogen replacement therapy on stroke incidence and bone fractures in a large cohort of 100,000 post-menopausal women in the United States. After 2 years of follow-up, it was reported that there was no association between estrogen replacement therapy and bone fractures (Risk Ratio = 1.0). What would be another explanation for the findings?

4. A case-control study examined the effect of prescription antibiotic use during pregnancy on childhood cancer. Cases were randomly chosen from children with cancer in a cancer registry in the United States, and controls were selected randomly from the U.S. population. Exposure to prescription antibiotics during pregnancy was determined from interviews with the child's mother. The study reported an odds ratio of 2.1 and suggested that there was a causal relation between antibiotics and childhood cancer. Give an alternative explanation for these findings.

ONLINE RESOURCES

Developing a Protocol for Observational Comparative Effectiveness Research: A User's Guide: http://www.effectivehealthcare.ahrq.gov/ehc/products/440/1166/User-Guide-to-Observational-CER-1-10-13.pdf

Epi Info: http://www.cdc.gov/epiinfo/

Open Source Epidemiologic Statistics for Public Health, Version 2.3.1: http://www.openepi.com/OE2.3/Menu/OpenEpiMenu.htm

Strengthening the Reporting of Observational studies in Epidemiology (STROBE): http://www.strobe-statement.org/

REFERENCES

1. Ray WA, Murray KT, Hall K, Arbogast PG, Stein CM. Azithromycin and the risk of cardiovascular death. *N Engl J Med.* 2012;366(20):1881–1890.
2. Sorensen HT, Lash Tl, Rothman KJ. Beyond randomized controlled trials: a critical comparison of trials with nonrandomized studies. *Hepatology.* 2006;44:1075–1082.
3. Selby JV, Beal AC, Frank L. The patient-centered outcomes research institute (PCORI) national priorities for research and initial research agenda. *JAMA.* 2012;307(15):1583–1584.
4. Sheets NC, Goldin GH, Meyer AM, et al. Intensity-modulated radiation therapy, proton therapy, or conformal radiation therapy and morbidity and disease control in localized prostate cancer. *JAMA.* 2012;307(15):1611–1620.
5. Kozma CM, Reeder CE, Schultz RM. Economic, clinical and humanistic outcomes: A planning model for pharmacoeconomic research. *Clin Ther.* 1993;15:1121–132.
6. Heinonen S, Silvennoinen H, Lehtinen P, Vainionpaa R, Ziegler T, Heikkinen T. Effectiveness of inactivated influenza vaccine in children aged 9 months to 3 years: an observational cohort study. *Lancet Infectious Diseases.* 2011;11(1):23–29.
7. Shannon J, Tewoderos S, Garzotto M, et al. Statins and prostate cancer risk: A case-control study. *Am J Epi.* 2005;162(4):318–325.
8. Shrier I, Platt RW. Reducing bias through directed acyclic graphs. *BMC Medical Research Methodology.* 8:70;2008.
9. Jurek AM, Greenland S, Maldonaldo G, Church TR. Proper interpretation of non-differential misclassification effects: expectations vs observation. *Int J Epidemiol* 2005;34:680–687.

© Bocos Benedict/ShutterStock, Inc.

OTHER OBSERVATIONAL STUDIES

JOEL F. FARLEY, PHD

CHAPTER OBJECTIVES

▸ Discuss commonly used other observational study designs
▸ Describe and interpret studies using other observational study designs
▸ Examine the potential strengths and limitations of other observational designs
▸ Understand strategies to strengthen other observational study designs

KEY TERMINOLOGY

Convenience sample
Cross-sectional studies
Ecological fallacy
Ecological study
Generalizability

Non-equivalent
   comparison group
Pre- and post-
   observational designs
Purposively sample

Random sample
Sampling
Stratified random
   sampling
Time series design

INTRODUCTION

Oftentimes it is not possible for researchers to conduct randomized trials or epidemiologic studies for various reasons. In such instances, other observational study designs may be considered to evaluate pharmaceuticals and pharmacist services. These study designs are less formal than traditional cohort or case-control studies and often lack important design features that may threaten the internal validity of the study. Understanding when to use these studies is as important as understanding how to interpret their findings. In this chapter, a number of unique observational study designs are described including cross-sectional studies, pre- and post-observational studies, ecological studies, and time series evaluations. Several examples from the literature and real-world examples are used to understand the role of these studies in making inferences between pharmaceutical exposures and outcomes.

CROSS-SECTIONAL STUDIES

As their name implies, **cross-sectional studies** examine population characteristics at a cross-section (one point) in time. These studies are most often used descriptively to capture information about a population, such as disease prevalence, but may also be used to examine associations between an independent (exposure) and a dependent (outcome) variable. Without exception, inferring causal relationships from cross-sectional studies is fraught with uncertainty.

STUDY DESIGN

One of the more common types of studies using a cross-sectional design is a survey. Surveys are standardized questionnaires used to describe a population at a given point in time. The following example describes the use of a survey to collect information in the community pharmacy setting. Consider an example of a community pharmacy owner deciding whether to purchase a bone densitometer. Before committing resources to the purchase of this densitometer, the owner may be interested in the number of patients who might use this service, the amount they would be reimbursed for this service, and their risk of osteoporosis. To better understand the need for this service, the owner may develop a questionnaire to collect information regarding demographics (age, gender, race, and ethnicity), exposure to medications that increase osteoporosis risk (e.g., bisphosphonates, corticosteroids, and proton pump inhibitors), family and clinical history of osteoporosis, willingness to use the service, willingness to pay for the service, and the amount they would be willing to pay.

Identifying the Target Population

One of the first steps in conducting a cross-sectional study is to determine the target population. This is the population with desired clinical and demographic characteristics that will ultimately benefit from generalization of the study findings. In the previous example, the owner would certainly be interested in current customers or patients. However, it is possible the owner may also be interested in patients frequenting competitor pharmacies. Limiting administration of the survey to patients at a particular pharmacy would also limit generalizability. **Generalizability**, as defined previously, refers to the extent to which observations in the study population extrapolate to the overall population of interest. Researchers conducting cross-sectional studies should carefully consider the effect that excluding groups of respondents may have on generalizability to the population of interest.

Once the researcher identifies the target population, the next step is to select individuals from that population to complete the questionnaire. The most complete means of obtaining a generalizable estimate of the target population would be to obtain information on every single person in that population. However, this is generally not feasible. Most cross-sectional studies are conducted in a subset (sample) of individuals from the overall population. One rare exception is a census, which is a complete accounting of a population. In the United States, a census of the entire population is taken every 10 years to appropriately apportion federal funding for social and economic programs and ensure fair representation in the U.S. House of Representatives. The collection of information on an entire population can be inefficient when estimates of the population are acceptable. The 2010 U.S. Census was estimated to cost $13 billion.[1] This cost may be appropriate given the importance of its findings in the decisions that are made on the basis of these findings. However, for most studies, a less precise estimate of the population will suffice. **Sampling** refers to selecting a subset of the target population to conduct a study. It increases efficiency by reducing respondent and researcher burden during the data collection process.

Representative sampling

The goal of sampling in most studies is to generate a representative sample of the target population from which study participants are selected. The most common method to select a representative sample is to select participants from the population through a random process. A **random sample** is a study population selected using a chance (random) process. The random selection of participants ensures that the characteristics of the people that comprise the study population are similar to the target population from which they are selected. It should be noted that even with random sampling, there is no guarantee that the sampled population will be completely representative of the target population. Similar to a coin toss, if one were to flip a coin 100 times, the coin flip would not always result in 50 head and 50 tail flips. The result could lead to 55 head and 45 tail flips or, alternatively, 45 head and 55 tail flips. However, over a sufficient number of iterations of this process, the average of these coin flips would result in a balance of 50% heads and 50% tails. This random variation in the chance process is similar to the variation that may be present in the random sampling process.

The response rate in cross-sectional surveys is another important consideration. Not all individuals who are sampled will ultimately participate in the study. Non-response is not problematic if it occurs randomly among the population. However, if this information occurs differentially on the basis of the characteristics being described, this could yield bias generalizability of the study. To illustrate, if 75% of older adults, 50% of working-aged adults, and 25% of families with children responded to a survey, there might be reason to believe that age is an important contributor to willingness and ability to complete a survey. This age variability in response means that the sample in which data was collected is not representative of the population from which the data were collected.

In general, a 60% response rate is considered a good benchmark in determining adequate survey response.[2] Although outside of the scope of this chapter, two references are available for individuals who wish to improve response rates in surveys.[3] Despite response rate, a researcher can take steps to compare whether the sampled population differs from the target population if information about the target population is available. For example, there may be information from previously collected data, such as a census, that would have neighborhood characteristics. This information would help determine whether the population studied is truly representative of the target population.

Another option available to the researcher would be to perform a random sample of individuals from strata (called **stratified random sampling**) on the basis of the underlying characteristics of the population such as age or gender. Strata are mutually exclusive and exhaustive levels of population characteristics like age. If the pharmacist knew that 50% of the patients were 65 years or older, 30% were aged 18–64, and 20% less than 18 years of age, then the pharmacist could randomly sample a number of patients from each age strata to reflect this distribution of ages found in the overall population. This requires a good understanding of the target population, which may not always be available. Stratified random sampling produces a representative sample from each stratum for comparative and/or representative reasons. Simple random sampling may or may not provide a sufficient sample in each stratum.

Non-representative sampling

In some instances, obtaining a representative sample of individuals from the target population may not be feasible or desirable. In such cases, a convenience sample may suffice. A **convenience sample** is a non-random sample of respondents available to a researcher at a given place or time. In the previous example, the pharmacist considering purchasing a bone densitometer may be tempted to provide the survey on his day off. Depending on the day of administration, the convenience sample selected by the pharmacist may differ from the overall population frequenting his pharmacy. If, for example, the pharmacist conducts the study on a Tuesday from 1PM–5PM, the patients completing the survey will be less likely to be employed full-time (since most full-time employees would be at work at this time), may over represent stay-at-home mothers, or may differ in other important ways from the overall customer base at the pharmacy. The population will therefore not be generalizable to all patients using the pharmacy.

In some cases, a researcher may not desire a broad representation of the overall population, but only be interested in results from a specific sample of patients. In these cases, the researcher may **purposively sample** respondents with desired characteristics non-randomly. In the densitometer example, it may be possible that the pharmacist only desires to understand the characteristics of patients aged 65 and older. One could see specifically how the pharmacist may not be interested in the characteristics of a pediatric patient population or less interested in a non-elderly adult population given that the risk of osteoporosis is highest in older adults. Therefore, the pharmacist may purposively (non-randomly) sample only adults aged 65 and older to complete the study. This purposive sample will provide the needed information about the elderly based on the non-random sample, but will not be representative of the entire patient population frequenting that pharmacy.

Data Collection

Data from cross-sectional studies may be collected either prospectively or retrospectively. Retrospective data may be used if previously collected to analyze a population at a point in time. Prescription records would be one example of a data source that may be available to a pharmacy researcher. Retrospective analyses are limited to data already captured or the questions asked by other researchers. As such, all information of interest may not be available to a researcher. Therefore, many researchers collect data prospectively by generating a standardized questionnaire. A number of sources are available to researchers generating study questions. Pharmacists interested in developing questionnaires are encouraged to seek additional sources when putting together survey instruments.[4,5]

Once the questions are formulated, information can be collected a number of different ways, such as telephone interviews, in-person interviews, and mailed or Internet surveys. The method of administration should be determined by the needs of the researcher. It is generally less burdensome on a researcher to collect information via a mailed survey or Internet survey than via in-person or telephone interviews. However, there are fewer opportunities in a mail or Internet survey to clarify issues that may arise in the process of completing the survey, which can lead to questions being answered inappropriately or not at all. A number of other considerations also are important in determining method of administration. Mail questionnaires, for example, may be difficult for individuals with lower levels of education or reading proficiency to complete. Internet surveys may be less likely to be completed if the population targeted is older and does not use the Internet. Finally, telephone surveys may not include individuals who only use cellular telephones and do not have phone numbers available otherwise.

ANALYSIS

The next step in a cross-sectional study is to analyze data. Most cross-sectional studies are purely descriptive. In such cases, data analysis simply consists of summarizing the characteristics of the population using means and percentages. However, sometimes a researcher may examine an association between two variables collected during the same cross-section in time. The analytical cross-sectional studies have potential biases that should be considered by researchers, and this type of analysis should be interpreted cautiously.

In the previous example, the pharmacist collected information on both risk factors for developing osteoporosis and information on rates of osteoporosis. If the pharmacist noted a 50% increased rate of osteoporosis in patients using corticosteroids, he may be tempted to attribute corticosteroid use as a cause of osteoporosis. Although this association is considered accurate according to the clinical literature, the design of a cross-sectional observational study prevents attributing this causal inference. Because this study collected information on the exposure and outcome simultaneously, it is unclear whether prior exposure resulted in the outcome. In fact, it is entirely possible that patients may have had osteoporosis and were later initiated on a corticosteroid. One of the requirements of making a causal association between an exposure and an outcome, as pointed out in Chapter 4, "Research Design and Methods," is that the exposure must occur before the outcome.

STRENGTHS AND LIMITATIONS

Cross-sectional studies are an efficient means of capturing information about a population at a given point in time and results from these studies are relatively simple to analyze. However, as indicated, cross-sectional studies have a number of potential limitations including non-response, which may limit generalizability. In addition, clinicians should be cautious when interpreting associations from cross-sectional studies given biases of temporality. Another limitation of cross-sectional studies is that they capture data on prevalence, not incidence of exposure or outcomes. Because data are collected at a single point in time, it is not possible to capture information about new (incidence) cases of a disease, only existing (prevalence) cases at the time these data were collected. If disease incidence is of interest to a researcher, longitudinally following patients over time would be necessary to rule out previously existing cases.

PRE- AND POST-OBSERVATIONAL STUDY DESIGNS

The major limitation of cross-sectional studies is the lack of information about a population over time, resulting in biases of temporality when making causal inferences. Two specific epidemiologic designs, cohort and case-control studies, address this limitation. However, the traditional cohort and case-control study designs are not always possible to conduct. In **pre- and post-observational designs**, a researcher examines the effect of an intervention by comparing observations occurring after the change to observations occurring before the change. This type of study design is frequently referred to as a one group pretest-posttest (or pre-post) or before-after study design.[6] In a pre-post study design, observations are collected both before and after a specific exposure, eliminating the aforementioned bias of temporal precedence from cross-sectional studies.

STUDY DESIGN

To better understand the pre-post study design, consider the following example based in part on a published study that examined a prior authorization program in the Georgia Medicaid program.[7] This step-therapy policy required any patient filling a prescription for olanzapine, risperidone, or clozapine to first fail at least two different regimens of a first-generation antipsychotic agent. The program was enforceable from November 1996 through September 1997. Although based on an actual study, the myriad examples presented below do not reflect the actual results from that study. The reader should refer to the actual study if interested in its results.

The most basic pre-post study design is the one-group pre-test post-test study design in which observations are compared before and after an intervention in the population of individuals affected by the intervention. In this design, information on each individual would be collected before the study (pre-test) by the researcher and compared to information collected after the study (post-test). The study design is presented diagrammatically as $O_1 \, X \, O_2$ where O_1 represents the first study observation which occurs before the intervention, X represents the intervention, and O_2 represents the second observation following the intervention.

Data Collection

Pre-post studies are often conducted retrospectively. The most common scenario in which a pre-post study design is conducted is when a natural and common phenomenon affects a population. In the previous antipsychotic restriction example, the researcher likely has no control over the policy being implemented and can only observe the effect of the policy on patients. However, in some instances, there may be advanced notification of the change, allowing data to be collected prospectively before the policy and after the policy.

ANALYSIS

In the prior example, the researcher might compare average antipsychotic expenditures in May 1996 (6 months before the policy) as a pre-test measurement to post-test expenditures in April 1997 (6 months after the policy). Given the restrictive nature of the policy, the researcher would anticipate a drop in antipsychotic expenditures following the policy. However, in this example, the researcher is surprised to find an increase in antipsychotic expenditures from $0.75 to $0.85 per beneficiary per month using this study design. Given that the outcome variable is continuous, this change can be tested for significance using a *t*-test to examine the change in the outcome between observation periods. Alternatively, additional variables could be included in the model to control for the association between the policy and the outcome using linear regression. If the outcome is dichotomous (such as might be the case if the researcher is interested in the probability that a person uses an antipsychotic medication before and after a policy), the researcher could use a chi-square test to examine the probability of the outcome after the intervention compared to the period before the intervention. Again, if additional variables are of interest to the researcher, an alternative to the chi-square test would be a multivariate logistic regression model.

STRENGTHS AND LIMITATIONS

The pre-post study design is a significant improvement over the cross-sectional study design because it eliminates the bias of temporality. However, this study design is prone to potential biases such as history and maturation, covered in Chapter 4, "Randomized Controlled Trials." As a reminder, maturation is defined as a natural change in an outcome over time outside of the influence of the exposure of interest. In the United States, the price of antipsychotic medications has increased over time, as has the use of these medications for new mental health conditions. Not accounting for these natural changes outside of the policy could lead a researcher to conclude that the policy increased prescription expenditures when in fact external influences of maturation were the contributing factor.

Another significant concern is biases of history. History is the effect of a second factor occurring between the pre-test and post-test that is confused for the effect of the exposure of interest. Examples of potential historical threats in pharmacy include the addition of new medications or a generic entry in the market. Not accounting for historical biases could lead a researcher to inappropriately attribute a causal association between an exposure and outcome when a competing variable is responsible for the change.

The one-group pre-post study design could also be biased by regression to the mean. Regression to the mean refers to extreme scores on a variable at pre-test, which leads to more room for a score to approach the mean value than might otherwise be expected. If antipsychotic prescribing by clinicians was particularly low in Georgia before the policy and these drugs were underused for mental health problems in the state, a researcher might anticipate greater uptake of these medications over time than might be expected in other states. This would make it look as though the policy increased antipsychotic use when in fact the uptake of these medications was appropriate to bring the state closer to accepted standards of practice.

There are a number of strategies a researcher can employ to improve the one-group pre-post study design and reduce the limitations just discussed, as highlighted in **Table 6-1**. One option available to a researcher is to add observational time points to the study. Adding additional time points before the study allows the researcher to examine patterns of maturation and control for it. In the previous example, examining antipsychotic expenditures both 6 months (O_1) and 12 months (O_2) prior to the policy (X) shows growth in this outcome before the policy. The change in this outcome prior to the policy from O_1 to O_2 can then be compared to the change from O_2 to the post-observation O_3 to see if it was a policy effect or normal change due to maturation.

		Antipsychotic Expenditures per Member per Month		
TABLE 6-1 Pre-Test/Post-Test Study Design Variations				
Study Design	**Core Design**	**Observation 1**	**Observation 2**	**Observation 3**
One-group pre-test/post-test	$O_1 X O_2$	$0.75	$0.85	—
One-group multiple pre-test/post-test	$O_1 O_2 X O_3$	$0.68	$0.75	$0.85
One group treatment switching	$O_1 X O_2 \cancel{X} O_3$	$0.75	$0.85	$1.20
Pre-test/post-test with non-equivalent comparator	$O_1 X O_2$	$0.75	$0.85	—
	$O_1 O_2$	$0.70	$1.70	—

In this specific example, antipsychotic expenditures grew from $0.68 to $0.75 before the policy, which is similar to, albeit smaller than, the change after the policy.

Another design enhancement is to either remove treatment or reintroduce treatment (X_2). The benefit of removing or reintroducing treatment relates to reproducibility of study results. If the treatment had a positive influence on the outcome, removing the treatment should have the opposite effect on that outcome. This can be seen in the previous example where the removal of the policy ($\cancel{X}$) causes a reversal in the effect of the policy from O_2 to O_3. In this study, the original treatment effect showed a slight increase in antipsychotic expenditures from $0.75 to $0.85 per member per month. However, eliminating the policy resulted in a sharp increase in antipsychotic expenditures to $1.20 per member per month, suggesting the policy may have slowed a bigger expenditure increase.

A common design enhancement to the one-group pre-post study is to add a **non-equivalent comparison group** of individuals who are not subjected to the intervention. This study design is similar to the cohort study in which outcomes are compared between a treatment group and a control group before and after an intervention. Comparing antipsychotic expenditures in Mississippi, which lacked any prior authorization restrictions, shows an increase from $0.70 to $1.70 per member per month in the absence of the policy. This dramatic increase in expenditures suggests that the policy in Georgia may have curbed a similar increase in the state had the policy not existed. This study design is generally considered minimally sufficient for attributing causal inference between an exposure and outcome.[6,8] However, researchers should carefully consider differences between groups (selection bias) when making causal inferences.

TIME SERIES ANALYSIS

One of the design features described to improve the one-group pre-test/post-test design is to add more observations to the study, particularly in cases where maturation may exist. In **time series design**, multiple observations are added over time, usually before and after an intervention. If enough time points are available, a researcher can track trends in an outcome over time, before and after a policy, using a time series analysis. Time series analyses have been described as one of the stronger observational study designs to attribute causal inference.[6,8] It is particularly useful when an intervention occurs at a specific point in time and applies to a population of individuals simultaneously. This study design is adept at examining trends in an outcome over time, the potential for an immediate treatment effect, and the sustainability of a treatment effect over time.

STUDY DESIGN

The example describing the effect of a prior authorization policy in the Georgia Medicaid program will be used to describe the core design features behind a time series analysis. As mentioned, the policy was implemented in November 1996 and discontinued in October 1997. Using data from 1996–1997, the study allowed for comparison of a 10-month pre-policy period to an 11-month policy period. The time series analysis is set up by allowing each month to be treated as a separate observation of antipsychotic expenditures per member per month.

Generally, a researcher begins by plotting the outcome of interest over time, as seen in **Figure 6-1**. Plotting the outcome reveals a sudden reduction in the rate of antipsychotic expenditures immediately following the policy followed by an increase in expenditures after the policy, similar to the period preceding the policy.

The observations from a time series can help to examine a number of different things that could not be evaluated by simply comparing average expenditures at a single point before and after the policy in the pre–post study design. In particular, the pre-post study design did not capture maturation prior to the policy as seen with the trend of increasing expenditures in the plot above. It also did not capture the sudden reduction in antipsychotic expenditures that occurred immediately following policy implementation. Finally, it did not capture the fact that despite this sudden decline, trends in antipsychotic spending increased at the same rate as the period preceding the policy, which suggests that the effect of the policy may be short lived. The advantage of the time series analysis is its ability to discern such effects resulting from an intervention.

ANALYSIS

Time series analysis is often performed retrospectively. Although this analysis can be performed prospectively, capturing data on the same population of individuals repeatedly over a prolonged period of time risks attrition of subjects from the study. Data are therefore summarized, usually over the population across periods of time, using previously collected or administrative claims data. Once these data are summarized for each observation period, the researcher can predict the outcome using a linear regression model where the predictor of interest is the observation time period

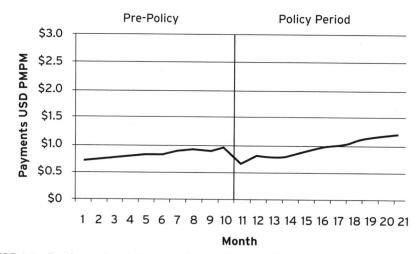

FIGURE 6-1 Trends in antipsychotic expenditures before and after the policy.

(ranging from 1 for the first observation to *n*, where *n* represents the last observation) with additional variables denoting whether the observation occurred before or after the policy. The specific function of this regression is out of the scope of this chapter. Readers interested in performing a time series analysis are encouraged to consult other resources.[9,10]

STRENGTHS AND WEAKNESSES

The time series analysis is a useful tool for capturing a more complete description of both immediate and sustained treatment effects that may occur after a change in treatment. This study design is also adept at controlling for changes that may occur in an outcome variable as a result of natural maturation. Despite these advantages, limitations of time series analyses persist. In particular, biases of history (outside influences occurring during the study period that may influence the outcome but are attributable to treatment) are still a threat. Similarly, attrition of subjects is a threat given that numerous observations are required to conduct this analysis. The more time points that a researcher needs to examine, the greater the potential for subjects to drop out of the study. Several additional features can improve the validity of the time series study design. One of the most compelling design features that can be added to a time series analysis is the inclusion of a non-equivalent comparison group similar to what was described in the pre-post study design. This is often considered the strongest quasi-experimental observational study design possible for evaluating programmatic changes across populations.[6,8]

Continuing with the example of the prior authorization policy in Georgia, one might compare antipsychotic expenditures to Mississippi, where this policy was not in place (**Figure 6-2**). The addition of the control group shows a rapid increase in antipsychotic expenditures in Mississippi around the time the policy went into place. This increase was due primarily to the introduction of olanzapine, which entered the antipsychotic market in September 1996. This represents a significant bias of history that was not captured well in the other study designs, showing the value of including a control group in these studies if possible. The inclusion of the control group allows the researcher to see the effect that this bias may have had in Georgia had the prior authorization policy not been in place.

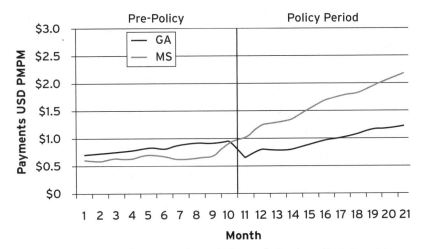

FIGURE 6-2 Trends in antipsychotic expenditures before and after the policy in two states.

ECOLOGICAL STUDIES

In some circumstances, a researcher may not have information from individuals when conducting a study, but may instead have information about groups of individuals. An **ecological study** is a study that makes comparisons between groups of individuals rather than between individuals themselves.[11] This group information may be available on either the treatment exposure or outcome of interest. There may be several reasons why a researcher would use aggregated information instead of individual information. These data may be easier to collect and less costly to acquire given that this information is often available in registries, censuses, or previously conducted surveys. In some instances, aggregated data may supplement data collected on individuals when this information does not exist in other data sources per individual. A common example in health research is the use of census information across a region or zip code to approximate education or income, which is not available in administrative claims data sets.

STUDY DESIGN AND ANALYSIS

A specific question that lends well to the ecological study design is research on whether pertussis cases are lower in states where pharmacists have the authority to vaccinate patients with tetanus diphtheria and pertussis (TDAP) vaccines. In this example, the unit of analysis is the state. The outcome of interest would be aggregated rates of pertussis within each state. A researcher might use previously collected data to compare pertussis cases within each state as tracked by the Centers for Disease Control and Prevention (CDC) to immunization laws available in board of pharmacy regulations. Once aggregate information is collected, rates of pertussis could be compared using *t*-tests to compare the mean number of pertussis cases in states with versus states without vaccination authority.

STRENGTHS AND WEAKNESSES

One of the primary advantages of ecological studies is that they usually rely on previously collected information, making them easy and inexpensive to conduct. However, they are subject to significant limitations. In the pertussis example, the researcher may be tempted to say that individuals that have access to pharmacist immunization services are more likely to receive TDAP vaccination and less likely to develop pertussis. However, since information is not available on individuals, but only across groups, this association is not valid due to a bias of ecological fallacy. The **ecological fallacy** refers to inappropriately inferring an association among individuals when observed in a group.

There are several factors that are not accounted for in the group study design that would prevent us from making an association at the level of the individual. Although pharmacist immunization authority may be thought of as the contributing factor leading to higher rates of vaccination within a state, it is unknown whether rates of immunization are being driven by pharmacists and not by a different medical provider. Suppose, for example, that states that have more immunizations have higher immunization rates because physicians in these states are screening and providing TDAP vaccines at higher rates. If an individual inference is made from group associations, it can lead to inappropriate inference of higher immunization rates with pharmacists when in fact it could be other providers that are the reason for the higher immunization rates.

SUMMARY AND CONCLUSIONS

The observational study designs covered in this chapter vary considerably in their conduct and purpose, as seen in **Table 6-2**. Each has a unique contribution to pharmacy literature, and there are a number of significant limitations that should be considered carefully by pharmacists when making clinical decisions on the basis of these studies. The potential limitations of these studies should be carefully considered when interpreting results. There are numerous study design enhancements that can increase validity in making causal inferences between a treatment exposure and outcome of interest in these studies. Of the study designs mentioned within this chapter, only pre-post with a non-equivalent comparator group, time series, and time series with a non-equivalent comparator group study design are considered strong enough to make causal inferences between an exposure and an outcome. However, even these study designs have important limitations. Careful consideration of study limitations will guide clinicians using these types of studies when making clinical decisions.

TABLE 6-2	Summary of Other Observational Study Designs, Use, and Limitations		
Study	*Design*	*Appropriate Use*	*Major Design Limitations*
Cross-Sectional	Data are systematically collected to describe a population at a given point in time.	Most appropriate for describing a population at a given point in time.	Unable to examine associations between an exposure and outcome given a bias of temporal precedence.
Pre-test/Post-test	Outcomes are compared before and after an intervention on a population affected by the intervention.	Used to describe a population both before and after an intervention to examine changes resulting from the intervention.	Biases of maturation, history, and regression to the mean prevent causal inference from this design unless additional design features are included.
Time Series	Outcomes are examined over numerous observations before and after an intervention.	Useful for describing a change in the trend (growth over time) or level (sudden disruption) of an outcome in a population affected by an intervention.	Biases of history may still influence changes in an outcome if present. Attrition concerns exist given the need to examine a population over an extended period of time.
Ecological	Aggregated data are used to examine associations across populations instead of individuals.	Used to compare group associations between populations when data is not available on the specific individuals comprising the population.	Group associations may not reflect associations between individuals due to the ecological fallacy.

REVIEW QUESTIONS

1. How does the pre-post study design reduce the bias of temporal precedence in a cross-sectional study?
2. Describe the value of adding a control group to both pre-post and time series evaluations when comparing outcomes among individuals.
3. Which of the study designs presented in this chapter is most appropriate for examining subtle changes in outcomes when maturation is a concern and why?
4. Which study design is more appropriate for examining effects of an intervention that may occur gradually over time and why?
5. What steps should a researcher take to ensure that respondents to a survey are generalizable to the source population that was surveyed?

ONLINE RESOURCES

Issues in Survey Research Design: http://ocw.jhsph.edu/index.cfm/go/viewCourse/course/survey researchdesign/coursePage/index/

National Center for Health Statistics: Surveys and Data Collection Systems: http://www.cdc.gov/nchs/surveys.htm

National Information Center on Health Services Research and Health Care Technology Finding and Using Health Statistics: http://www.nlm.nih.gov/nichsr/usestats/index.htm

REFERENCES

1. Government Accountability Office. *Additional Actions Could Improve the Census Bureau's Ability to Control Costs for the 2020 Census*. Available at: http://www.gao.gov/products/GAO-12-80. Accessed on January 14, 2013.
2. Johnson TP, Wislar JS. Response rates and nonresponse errors in surveys. *JAMA*. 2012;307 (17):1805–1806.
3. Dilman DA, Smyth JD, Christian LM. *Internet, Mail, and Mixed-Mode Surveys: The Tailored Design Method*. 3rd ed. Hoboken, NJ: Wiley and Sons; 2008.
4. Day LA, Cornelis LJ. *Designing and Conducting Health Surveys: A Comprehensive Guide*. San Francisco, CA: Wiley and Sons; 2006.
5. Streiner DL, Norman GR. *Health Measurement Scales: A Practical Guide to Their Development and Use*. 3rd ed. Oxford, England: Oxford University Press; 2008.
6. Shadish WR, Cook TD, Campbell DT. *Experimental and Quasi-Experimental Designs for Generalized Causal Inference*. Boston, MA: Houghton Mifflin Company; 2002.
7. Farley JF, Cline RR, Schommer JC, Hadsall RS, Nyman JA. Retrospective assessment of Medicaid step-therapy prior authorization policy for atypical antipsychotic medications. *Clin Ther*. 2008;30(8):1524–1539.
8. Soumerai SB, Ross-Degnan D, Fortess EE, Abelson J. A critical analysis of studies of state drug reimbursement policies: research in need of discipline. *Milbank Q*. 1993;71(2):217–252.
9. Neter J, Kutner MH, Nachtsheim CJ, Wasserman W. *Applied linear statistical models*. 4th ed. Boston, MA: WCB/McGraw-Hill, 1996.
10. Wagner AK, Soumerai SB, Zhang F, Ross-Degnan D. Segmented regression analysis of interrupted time-series studies in medication use research. *Med Care*. 2002;27(4):299–309.
11. Morgenstern H. Ecological studies in epidemiology: concepts, principles, and methods. *Ann Rev Pub Health*. 1995;16:61–81.

CASE REPORTS AND CASE SERIES

JANE R. MORT, PHARMD

OLAYINKA O. SHIYANBOLA, PHD

CHAPTER OBJECTIVES

- ▸ Discuss the objectives of case series and case reports
- ▸ Outline the necessary components of case reports
- ▸ Describe design and methodology of case series studies
- ▸ Evaluate strengths and weaknesses of case reports and case series
- ▸ Evaluate the results reported in case reports and case series

KEY TERMINOLOGY

Case report
Case series
Publication bias
Reliability
Validity

INTRODUCTION

Case reports and case series are descriptive studies that recount a patient scenario complete with pertinent medical information such as laboratory values, medications, and diagnosis.[1,2] The case report includes a detailed discussion of a unique medical scenario of a single case or event in light of the currently available literature and provides an evaluation of the findings.[3] Case series describe "a group of patients with similar diagnoses or undergoing the same procedure followed over time."[4] Although case reports and case series are at the lower end in the hierarchy of evidence, they provide valuable information to practitioners and policy makers.[1] In fact, five of the "51 Landmark Articles in Medicine" identified over a 150-year period were case reports.[5–7]

With increasing emphasis on randomized studies for evidence-based medicine, some have come to question the need and utility of case reports and case series.[8,9] Over the last several years, the number of published case reports has declined due to the perception that they are anecdotal and limited in their ability to be generalized.[5] In addition, publication costs, limitations in print space, need for peer reviewers, journal competition, and emphasis on the impact factor have brought about a decrease in number of case reports published.[5,10] Despite the need for well-designed studies, case reports have provided significant information that has helped to advance medical treatment.[5–7] Case reports have been found to be a viable source for identifying unexpected or uncommon occurrences, previously unknown conditions, new adverse drug reactions (ADRs), and innovative indications for medications.[9] This chapter will provide a description of case reports and case series including, for each, a definition, characteristics, study design features, writing guidelines, strengths/limitations, and points for critical evaluation.

CASE REPORTS

CASE REPORT DEFINITION

Case reports are the most basic form of medical evidence that often provides the first suspicion that an issue exists.[9–11] A **case report** is a brief report of clinical characteristics or course from a single clinical subject or event without a comparison.[3,6] This form of literature only serves to provide a description of a situation and is not intended to lead to a conclusion or answer a hypothesis.[1,12] Case reports may be organized according to their objectives in describing a specific type of situation such as identification of a new condition or presentation, an unknown adverse effect, or a new use for a medication.[9,12] Each type of case report will be described in greater detail.

CASE REPORT TYPE BASED ON OBJECTIVES

Case reports may be used to describe uncommon diseases, unique variants of known conditions, or unknown conditions (**Table 7-1**). For example, a unique variant of diabetes involving mitochondrial differences is associated with fewer neurologic and vascular changes and was identified via a case report.[9] However, care must be taken in the clinical application of the identification of rare conditions given the extreme infrequency of the situation in common everyday practice.[12]

Case reports may be used to identify ADRs. In fact, serious ADRs have been identified via case reports more often than any other research approach, and removal of most medications from the market due to ADRs emanate from case report evidence.[11,13] The latter is likely due to limitations of the evidence required by the Food and Drug

TABLE 7-1	Types of Case Reports
Type	**Feature**
Disease Identification	• Previously unknown or variant of known condition • Reader must avoid generalization of the rare condition
Adverse Drug Reaction (ADR) Reporting	• Most common source of information for drug removal • Excellent in identifying rare and serious ADRs • Utility in identifying ADRs in special populations
New Treatment Approach	• Generally used to generate a hypothesis for further testing with a more resource-intensive design • May lead to unsubstantiated use of medications for unapproved indications
Educational	• Present a scenario to help clinicians improve practice skills
Quality Assurance	• Practice errors can illustrate problems to avoid by other practitioners

Administration (FDA) for market approval.[13] The pre-marketing evidence supplied to the FDA is of limited duration and, therefore, if an adverse effect is delayed, then it will not be reported. In addition, adverse effects that occur as rarely as 1 in 10,000 patients or less would not be identified in pre-marketing studies simply due to the small sample size in pre-market studies. Finally, ADRs that occur in special populations are frequently not identified because these patients are often excluded from research. The effect of a reduction in publication of ADR case reports on recognition of serious reactions is of concern. In addition, the tendency to only publish previously unreported ADRs minimizes the production of a body of evidence supporting the occurrence of a unique ADR.[14] Reporting of ADRs through MedWatch, however, continues to provide a mechanism for ADR tracking.[13]

Case reports may be used to document previously unknown effectiveness of an agent in the management of a condition.[9] An interesting example involves the presentation of hypoglycemia in a patient with an infection that was treated with a sulfa drug. This information led to the development of sulfonylurea agents for diabetes.[9] Similarly, sildenafil was created based on reports of erectile effects from specific antihypertensive agents.[11] Evidence for new uses of medications is often not as dramatic and clear-cut as these examples and may lead to off-label use of medications, which is not substantiated. Specifically, a study examining dermatologists' prescribing practices found that 14% of medications were used for off-label indications and 70% of this use was supported by limited data.[10] Care must be taken in interpreting case-based findings that suggest an agent is effective in treating a condition.

In many instances, the case report leads to a study that tests a hypothesis. This is based on the theory that the case report represents an unexpected occurrence, which brings about theorizing and then testing of the hypothesis.[9] Case reports can be used to guide the more time consuming and resource-intensive research approach to determine the validity of results.[6] For example, case reports suggested the occurrence of liver tumors in patients taking oral birth control pills.[1] This information led to a case-control study demonstrating a strong relationship between continued use of high-dose oral birth control pills and hepatocellular adenomas. A project examining case reports in the journal *Lancet* found that 103 case reports led to 24 randomized controlled trials.[10] Conversely, a study looking at 63 previously unreported ADRs in five journals found that only 17% were evaluated further.[15] The latter may be a more conservative report of the impact of case reports on subsequent research activities due to the project requirement that the case had not previously been reported. Often, multiple reports are needed to substantiate an issue and lead to a well-designed study.

Case reports may be published to educate clinicians in a variety of ways such as recognizing common or unique clinical situations, developing patterns of clinical thinking, and gaining knowledge through a short overview of the literature that ties information directly to patient care.[6,9] Case reports can also serve as a quality assurance tool, helping others avoid similar mistakes. For example, a case study published in the *New England Journal of Medicine* guided the reader through the problem-solving process in a complex case of methotrexate toxicity due to a medication error (methotrexate administered daily instead of weekly due to a transcription error) and helped practitioners recognize the need to consider medication errors as the source of complex life-threatening illness.[16]

CASE REPORT STUDY DESIGN AND WRITE-UP

Design

Case reports may be either prospective or retrospective.[6,17] The retrospective design is more common and involves reporting an observed occurrence after the event. The retrospective design is limited by the information and outcome measures recorded during the actual event. Conversely, the prospective case report entails pre-planning the proposed treatment approach and measurements of impact. Subsequent patient management follows the prescribed plan. This approach involves more preliminary work but facilitates the write-up of the case report by clinicians. Because the strength of a case report is its written description, the report or write-up is critical in the conduct and design of the case report.

Identification and Preparation

Because the strength of case reports is in describing the novel occurrence, the first step in writing a case report is to recognize a unique situation.[18] To ensure that the case is truly unique, clinicians must review the literature to determine if the case will add to the body of knowledge on the topic in question. In addition, clinicians should talk with the other providers to make sure no one else is working on the project.[18] Selection of the proper journal is an important step and may influence the manuscript and consent form. Clinicians should consider journals for publication based on the nature of the case and carefully review the instructions for authors in the specific journal.[18] Consent must be obtained from the patient or next-of-kin if the person has passed away. Preparation for the case study write-up involves obtaining patient information including demographic information, history, test results, treatments, and time course.[18]

Overview of Write-Up

The case report typically contains a structured abstract, an introduction containing background on the main point of the case, a description of the patient case, a discussion of the case in the context of available literature, and a conclusion highlighting the main point of the case.[6] Important characteristics of the case report include emphasizing a salient point, providing the information in an objective manner, and not attempting to draw conclusions that go beyond the uncontrolled reporting of a case (e.g., causality).[3,6]

Case reports should have a clear title that optimizes access via literature searches. In general, the introduction should include a sufficient review of the topic to allow the reader to recognize the importance of the issue and the relevance of the case.[3,6] The case should include all of the necessary information (diagnosis, treatment, medications, laboratory values, outcome measures) and time course to allow the reader to fully evaluate the case.[3,6] Identifying information such as patient initials, date of birth, and even specific dates of admission should be removed.[3] The patient's medication history should include dosages, routes, dosage forms, start and stop dates, and blood levels if available. Description of the time course is important in understanding the event and evaluating the possible causal relationship. Despite the desire to include a complete description of all aspects of the case, the report must be free of extraneous information. Conclusions should not be stated in this section.

The discussion section should include an evaluation of the situation in light of the information available. The report should clearly state what is unique and the relevant clinical issues learned from the reported case.[3] For example, if a case report focused on an off-label use, the typical management options for the condition in question would be presented along with their efficacy data.[6] The discussion should examine the validity of the proposed relationship including an objective evaluation of other potential causes or unique patient variables.[3,6] This is necessary because there is no means to control for patient variables in a case report.[6] The discussion section should conclude with a summary of the important aspects and direction for future work, not just "additional research is needed in this area."[6] Figures or tables are used to present information from the case or to support the discussion but should avoid repetition of the text.[6] The figure or table should stand on its own without requiring the text to explain the information. The case report should also contain acknowledgment of work done by others. Informed consent should also be stated in the case report.[10] The conclusion should state in a concise manner what is to be gleaned from the evidence of the case report.[6] Care must be taken to ensure that the conclusions do not go beyond the facts of the case.

CHARACTERISTICS OF A GOOD CASE REPORT

A good case report must clearly make a unique and novel point.[9,11] There needs to be sufficient background description for the reader to understand the unique aspect being reported. The time frame of condition onset and means for diagnosis or identification should be stated. The patient characteristics should include aspects such as age, sex, race, conditions, and family history. A detailed clinical course of the event and outcome should be provided. The case must describe concisely the patients' medications including prescription, over-the-counter, and natural products with relevant start and stop dates, dosages, routes, and schedules. The impact of a medication dechallenge (taking the medication away) and rechallenge (restarting the medication) should be recorded if available.[19] Patient outcomes, diagnostic work, and laboratory results should be reported along with their time course. The case report should provide convincing evidence by itself.[9] The description and discussion of the case should provide scientific evidence to explain the findings.[3]

Use of widely accepted tools to evaluate the event will help to analyze the strength of the relationship being described. For example, the Naranjo scale helps to grade the relationship between an event and a medication as a cause of the event.[20,21] This scale contains 10 items that are scored based on yes or no answers, with a possible score range of −4 to 13. A definite ADR is ≥9, probable is 5 to 8, possible is 1 to 4, and doubtful is ≤0. The 10 questions evaluate whether the occurrence has been reported previously, the event started with the drug, the problem improved on discontinuation, the event recurred with rechallenge, other possible causes exist, the problem occurred with placebo, toxic levels were present in body fluids, the event worsened with increasing doses or improved with decreasing doses, the patient reacted previously to a medication in the drug class, and the event was demonstrated with objective results. Similarly, the Drug Interaction Probability Scale (DIPS) uses a 10-question evaluation with "highly probable" scores of >8 to "doubtful" of <2.[22] These tools provide objectivity in the evaluation of the case's facts and can be used by readers, authors, reviewers, and editors to evaluate the validity of the relationship between a medication and an adverse event.[20]

The Guideline for Good Clinical Practice by the International Conference on Harmonisation (ICH) has differentiated ADRs and adverse events on the basis of the relationship between a medication and an adverse event.[23] According to the ICH, ADRs should have a "causal relationship" or at least "reasonable possibility" of a relationship between a medication and an adverse event. An adverse event is any "untoward medical occurrence" that is not necessarily associated with a medication.[23] It can include any untoward observations in disease, symptom, or laboratory findings. Consequently, the Naranjo scale and DIPS are very useful tools in reporting ADRs in case reports.

CASE REPORT STRENGTHS

The greatest strength of the case report is the utility to identify rare or novel events (**Table 7-2**). This descriptive form of research provides a screening mechanism for identifying unique events in the general population based on the large sample and extended time frame.[13] This allows for the identification of rare events, problems specific to unique populations, and even common events occurring after an extended period of time. All of these are challenges to many other research designs. Although case reports are the weakest in the hierarchy of evidence, they are strongest in generating new ideas for future research. It has been suggested that the way to advance knowledge is through new ideas.[9] Case reports, therefore, serve an important role in generating new theories/hypotheses and identifying potential new issues for more rigorous evaluation.

Additional strengths of the case report focus on its simplicity and economy. The information necessary for the case report is already present and, therefore, this design requires no additional resources (e.g., dollars, facilities) except author time.[1] There are limited ethical issues (e.g., consent and anonymity of the patient) because the event has

TABLE 7-2	Strengths and Weaknesses of Case Reports and Case Series Design	
	Strengths	**Weaknesses**
Case Reports	Identifies rare occurrences	No causal inference can be made
	Identifies delayed ADRs	Potential reporting bias
	Hypothesis generation	No statistical analysis
	Requires minimal resources	Potential for reporting false results
Case Series	Study results are closer to those of routine clinical practice	No causal inference can be made
	May be useful when a randomized controlled trial is challenging to conduct	Susceptible to selection and measurement bias
	High external validity	Absolute risk cannot be calculated
	Cost-effective and time-saving design	Data collection may be incomplete

already taken place.[1,9] Because these reports often generate a hypothesis, the case report provides an economical way to guide the more expensive research approaches such as a placebo-controlled, randomized trial. These real-world experiences are also useful in showing an educational issue or guiding an improved practice.[9] Practitioners can use this information to gain unique insight into a practice that might have otherwise remained unrecognized, creating a "teachable moment."

CASE REPORT LIMITATIONS

Proving causality in case reports is limited due to significant concerns of internal validity and confounding factors such as variation in disease progress, co-occurring treatments and conditions, and treatment selection.[10,17] Significant biases may also exist as the findings are based on a single event/patient without any comparison group; therefore, statistical significance cannot be evaluated in a case study report. Consequently, the case reports are considered the weakest designs to generate evidence due to these methodological and design concerns.[9] Thus, the findings from case reports are difficult to use for clinical decision making.[24]

Reporting bias can also pose a problem. Case reports of new approaches to treatment most often describe successful situations. In one study, 90% of case reports and case series reported positive outcomes and only 10% reported unsuccessful findings.[10] There exists a potential for manipulation in reporting novel occurrences to support the effectiveness of an agent for off-label indications by manufacturers or those interested in the success of the medication. This is especially relevant in the publication of manufacturer-sponsored educational supplements to journals that focus on a specific issue.[10] Because the case report describes novel occurrences, it has a high level of sensitivity;[9,11] however, it has a chance of reporting false results and thus has a lower level of specificity.[11] Research examining the correctness of 47 case reports found 74.5% (35 cases) to be "clearly correct."[11] Although this reminds the reader to be cautious in assuming the case report has drawn the correct conclusion, the authors note "the predictive record of such unstructured observations is amazingly good."[11]

Recurrent case reporting may help to strengthen the evidence of a case report. For example, sleep attacks in patients taking dopamine agonists were examined through a review of case reports and identified 124 patients in 20 publications.[25] This information helped to characterize the current understanding of the adverse event and promote further studies. Some journals, however, are considering publishing only previously unreported case occurrences.[14] This limits the ability to use case reports as a body of evidence to strengthen a hypothesis or evaluate the magnitude of concern.

CRITICALLY EVALUATING CASE REPORTS

Case reports must be read in an evaluative manner to determine the validity and utility of the information.[26] Pierson has created a tool to examine case reports using a simple set of five criteria: quality of documentation, uniqueness, educational value, objectivity, and interpretation of the situation.[26] Each item is scored on a scale from 0 to 2 with a summated score of up to 10 points. First, "documentation" examines aspects of the case report from insufficient evidence supporting the critical point of the report to the presence of all necessary information. "Uniqueness" is determined by the evidence of a complete literature review. Results may range from the case being reported in the same journal to no previously reported occurrences. "Educational value" focuses on the ability to apply the information to other situations. For example, is the description sufficiently clear and classic to apply to other cases? "Objectivity" centers on the biased or unbiased reporting of information in the case report itself. "Interpretation" examines the support for the conclusions and recommendations made in the discussion. This includes the quality and use of the literature review. A complete description of this tool can be found in the article by Pierson. A checklist for evaluating the validity and educational value of a case report is also described in this resource.[26] This checklist includes specific items to consider for each portion of the case report from the title to the references.

CASE SERIES

CASE SERIES DEFINITION

Case series study consists of a group of patients who have been diagnosed with the same condition or are following similar procedures over a period of time.[4,27] It does not include a comparison group. A case series puts together single specific cases (two cases up to thousands) and includes them in one report.[1,4] This descriptive study design is comprised of individuals whose inclusion is based on the occurrence of a definite illness or illness-related outcome.[28] A case series can be used in certain scenarios including the preliminary report of a new and emerging condition or treatment, the report of outcomes by a health professional or institution, or in a multi-institutional registry.[4]

PURPOSE OF A CASE SERIES

The primary purpose of a case series is similar to case reports including evaluation of disease course, ADRs, and effectiveness; however, the findings of case series are stronger than case reports mainly because of sample size. The case series serves to produce assumptions that can be further examined in stronger and more robust methodological studies.[27]

CASE SERIES STUDY DESIGN AND WRITE-UP

Design

The study question should be clearly defined and appropriate for a case series. Specifically, the question should typically not examine efficacy. The study question should always include the population being studied, the intervention/treatment, and the main study outcomes.[27]

The inclusion and exclusion criteria for the study population must be mentioned and well described. Specific clinical criteria should be used in the description of the case series so that any reader can accurately examine a relationship between their patients and those included in the case series.[4] A case series should define the case in question. For example, if the researcher is investigating a series of patients with migraines, a definition of a migraine should be provided. Important information that clearly describes the patient such as demographic features (e.g., age, gender) and relevant clinical aspects (e.g., disease, illness stage, and duration of illness) should also be included. The nature of the patient population may be impacted by the setting. For example, a case series from a tertiary care center will likely be composed of patients who are more difficult to treat (e.g., refractory to first-line therapy).[4] Therefore, including a detailed description of the setting and the population will allow a community practitioner to determine if the patients in the study can be compared to those seen in their own practice, hence, increasing the external validity of the study.[4,27] In addition, the number of patients in the case series should be included along with the length of time it took to reach the exact sample size needed. Elimination of patients from the case series should be described for the reader to evaluate the potential occurrence of selection bias. Finally, there should be a description of the follow-up including attrition of patients during follow-up or if some patients decided to reject the intervention.[4]

A thorough description of all interventions must be included with sufficient clarity for replication. In addition, co-intervention clarity is also required because these approaches and therapies may significantly affect patients' outcomes and vary greatly depending on the practice setting (e.g., referral center, primary care setting).[4,27]

All outcome measures used in case series should be valid and reliable. **Validity** is the extent to which the instrument measures what it is intended to measure, whereas **reliability** is the degree to which repeated measurements produce consistent results.[27] There should be references to show how the outcomes were validated. All procedures for outcome measurement should be standardized and continued long enough for the measured outcomes to have occurred.[4,27]

There should be blinding of the investigators assessing the outcomes. Preferably, the evaluator of the outcome should not be aware of whether the participant has received the intervention or not.[4] In some cases, the investigator may only collect the outcome data and not collect patient information. Because there is a strong possibility of bias depending on the data collection method/source, it is important that the data collection steps be adequately described. This also will allow replication of the work.

Analysis

Because there is no comparison group, only descriptive statistics such as a mean or the prevalence of a disease should be used, especially because the case series is a descriptive study. In these studies, no probability statistics and comparative tests (like a *t*-test, *chi*-square, or ANOVA) with *p*-values should be included.[27] Some case series may compare their patient outcomes with those of other past case series. This scenario, called using historical controls, needs to be used with caution as certain co-interventions may change over the course of the years. In another design approach, a patient may serve as his or her control in a pre-post analysis. In this case, the paired nature of the data allows for statistical comparison but care must be taken due to variables that may confound this longitudinal comparison (e.g., disease fluctuations, patient optimism with new treatment).[4]

Reporting

The external validity should be discussed including the characteristics of the patients, features of the follow-up, and any potential bias.[27] Specific data on patient follow-up (rates, reason for dropout) should be included. Comparison of case series studies is difficult due to significant variations in follow-up; therefore, caution should be taken in comparing findings. Because no hypothesis is being tested, descriptive data constitute the only conclusions that can be made. For example, "our patients treated by treatment X showed good outcome Y after Z months of follow-up."[27] If additional information is used to support the conclusions, the author should clearly state and cite this information appropriately. Also, study limitations and a description of future research steps should be stated. Based on the strength of evidence, randomized controlled trials may be recommended.[4]

The sources of funding or sponsorship should be stated. Evidence has shown a relationship between studies that demonstrate treatment improvements and certain types of funding, especially privately or industry-funded studies. The reasons for this may include the use of multiple publications of the same data and the potential for publication bias. **Publication bias** refers to the preferential publication of positive results.[4] In addition, authors should disclose consulting or board appointments with a pharmaceutical manufacturer that might possibly create a conflict of interest and potentially influence reporting of results.[4]

GENERAL GUIDELINES AND EVALUATION OF A CASE SERIES

All key features that should be addressed when designing and carrying out a case series study are listed in **Table 7-3**. The characteristics of a good case series are illustrated in the guidelines for writing a case series. A good example of a case series report is Auerbach et al.[29] The criteria for evaluating the quality of a case series report are reflected in the description of the key features of this study design (Table 7-3).

STRENGTHS AND WEAKNESSES OF A CASE SERIES

Strengths

Despite the small sample size, case series studies are of utility to clinicians primarily based on their close approximation to the patient population seen in actual practice, which helps clinicians use the findings. Careful study design can minimize the bias and issues with small sample size.[8,30] Additional advantages of the case series design include a high precision in identifying unanticipated innovative occurrences

TABLE 7-3 Key Features of a Case Series Report	
Aspect for Evaluation	**Desired Features**
Research Question	Clearly defined Does not involve comparative efficacy
Study Population	Well-defined inclusion/exclusion Clearly described patient population Description of patients not included or lost to follow-up Description of the practice setting
Interventions	Thorough description of primary intervention Complete presentation of all co-interventions
Outcome Measures	Information on validity and reliability of measures Description of what constitutes improvement Outline of time frame for follow-up Blinding of those collecting outcome measures from knowledge of the specific intervention Source and method of data collection
Statistical Analyses	Descriptive statistics Individual patient pre- versus post-intervention measures may be used and are the only reason for comparative statistical analysis May compare to historical data
Discussion/Conclusions	Statements are consistent with the nature of the data reported
Funding Source/Conflicts	Acknowledgment of funding source or other potential conflicts of interest

(especially advanced medical outcomes),[8,11] simple methods, and straightforward data analysis.[30]

A case series is useful when a randomized controlled trial (RCT) is not appropriate despite RCT's high quality of evidence. For example, an RCT may be inappropriate due to ethical issues or the need to identify rare adverse effects of treatments.[4,26,31] Case series studies are very good at identifying unique occurrences and serving as "hypothesis generating" studies.[4,9] This is similar to case reports.[1,12] Case series studies, however, are explorative and provide descriptive findings in a group of patients with an explicit condition who are managed with a specific intervention.[4] Incidences, means, and confidence intervals of key measures of interest can be calculated as multiple cases are selected, unlike a case report.

Clinicians find the results of case series studies to be relevant to their practice based on the sampling approach. While RCTs specifically exclude and include patients, studies using the case series design typically include consecutive patients, all of whom have additional conditions and treatments that make the sample similar to the typical practitioner's patient. This increases what is referred to as external validity—generalizability of study findings.[27]

Case series studies are efficient and cost-effective. These benefits are achieved through the simplicity of the study design, which does not include a comparison group and therefore does not involve randomization.[27] Furthermore, minimal resources are needed to obtain and analyze data for a group of patients.

Weaknesses

The case series design does not involve randomization or a control/comparison group, which are required to evaluate actual causality.[27] Furthermore, improvements in study endpoints can be due to either the treatment, the natural course of the condition, or other extraneous variables. Due to the lack of a control group, the researcher is unable to control for these variables; therefore, causality cannot be evaluated. On the other hand, a case series study that reports negative results may help to avoid more rigorous study designs.[4]

Similar to case reports, significant concerns of internal validity, such as selection, history, maturation, testing, and instrumentation, exist in case series reports.[32] Case series do not provide strong evidence such as other observational or randomized research.[9] In addition, temporal sequence for exposure and outcome manifestation is not always clear.

Often, the data obtained in a case series are based on past observations of patients. Because of this retospective approach, the completeness of the data including follow-up in a case series may be limited, not examined in a consistent manner, or subject to measurement variability. Consequently, retrospective case series designs create difficulty in interpreting results. This is in contrast to an RCT, where there are strict and detailed prospective protocols for the study design.[27]

Bias is a major problem for case series studies, especially selection and measurement bias.[27] Selection bias occurs in a case series because follow-up data may be obtained from individuals with the best outcomes. Measurement bias is most often due to variations in measure approaches or process. To reduce measurement bias, the individual who is assessing the outcomes should be blinded to the intervention.

Relative risks cannot be quantified with case series data due to the lack of a comparison group.[28] Conversely, in a cohort study, patients are selected based on their exposure to a risk factor (such as smoking) or an intervention (such as a hip replacement). Given a particular exposure, an absolute risk (or rate) for an outcome can be calculated, including a relative risk.

SUMMARY AND CONCLUSIONS

Though no causal inferences can be made from a case report or case series, these reports are effective in recognizing a potential novel occurrence and generating new hypotheses about the safety and efficacy of treatments. They are usually the "first form of evidence" in clinical medicine and have played an important role in medical literature. These designs are also easy to implement and are cost-effective. However, there are significant limitations to these approaches due to such factors as lack of a control group, confounding factors, and potential biases. Therefore, typically more evidence must be obtained from stronger observational studies and RCTs controlled trials before treatment conclusions can be made. Although these designs are the weakest in the hierarchy of evidence, they are strongest in generating new ideas for future research.

REVIEW QUESTIONS

1. What is the role of case reports in advancing medical knowledge?
2. Should case reports continue to be included in journals? Explain your answer.
3. Why is a case series important in evidence-based medicine?
4. What are important criteria for evaluating a good case series report?

ONLINE RESOURCES

BMJ Case Reports Guidelines: http://casereports.bmj.com/site/about/guidelines.xhtml
BMJ Case Reports Template: http://casereports.bmj.com/site/about/june2011fullcases_template.doc
National Cancer Institute. NCI Best Case Series Criteria for Optimal Case Studies: http://cam.cancer.gov/new_bestcase_protocol.html

REFERENCES

1. Grimes DA, Schulz KF. Descriptive studies: what they can and cannot do. *Lancet*. 2002;359:145–149.
2. Kelly WN, Arellano FM, Barnes J, Bergman U, et al. Guidelines for submitting adverse event reports for publication. *Pharmacoepidemiol Drug Saf*. 2007;16:581–587.
3. Cohen H. How to write a patient case report. *Am J Health-Syst Pharm*. 2006;63:1888–1892.
4. Carey TS, Boden SD. A critical guide to case series reports. *Spine*. 2003;28:1631–1634.
5. Kasim NHA, Abdullah BJJ, Manikam J. The current status of the case report: terminal or viable? *Biomed Imaging Interv J*. 2009;5(1):e4.
6. Green BN, Johnson CD. Writing patient case reports for peer-reviewed journals: secrets of the trade. *J Sports Chiropr & Rehabil*. 2000;14(3):51–59.
7. Pace BP, Lundberg GD. Celebrating 150 years of the AMA and the first 100 years of JAMA. *JAMA*. 1996;276:833.
8. Albrecht J, Meves A, Bigby M. Case reports and case series from *Lancet* had significant impact on medical literature. *J Clin Epidemiol*. 2005; 58: 1227–1232.
9. Vandenbroucke JP. Case reports in an evidence-based world (Editorial). *J R Soc Med*. 1999;92:159–163.
10. Albrecht J, Werth VP, Bigby M. The role of case reports in evidence-based practice, with suggestions for improving their reporting. *J Am Acad Dermatol*. 2009;60:412–418.
11. Vandenbroucke JP. In defense of case reports and case series. *Ann Intern Med*. 2001;134:330–334.
12. Hoffman JR. Rethinking case reports. Highlighting the extremely unusual can do more harm than good. *WJM*. 1999;170:253–254.

13. Brewer T, Colditz GA. Postmarketing surveillance and adverse drug reactions. Current perspectives and future needs. *JAMA*. 1999;281:824–829.

14. Khan KS, Thompson PJ. A proposal for writing and appraising case reports. *BJOG*. 2002;109: 849–851.

15. Loke YK, Price D, Derry S, Aronson JK. Case reports of suspected adverse drug reactions–systematic literature survey of follow-up. *BMJ*. 2006;332:335–339.

16. Kalus RM, Shojania KG, Amory JK, Saint S. Lost in transcription. *NEJM*. 2006;355:487–491.

17. Green BN, Johnson CD. How to write a case report for publication. *J Chiropr Med*. 2006;5:72–82.

18. Kirthi V. How to write a clinical case report. *RCP Insight*. 2011.

19. US Department of Health and Human Services. Good pharmacovigilance practices and pharmaco-epidemiologic assessment. *Guidance for Industry*. 2005; March.

20. Author guidelines. *The Annals of Pharmacotherapy*. http://www.sagepub.com/upm-data/57856_AOP_Author_Guidelines.pdf. Accessed October 28, 2013.

21. Naranjo CA, Busto U, Sellers EM, et al. A method for estimating the probability of adverse drug reactions. *Clin Pharmacol Ther*. 1981;30:239–245.

22. Horn JR, Hansten PD, Chan LN. Proposal for a new tool to evaluate drug interaction cases. *Ann Pharmacother*. 2007;41:674–680.

23. International Conference on Harmonisation of Technical Requirements for Registration of Pharmaceuticals for Human Use. Good Clinical Practice E6 May 1996. http://www.ich.org/fileadmin/Public_Web_Site/ICH_Products/Guidelines/Efficacy/E6_R1/Step4/E6_R1__Guideline.pdf. Accessed October 9, 2012.

24. Etminan M, Wright JM, Carleton BC. Evidence-based pharmacotherapy: review of basic concepts and applications in clinical practice. *Ann Pharmacother*. 1998;32:1193–1200.

25. Homann CK, Wenzel K, Suppan K, et al. Sleep attacks in patients taking dopamine agonists: review. *BMJ*. 2002;324:1483–1487.

26. Pierson DJ. How to read a case report (or teaching case of the month). *Respiratory Care*. 2009;54: 1372–1378.

27. Kooistra B, Dijkman B, Einhorn TA, Bhandari M. How to design a good case series. *J Bone Joint Surg Am*. 2009;91(suppl 3):21–26.

28. Dekkers OM, Egger M, Altman DG, Vandenbroucke JP. Distinguishing case series from cohort studies. *Ann Intern Med*. 2012;156:37–40.

29. Auerbach DM, Darrow WW, Jaffe HW, Curran JW. Cluster of cases of the acquired immune deficiency syndrome. Patients linked by sexual contact. *Am J Med*. 1984;76(3):487–492.

30. Jabs DA. Improving the reporting of clinical case series (Editorial). *Am J Ophthalmol*. 2005;139: 900–905.

31. Kempen JH. Appropriate use and reporting of uncontrolled case series in the medical literature. *Am J Ophthalmol*. 2011;151:7–10.

32. Shadish WR, Cook TD, Campbell DT. *Experimental and Quasi-Experimental Designs for Causal Inference*. Boston, MA: Houghton Mifflin; 2001.

STATISTICAL PRINCIPLES AND DATA ANALYSIS

MEASUREMENT AND DESCRIPTIVE ANALYSIS

KAREN BLUMENSCHEIN, PHARMD

AMIE GOODIN, MPP

CHAPTER OBJECTIVES

▸ Identify and describe the two general functions of statistics

▸ Describe measurement and variable classification schemes

▸ Describe and use measures of central tendency and dispersion

▸ Organize and present data in a scientifically meaningful way

▸ Differentiate between proportions and rates, including prevalence and incidence

▸ Describe performance measures for diagnostic tests, including sensitivity, specificity, and predictive value

▸ Describe receiver operating characteristic curves and their role in diagnostic tests

KEY TERMINOLOGY

Arithmetic mean
Bar chart
Box and whisker plot
Coefficient of variation
Continuous variables
Control variables
Dependent variable
Descriptive statistics
Discrete variables
False negative rate
False positive rate
Frequency table
Histogram
Incidence
Independent variable
Inferential statistics
Interquartile range

Interval data
Mean
Measures of central tendency
Measures of dispersion
Median
Mode
Negative predictive value
Nominal data
Ordinal data
Pie chart
Positive predictive value
Prevalence
Proportion
Qualitative data
Quantitative data
Range

Rates
Ratio data
Receiver operating characteristic (ROC) curve
Sensitivity
Skewness
Specificity
Standard deviation
Statistics
True negative rate
True positive rate
Variable classification schemes
Variance

INTRODUCTION

In research, measurement is the process of collecting and recording observations about the variables that are of interest in a specified project. These collected observations are called data. There are a variety of tools that researchers can employ to collect observations. Some examples of measurement tools include stadiometers (height), sphygmomanometers (blood pressure), enzyme-linked immunosorbent assays (antibodies in serum), and questionnaires (health status). Once observations are collected, these measurements about the variables of interest (i.e., data) are used to inform the research question, and this occurs through the use of **statistics**. A recent editorial in *Science* defined statistics as ". . . the science of learning from data, and of measuring, controlling, and communicating uncertainty."[1] Thus, functions of statistics include summarizing, organizing, presenting, analyzing, and interpreting data.[2]

This chapter is devoted to the summarizing, organizing, and presenting functions of statistics, commonly referred to as **descriptive statistics**. Analytic (e.g., hypothesis testing) and interpretation functions, which are collectively referred to as **inferential statistics**, will be covered later in this text. The chapter begins by introducing various schemes that can be used to classify and summarize variables so that collections of information can be simplified and communicated in a manner that is both straightforward and standardized. This is followed by a discussion of how to visualize and optimally present data so that it is logical and comprehensible. The chapter concludes with a discussion of summary measures used to convey morbidity and mortality information and summary measures used to describe diagnostic tests.

VARIABLE CLASSIFICATION SCHEMES

At the most fundamental level, data can be described as having either a qualitative or quantitative nature. **Qualitative data**, or meaningful information that is collected in words,[3] may provide valuable insight into the condition of individual patients, but are not typically used for the purposes of healthcare research with large populations of patients.[a] Written observations or notes found in medical records are examples of qualitative data. This chapter will focus on **quantitative data**, which are data that are collected as numerical or countable information. Any type of data that is countable in nature is quantitative, such as age, weight, and blood pressure.

Quantitative data can further be described as being either discrete or continuous. **Discrete variables** (or categorical variables) usually have only a few possible values and are often defined as "counts." Many types of healthcare data are collected as discrete variables, such as sex (male or female), number of hospitalizations, and variables that only take a value of either "yes" or "no." While discrete variables may take on few values, **continuous variables** may take an infinite number of values within a given range.[4] Continuous variables can be thought of as existing on some defined scale; for example, age, body temperature, and weight are all continuous variables. Both discrete and continuous variables are commonplace in medical literature and in healthcare practice.

---

[a] "Qualitative data" may also refer to discrete or categorical variables, and "quantitative data" may also refer to continuous variables. For example, the sex of a patient (e.g., male or female) is a discrete variable with a limited number of possible values, but sex may also be used to provide description in a qualitative context.

Identifying the appropriate **variable classification schemes** can help determine what types of statistical methods are appropriate for describing data or for making inferences. After determining the continuous or discrete nature of the variable in question, it is then helpful to determine the level of measurement. Each of the four levels of measurement is discussed in the following section. Refer to **Table 8-1** for a summary of levels of measurement.

LEVELS OF MEASUREMENT

Data that can be placed into narrowly defined categories that are not in any particular order are known as **nominal data**. Nominal data are discrete because they must take on one of a few possible, mutually exclusive, values. For example, the variable "sex" is nominal because it can take on two possible values: male or female. Because these two values are discrete, they cannot be handled in a meaningful way using mathematical operations (e.g., if you were to take an average of two observations—one male and one female—with male coded as 1 and female coded as 2, then you would be pursuing a nonsensical result of 1.5); however, it is possible to count the frequency of these values.

Ordinal data also consist of narrowly defined categories, but these categories may be ranked. Ordinal data are typically discrete because they must take on one of a few possible values but there are some instances when a large number of categories implies an underlying continuous scale. Many examples of discrete ordinal data can be found in patient assessment questions that ask the respondent to select an answer from a list that most closely represents their thoughts or feelings on the subject in question. For example, a patient assessment of healthcare service satisfaction may ask, "How often does your healthcare provider listen carefully to you?" and the patient answers by selecting one response from the following list: always, usually, sometimes, rarely, or never. Those response categories are narrowly defined and discrete, yet they describe different amounts or frequency of occurrence (i.e., there is a rank order).

Ordinal data are often collected through Likert scale–type questioning. A patient assessment question that employs Likert-type questioning will ask the patient to select their level of agreement with a presented statement.[5] For example, a Likert-type question may ask, "I experience frequent shortness of breath," and the patient must select from response options such as: strongly disagree, disagree, unsure, agree, or strongly agree.

TABLE 8-1	Levels of Measurement Summary		
Level of Measurement	**Discrete/ Continuous**	**Examples**	**Possible Mathematical Operations**
Nominal Data	Discrete	Male or female, race, does the patient have insurance? (yes or no)	Counts (frequency)
Ordinal Data	Discrete*	Likert-type questions, pain scales	Counts, median, percentiles
Interval Data	Continuous†	Body temperature in degrees (Fahrenheit or Celsius)	Same as ordinal data plus addition, subtraction, mean, standard deviation
Ratio Data	Continuous†	Age, weight, height, income	Same as interval data plus ratios

*Ordinal data may imply an underlying continuous scale when large numbers of categories are present.
†Interval/ratio data may be discrete if the variable can only take on integer values.

This type of ordinal data consists of defined categories that may be ranked, but the distance between each of the responses is unclear.

One example of ordinal data that implies an underlying continuous scale is a measure that healthcare providers use to assess pain as reported by their patients. A healthcare provider may ask the patient, "On a scale from 1 to 10, where 1 is little or no pain and 10 is the most severe pain imaginable, how much pain are you experiencing?" The patient would answer with one of the values in this scale, and the placement of that value is meaningful. For example, the response of "8" signifies more pain than "2," but the distance between these two values is not meaningful because the unit of measurement for pain is not defined. The lack of a defined and meaningful zero point prohibits certain mathematical manipulations of these values, so a pain rating of "8" is not equal to 4 times the pain rating of "2."

When the scale of ranked data represents meaningful differences between numbers, but still lacks a defined and meaningful zero point, it is classified as **interval data**. An example of interval data is body temperature measurements in degrees. If a patient's body temperature changes from 98.2°F to 102.2°F, then it has increased 4°F, and this 4°F difference is the same as a change from 98.9°F to 102.9°F. This change can be calculated because a Fahrenheit degree is measured on a defined scale, where the distance between each degree is constant. Interval data are usually considered to be continuous and, therefore, may be compared using simple mathematical operations, such as addition and subtraction, in a meaningful way.

Ratio data have all of the properties of interval data, but there is an absolute minimum or zero point to the scale; in other words, there is a defined and meaningful zero point that denotes "none of" the property being measured (i.e., a value of a drug concentration in the blood of 0 means that there is no drug in the blood). Ratio data are usually continuous, and these data may be mathematically manipulated in various ways to yield descriptions of the data. For example, patient weight in pounds may be added, subtracted, or averaged and the distance between the units of measurement, in this case pounds, is measured on a defined scale with a meaningful zero point (i.e., a patient cannot weigh less than zero pounds). Because of the absolute zero point, ratio data allow for ratio calculation. Returning to patient weight as the example, a patient who weighs 210 pounds weighs twice as much as a patient who weighs 105 pounds. This ratio comparison (210/105) is not possible with data from other levels of measurement, so, for example, it would be inappropriate to say that 80°F is twice as hot as 40°F.

CASE STUDY 8-1 **Medical Literature Connection**

A paper published in *Clinical Therapeutics* by Kim, Lee, Koh, et al. describes measuring pain in a sample of patients using a visual analog scale. Patients were asked to rate their pain on a scale of 0 to 100, where 0 was no pain and 100 was the most severe pain imaginable. This type of data is ordinal because the distance between values is not defined, but implies an underlying continuous scale. Although technically ordinal and discrete, it is fairly common to treat such a variable as continuous during data analysis, which is essentially what Kim et al. do.

Data from Kim J, Lee EY, Koh E-M, et al. Comparative clinical trial of S-adenosylmethionine vs. nabumetone for the treatment of knee osteoarthritis: an 8-week, multicenter, randomized, double-blind, double-dummy, phase IV study in Korean patients. *Clin Ther.* 2009;31(12):2860–2872.

THE CONCEPTUAL ROLE OF VARIABLES IN RESEARCH QUESTIONS

In research, one variable is hypothesized to explain an observed clinical phenomenon. This explanatory variable is designated as the **independent variable** in research terminology, because the values that the independent variable take are not influenced by other variables in the model. The independent (explanatory) variables explain or predict the values that the **dependent variable** will take. For example, suppose that a new hypertension medication is being compared to a placebo to test the hypothesis that the new medication leads to a reduction in blood pressure. The drug (new medication or placebo) would represent the independent variable because it is proposed to explain any reduction in blood pressure, which is the dependent variable in this scenario.

Other variables that are related to the dependent variable are typically included in most research designs. These other explanatory variables, or **control variables**, are also presumed to influence the dependent variable. Control variables hold external conditions constant so that the effect of the independent variable may be measured using statistical testing.[b] Revisiting the previous hypothesis that a new hypertension medication is related to reduced blood pressure may prompt the decision to include other measures such as age, race, and sex as control variables. All of these proposed control variables may impact the dependent variable (blood pressure) in some way, but controlling these values allows researchers to isolate and assess the effect of the independent variable of interest (new hypertension medication or placebo).

MEASURES OF CENTRAL TENDENCY (MEASURES OF CENTRAL LOCATION)

Measures of central tendency (also called measures of central location) are used to provide information about the center or "typical value" of a set of numbers. There are three common methods for measuring the central location of a variable: mean, median, and mode. Each of these methods and the appropriate usage of each of these measures are discussed in this section.

The **mode** is not reported as often in clinical research as other measures of central location. Mode is calculated by counting the occurrence of each value of the variable and is assigned as the value that appears most often. For example, given the information about the variable "Patient Age" in **Table 8-2**, the occurrence of each age can be counted: age 20 appears 3 times, age 42 appears 2 times, and ages 68, 51, and 38 each appear once. The age 20 appears most often; thus, 20 is the mode for this variable.

The mode may best be used in situations that describe the central location of a variable if its values are non-numerical qualities or attributes. For example, if the variable were measuring sex, with values being either male or female, the modal count would be an appropriate description of central tendency. A variable may be multimodal if two or more values of the variable appear equally most often.

The **median** is calculated by listing the values of a variable in ascending or descending order and reporting the value that lies in the middle of this list. If a list has an even number of values, then the arithmetic mean between the two middle values is calculated and reported as the median. The patient age example from Table 8-2 can be ordered by value as follows: 20, 20, 20, 38, 42, 42, 51, and 68. The two middle values in this

---

[b] See Chapter 11, "Simple and Multiple Linear Regression," for more information.

TABLE 8-2   Patient Age and Measures of Central Tendency

Original Data		Frequency Table		Measures of Central Tendency	
Patient	Age	Value	Frequency	Measure	Value
Ken	20	20	3 times	Mode	20
Sally	38	42	2 times	Median	40
Nate	42	38	1 time	Arithmetic Mean	37.63
Mary	20	51	1 time		
Min	20	68	1 time		
Will	42				
Sarah	68				
Jacob	51				

list are 38 and 42. When an arithmetic mean for these two middle values is calculated ((38 + 42)/2), a median of 40 is obtained.

The median is most appropriately used in situations where a few values of a variable are noticeably larger or smaller than most of the rest of the values. These values are known as outliers. In these situations, a median is preferable to the mean because it is a more accurate representation of the majority of values present in the data. For example, imagine trying to accurately describe the typical annual income of a group of people who made $25K, $30K, $27K, $31K, $28K, and $60 million. The person making a substantially higher income than the rest of the group would cause the "average" annual income of the group to appear much higher, thus distorting the measure to reflect disproportionately more of the outlier's income.

The **arithmetic mean** is known to most people as simply the "average" of a set of values. As all of the described measures of central tendency may be thought of as averages, the formal terminology will be used here when calculating the arithmetic mean. The algebraic definition of the **mean** is $\dfrac{\sum x_i}{n}$, which can be interpreted in words as the sum of all the values of a variable divided by the total number of observations. When this definition of the arithmetic mean is applied to the patient age example from Table 8-2, the calculation is as follows:

$$\frac{20+20+20+38+42+42+51+68}{8} = \frac{301}{8} = 37.63 \text{ years.}$$

The arithmetic mean is the appropriate tool to use when describing the typical value of variables at the interval and ratio levels of measurement. A notable exception occurs when describing data that have apparent outliers.

MEASURES OF DISPERSION

Measures of dispersion are used to describe how data are spread and provide information about the variability in a distribution of observations. Combining measures of central tendency and dispersion yield a detailed illustration of what the data represent. The most basic measure of how data are spread is the **range**. The range is calculated by taking the difference between the lowest value in the data and the highest value in the data. Returning to the patient age data in Table 8-2, the range of patient ages is calculated by subtracting 20 from 68 to yield a range of 48 years. **Interquartile range (IQR)** is similarly calculated, but is restricted to values that lie within the middle 50% of the distribution, so IQR is equal to the upper quartile value minus the lower quartile value. Quartiles divide the range of a variable's values into four equal sections. A simple way to visualize quartiles is to imagine a dollar bill that has been exchanged for four quarters. The first quarter is analogous to the first (25%) quartile, the second quarter to the second quartile (50%, which is also the median value), the third quarter to the third quartile (75%), and the fourth quarter will make the dollar whole (100%). Range and IQR are useful tools when describing the qualities of any type of numerical data.

The two most common methods for describing the dispersion of a variable are **variance** and **standard deviation**.[c] Variance shows how far the values of a variable lie from the mean with the measure σ^2, which is mathematically defined as the average squared distance of values from their mean:[4]

$$\sigma^2 = \frac{1}{N}\sum_{i=1}^{N}(x_i - \text{mean})^2$$

The standard deviation is the square root of the variance:

$$\sigma = \sqrt{\frac{1}{N}\sum_{i=1}^{N}(x_i - \text{mean})^2}$$

where N refers to the total number of values.

The standard deviation tends to be reported more often than variance because it is expressed using the same units as the original data. Variance and standard deviation are measures of variability that may be calculated for continuous data and some types of discrete data (e.g., a yes/no or dichotomous variable).

The **coefficient of variation** is a useful descriptive tool for visualizing the extent of variability in data once the standard deviation and mean have been calculated. The coefficient of variation (CV) is mathematically defined as:

$$CV = \frac{\text{standard deviation}}{\text{mean}}$$

The CV is sometimes multiplied by 100% to provide a more straightforward interpretation. The use of this statistical tool is only appropriate for ratio-level data and is most often employed when comparing two or more groups that have different arithmetic means.[4]

Skewness is another important characteristic to consider when describing data. Skewness indicates that the data are not evenly distributed around the mean; in other words, more of the data are concentrated to either the right or the left of the mean value, and the "tail" on the opposite side of the mean is longer. Consider **Figure 8–1A**. In this example, the variable is right, or positively, skewed. Graphically, most of the data lay to the left of the mean, but the right tail is quite long and the mean is greater than the median. Left, or negatively, skewed data follow the opposite pattern, where more data fall to the right of the mean but the left tail is extended, as shown in **Figure 8–1B**. With negatively or left skewed data, the median is greater than the mean.

---

[c] The formulas for variance and standard deviation shown here are in "population" notation. For a "sample" of size n, $n-1$ is used in the denominator rather than N, the total number of values in a finite population, in these formulas. Chapter 9, "Interpretation and Basic Statistical Concepts," provides a distinction between samples and populations. Dividing by $n-1$ rather than n is necessary so that the sample variance can be used in statistical inference procedures.

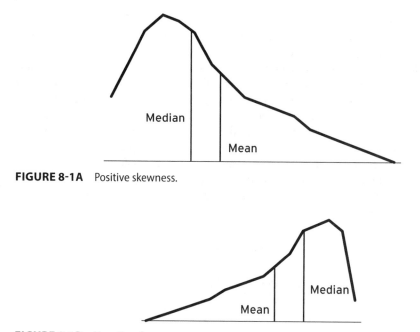

FIGURE 8-1A Positive skewness.

FIGURE 8-1B Negative skewness.

ORGANIZING AND VISUALIZING DATA

Descriptive statistics like measures of central tendency and dispersion are useful tools for explaining data, but visual representations of data are powerful demonstration aids when used effectively. Visual representations of data can be categorized as tables, plots, graphs, and charts. The simplest form of visual representation is the **frequency table**, which can be used to organize discrete or continuous data at any level of measurement. Frequency tables are used to present counts, or frequencies, of each value category within a variable. A well-constructed frequency table will include a clear title, appropriate column names, and adequate space and row/column delineation for easy reading. Tally marks should be avoided when displaying count data. Instead, use value category names and numerical counts with clearly marked units of measurement.

CASE STUDY 8-2 **Medical Literature Connection**

Return to the Kim, Lee, Koh, et al. paper in *Clinical Therapeutics* for an example of good frequency table construction. Table I from these authors provides the reader with all of the key information necessary to interpret the data and is organized in such a way as to not appear overcrowded or difficult to read.

Data from Kim J, Lee EY, Koh E-M, et al. Comparative clinical trial of S-adenosylmethionine vs. nabumetone for the treatment of knee osteoarthritis: an 8-week, multicenter, randomized, double-blind, double-dummy, phase IV study in Korean patients. *Clin Ther.* 2009;31(12):2860–2872.

Table 8-3A is an example of a poorly organized frequency table. The categories are difficult to interpret based upon the lack of labels and description of units, as well as poor spacing and formatting choices. **Table 8-3B** presents the same data, but offers helpful descriptions and clear organization that make it easy for the reader to interpret.

The **box and whisker plot**, or box plot, is a visually meaningful way of presenting the range or spread of data. This simplified plot allows the researcher to pinpoint the minimum and maximum values in the data and highlight the IQR and median. The IQR makes up the "box" part of the graph with the median denoted by a line inside the box, whereas the minimum and maximum values typically mark the "whiskers" (**Figure 8-2**). Occasionally, the mean value may also be indicated on a box plot (in Figure 8-2, the mean values appear as diamonds). It is important to note that only one axis of this "graph" is labeled with mathematically meaningful units, which is why it is referred to as a plot rather than a formal graph.

This type of visualization is useful when making comparisons across different groups that may not have equivalent underlying distributions. Figure 8-2 compares mammography screening across patient care venues. This box plot shows the distribution of breast exams in all facilities (on the left) followed by the distribution of breast exams in selected types of healthcare facilities. The distributions underlying the measurement of exams per year from each healthcare venue are not necessarily equivalent, and the box plot is an effective method of organizing the data without making that assumption.

A **bar chart** is used to graph discrete, categorical data and is typically aligned horizontally. Though visually similar, a **histogram** is used to graph continuous data that have been apportioned into discrete categories. The columns of a bar chart do not touch, whereas the columns of a histogram typically connect to illustrate the underlying continuity of the variable. A good histogram or bar chart will include a descriptive title, labeled axes with well-defined units of measurement, and appropriate divisions of continuous data into discrete categories. Histograms and bar charts are appropriate for

TABLE 8-3A Example of a Poorly Organized Frequency Table	
Patient Characteristic	**Frequency**
M	55 (35.5)
F	100 (64.5)
<18	3 (1.9)
18–64	120 (77.4)
>65	32 (20.6)

TABLE 8-3B Example of a Well-Organized Frequency Table	
Patient Characteristic	**Frequency (% of Patients)**
Sex	
Males	55 (35.5%)
Females	100 (64.5%)
Age in Years	
<18	3 (1.9%)
18–64	120 (77.4%)
>65	32 (20.6%)

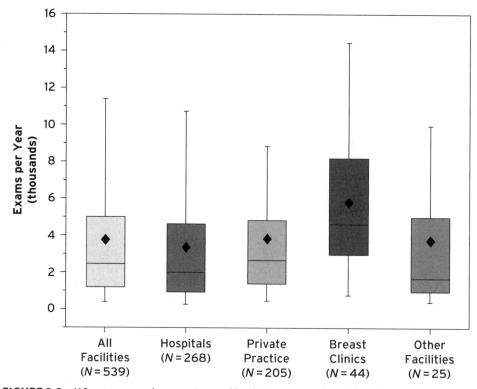

FIGURE 8-2   U.S. mammography screening workloads (January 2006–October 2006).

visualizing frequencies and distributions, but bar charts are not the best tool to illustrate trend data (i.e., a variable that changes over time).

Figure 8-3A is an example bar chart that graphs responses for a question that employed a Likert-type scale. **Figure 8-3B** is an example histogram that graphs mammography screenings by venue for the years 1997 through 2006. Notice the characteristics of each type of chart that make them the appropriate choice for the type of information being presented. The data presented in the bar chart in Figure 8-3A are categorical and discrete, whereas the data presented in the histogram[d] in Figure 8-3B are continuous and presented as a variable that changes over time.

The **pie chart** is intuitively simple to read when constructed well. This type of chart is used to represent proportions or relative quantities of values. There are several hazards when using this type of visual aid to present data. First, the pie chart display should be limited to a small number of categories to promote readability. Each category, or pie slice, needs to be clearly labeled and colored to show contrast with other categories. A legend may be used in place of labels for individual slices, but the

---

[d] A histogram, in essence, is used to display the frequency distribution of a single interval or ratio variable. In this particular histogram (Figure 8-3B), the frequency distribution for the variable "Year" is displayed, but histograms may also be used to display frequency distributions for a variable whose values were observed at one point in time. For example, a histogram could be used to display the distribution of cholesterol levels from a sample of 300 individuals.

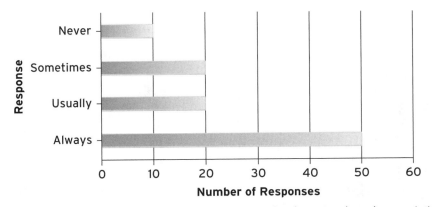

FIGURE 8-3A   How often does your pharmacist offer to provide information about the prescriptions you fill? (*N* = 100).

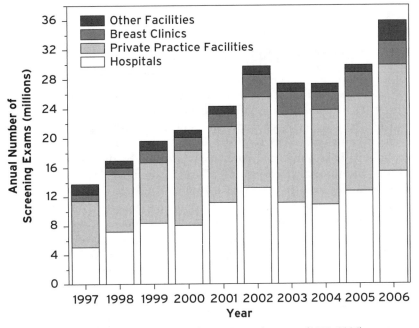

FIGURE 8-3B   Annual number of mammography screenings by venue (1997–2006).

presence of several small slices is a good indicator that a pie chart is not the best tool for presenting the data at hand. Also, it is important to consider that the data can be divided up proportionally in a logical way. **Figures 8-4A** and **8-4B** show pie charts that present the same data on blood type distribution in the United States. Which of these two charts is the more appropriate presentation, based upon the criteria described previously?

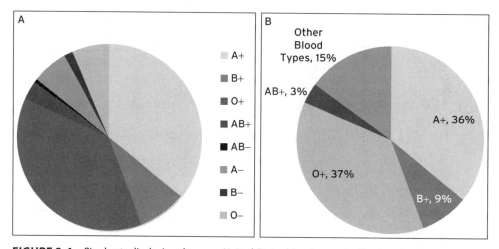

FIGURE 8-4   Pie charts displaying the same United States blood type distribution data (2012).

Source: Data from Stanford School of Medicine Blood Center: 2012. http://bloodcenter.stanford.edu/about_blood/blood_types.html.

COMMONLY ENCOUNTERED PROPORTIONS AND RATES

Characteristics measured on a nominal scale exist as counts or frequencies of occurrence. For such items, it is often useful to use proportions to describe a data set based on the number of times a specific characteristic is observed. A **proportion** is the number of observations with a given characteristic divided by the total number of observations in a given group. Thus, proportions are "parts" divided by the "whole." For example, the nominally measured characteristic "sex" can be used to calculate the proportion of females within a class of first-year pharmacy students, where the numerator (females) is a subset of the denominator (all students). Proportions are commonly reported as percentages, which is simply the proportion multiplied by 100%. **Rates** are similar to proportions with two added properties: they are computed over a specific time period (for example, per year) and they use a multiplier (for example, 1,000, 10,000, or 100,000). The multiplier is called the base. Examples of rates will be described in the next section.

MORTALITY AND MORBIDITY RATES

Both mortality and morbidity rates are used to describe the health status of populations. Death and disease rates are important both as a clinical concept and as a tool for conducting research. Assessing changes in disease rates over time is a vital component of evaluating the impact of interventions aimed at diseases, symptoms, or problems. The mortality rate is represented as:

$$\text{Mortality Rate} = \frac{\text{Number of individuals who died during a given period of time}}{\text{Number of individuals who were at risk of dying during the same time period}}$$

An overall mortality rate for the United States can be computed by examining the Centers for Disease Control and Prevention's National Center for Health Statistics Data. According to this data, there were 2,437,163 deaths in the United States in 2009.[6] A total U.S. population of 307,024,820 yields a mortality rate of 793.8 deaths per 100,000 population in the United States in 2009.

Morbidity measures, such as incidence and prevalence, can apply to diseases (e.g., diabetes), symptoms (e.g., lower back pain), or problems (e.g., adverse events due to a drug). These measures are commonly used in epidemiology as the basis for planning and evaluating health programs.[7] Both measures are used to convey the extent of disease, symptoms, or problems in a population. Intuitively, the concepts of incidence and prevalence are relatively straightforward; however, in practice, defining the incidence of a specific disease or the prevalence of a side effect can be challenging. A brief description of these measures is provided below.

INCIDENCE

Incidence is the term used to describe the risk of developing a new disease, symptom, or problem. The incidence proportion measures the number of new cases of a disease (or symptom or problem) that develop in a population at risk within a given period of time. Mathematically, this equates to:

$$\text{Incidence Proportion} = \frac{\text{Number of new cases of a disease}}{\text{Total number in the population at risk}}$$

Population at risk means all individuals in the population who do not have the disease at the beginning of the observation period, but were capable of developing the disease. For example, if the disease is prostate cancer, the denominator would only include men in the population who do not have prostate cancer but are capable of developing it during the observation period. In epidemiology, the incidence rate (also called incidence density) rather than the incidence proportion is often the preferred measure for describing new events, as it accounts for the total *time* that people are at risk of the disease and other important epidemiologic factors.

PREVALENCE

Prevalence measures the probability of having a disease at a point in time. Prevalence reflects existing disease in a population. Mathematically, prevalence is:

$$\text{Prevalence} = \frac{\text{Number of individuals who have the disease at a given point in time}}{\text{Number of individuals at risk for the disease in the population at the same point in time}}$$

Technically, the formula shown above provides what is called the point prevalence. The term "prevalence rate" is frequently encountered; however, prevalence is not a true rate because there is no unit of time in the denominator—prevalence is a proportion.

Prevalence typically represents the best estimate of the probability of the presence of disease before evaluating an individual's history, physical exam or lab tests.[8] To further clarify the presence of disease, clinicians employ diagnostic tests, which will be discussed in the following section.

DIAGNOSTIC TESTS

To have useful measures of incidence and prevalence, correct classification of individuals as either diseased or non-diseased is necessary. Diagnostic tests are tools that help clinicians determine whether individuals are apt to have a specific disease.

Unfortunately, diagnostic tests are not perfect and misclassification is unavoidable. Gold standard diagnostic tests (i.e., ones that provide a definitive diagnosis) are generally impractical either due to cost or complexity. Thus, there is a trade-off between identifying disease in individuals who really have the disease (true positives) and avoiding detection of disease in individuals who are actually disease-free (false positives).

PERFORMANCE MEASURES FOR DIAGNOSTIC TESTS

There are a number of summary measures (also called performance measures) for diagnostic tests. The commonly encountered performance measures are sensitivity, specificity, and predictive value. Performance measures provide a standard mechanism for quantifying the ability of a test to correctly classify individuals as either "diseased" or "not-diseased." They are important components for making clinical decisions as well as evaluating results of published studies. **Figure 8-5** presents a standard two-by-two table for evaluating diagnostic tests along with brief definitions for each of the concepts described in this section. Readers may find it helpful to refer back to Figure 8-5 as each new concept is introduced.

Sensitivity

Sensitivity is the ability of a diagnostic test to correctly identify individuals with disease. Mathematically, sensitivity is the proportion of individuals with the disease who are correctly identified by the test (Figure 8-5, I). Sensitivity is also called the **true positive rate**, indicating the probability that the diagnostic test is positive for a patient who truly has the disease. Tests with high sensitivity have low **false negative rates** (Figure 8-5, H). In other words, highly sensitive tests do not miss identifying many patients who actually do have the disease. Mathematically, sensitivity (true positive rate) and the false negative rate sum to one. Thus, if the sensitivity of a test increases, the false negative rate decreases.

Specificity

Specificity is the ability of a diagnostic test to correctly identify individuals without disease. Mathematically, specificity is represented as the proportion of individuals without the disease who are correctly identified by the test as disease-free (Figure 8-5, J). It is also called the **true negative rate**, indicating the probability that the diagnostic test is negative for a patient who does not have the disease. Tests with high specificity have low **false positive rates** (Figure 8-5, G). In other words, highly specific tests do not identify many patients as having a disease when they are actually disease-free. Mathematically, specificity (true negative rate) and the false positive rate sum to one. Thus, if the specificity of a test increases, the false positive rate decreases.

Predictive Value

Predictive values provide information about how likely it is that the individual does, or does not, have the disease given his/her test result. **Positive predictive value** is the probability that a patient has the disease given that a positive test result was obtained (Figure 8-5, K), and **negative predictive value** is the probability that a patient does not have the disease given that a negative test result was obtained (Figure 8-5, L). Predictive

	True Condition of Disease		
Diagnostic Test Result	**Disease Present (+)**	**Disease Absent (−)**	**Total**
Positive (+)	w	x	$w+x =$ All testing positive
Negative (−)	y	z	$y+z =$ All testing negative
Total	$w+y =$ All patients with the disease	$x+z =$ All patients who do not have the disease	$w+x+y+z = n$ (Total number of patients)

Notes:

A. w: Patients who have the disease and have positive test results; **true positives**.
B. x: Patients who do not have the disease but have positive test results; **false positives**.
C. z: Patients who do not have the disease and have negative test results; **true negatives**.
D. y: Patients who have the disease but have negative test results; **false negatives**.
E. **Prevalence** of the disease = Total number of patients with disease divided by the total; $\dfrac{(w+y)}{(n)}$.
F. **Accuracy** of the diagnostic test: Proportion of all tests that are correct classifications: $\dfrac{(w+z)}{(n)}$.
G. **False positive rate:** Number of false positives divided by all patients who do not have the disease; $\dfrac{(x)}{(x+z)}$.
H. **False negative rate:** Number of false negatives divided by all patients with the disease; $\dfrac{(y)}{(w+y)}$.
I. **Sensitivity:** Proportion of individuals with the disease who are correctly identified by the test; $\dfrac{(w)}{(w+y)}$. Also called the **true positive rate**.
J. **Specificity:** Proportion of individuals without the disease who are correctly identified by the test; $\dfrac{(z)}{(x+z)}$. Also called the **true negative rate**.
K. **Positive predictive value:** Proportion of positive tests that correctly identify diseased persons; in other words, the proportion of individuals with a positive test who have the disease; $\dfrac{(w)}{(w+x)}$.
L. **Negative predictive value:** Proportion of negative tests that correctly identify non-diseased persons; in other words, the proportion of individuals with a negative test who do not have the disease; $\dfrac{(z)}{(y+z)}$.

FIGURE 8-5   Summary of diagnostic test performance measures.

values are affected by the prevalence of the disease in the population of interest. When disease prevalence is high, the positive predictive value increases; when disease prevalence is low, the positive predictive value decreases. For negative predictive value, the converse is true. In practice, the combination of sensitivity, specificity, and prevalence will determine the practical utility of a diagnostic test. The relationship between these measures is further detailed in other resources.[9,10]

Utility of Performance Measures for Diagnostic Tests

Ideally, diagnostic tests would be 100% sensitive and 100% specific. This would mean that all patients with disease would be identified (100% true positive rate), no patients with disease would be missed (0% false negative rate), and patients without disease would never be misclassified as having disease (0% false positive rate). Unfortunately, such a scenario is typically impossible or impractical; sensitivity is gained at the expense of specificity and vice versa.[11] There is a trade-off between sensitivity and specificity.

In practice, tests used to diagnose disease commonly have a sensitivity of 80% and a specificity of 90%;[8] however, the risk associated with a test must be considered when selecting diagnostic tests. For example, some diagnostic tests require invasive procedures that may result in serious complications. Furthermore, the implications of false negative or false positive results may vary depending on the disease at hand.[11] Selecting the test with the greatest specificity is preferred when using diagnostic tests to rule in a disease, when screening for disease in low-risk populations, or when testing for diseases that have a poor prognosis with few, if any, beneficial treatment options.[8,12] Similarly, selecting the test with the greatest sensitivity is common when screening for disease in high-risk populations and for ruling out a disease.[8,12]

RECEIVER OPERATING CHARACTERISTIC (ROC) CURVES

Results of diagnostic tests are classified as either positive or negative. A threshold, or cut-off value, must be selected that discriminates between a test result that is classified as positive vs. negative. For example, any test result below some specified value is classified as negative, and any result that exceeds this value is classified as positive. How is this threshold selected? Does changing the threshold affect the sensitivity and specificity of the test? These are important questions that have meaningful implications for patient care.

Receiver operating characteristic (ROC) curves are used to illustrate the trade-offs between sensitivity (true positive rate) and the false positive rate (recall that the false positive rate equals 1 − specificity). Each point on the ROC curve represents the sensitivity and false positive rate at a different decision threshold.

In **Figure 8-6**, sensitivity (true positive rate) is plotted on the vertical axis and the false positive rate (1 − specificity) is plotted on the horizontal axis. The (0,0) coordinate represents 0% sensitivity and 0% false positive rate. This is the extreme decision threshold where all test results are negative for the disease. The other extreme decision threshold is found at the (1,1) coordinate, where both the sensitivity and false positive rate are 100%—meaning that all test results are positive for the disease. The diagonal line connecting these two extremes represents the ROC curve of a hypothetical diagnostic test that has no ability to discriminate between patients with disease vs. those without disease. It is aptly named the "chance diagonal."[13] Any ROC curve that lies above this chance diagonal has some diagnostic ability.[13,14] Both ROC-1 and ROC-2 in Figure 8-6 represent tests that have useful diagnostic capabilities.

The area under the ROC curve allows for comparisons of different diagnostic tests. The area under the chance diagonal ROC curve is 0.5; the area under the ROC curve for a perfect diagnostic test is equal to 1. Thus, diagnostic tests that result in ROC curves with areas under the curve that are close to 1 indicate better tests.[13,14] Looking again at Figure 8-6, if the diagnostic tests generating ROC-1 and ROC-2 are both used for the same purpose, the test corresponding to ROC-1 would be preferred, as the area under the ROC-1 curve exceeds the area under the ROC-2 curve. The farther the curve is from the chance diagonal, the greater the discriminating power of the test.[13,14]

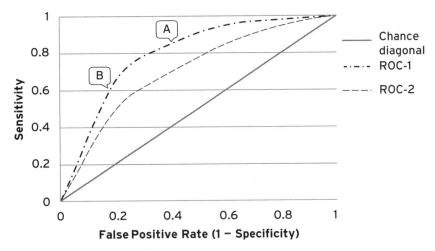

FIGURE 8-6 Receiver operating characteristic (ROC) curves.

The cutoff point between positive and negative test results can be selected based on the willingness to make trade-offs between sensitivity and the false positive rate. For example, at point A in Figure 8-6, a larger proportion of truly diseased patients will be detected (i.e., high sensitivity), but there will also be a larger number of false positives. At point B, the number of false positives is lower, but there is also less ability to detect patients who truly have the disease (i.e., lower sensitivity). So while ROC curves provide useful information, they do not circumvent the tradeoff that must be made between false negative and false positive test results and the resulting implications of such errors.

SUMMARY OF DIAGNOSTIC TESTS

This section has briefly introduced a few of the more common measures that can be used to summarize diagnostic accuracy. An important principle that must be kept in mind when applying the concepts of sensitivity and specificity is that the number of false positive and false negative results depends on the probability of the disease in the population of interest (i.e., the prevalence); thus, these measures cannot be viewed as fixed indicators. The definition of disease, disease prevalence, and the spectrum of disease in the population of interest impact diagnostic test results.[14]

SUMMARY AND CONCLUSIONS

Descriptive statistics are used in the summarizing, organizing, and presenting functions of statistics. Variables can be qualitative or quantitative, and quantitative variables can be measured on different levels (nominal, ordinal, interval, or ratio). Standard summary measures allow researchers to distill large and complicated collections of information into concise, effective, and meaningful descriptions of the data. Several formats are available for visualizing and presenting data. Proportions and rates are effective in providing morbidity and mortality information. Performance measures for diagnostic tests, including sensitivity, specificity, and predictive value, provide a standard mechanism for quantifying the ability of a diagnostic test to correctly classify individuals.

All of these measures provide the researcher with the tools to organize and describe data, a necessary step in the research process that precedes testing hypotheses and drawing conclusions. Subsequent chapters in this text will explore inferential statistics, which include the analytic and interpretation functions of statistics that are used to answer research questions.

REVIEW QUESTIONS

1. Identify and describe the two general functions of statistics.
2. For this question, use the human body measurements page available at http://www.wolframalpha.com/examples/HumanBodyMeasurements.html. If our patient is a 5'10" male weighing 200 pounds, is the patient's weight above or below the mean body weight for males?
3. You are the principal investigator for a small pilot study that is testing the impact of a medication therapy management program for patients with hypertension. Your patients have the following blood pressure measurements (systolic/diastolic) at the onset of the program: Male 125/80; Female 135/90; Female 135/100; Male 155/105; Female 165/95; Male 165/115; Female 150/100; Female 145/95; Male 195/130.
    a) Summarize these data visually. Organize and present them as a graph, chart, or table.
    b) Calculate the mean and median systolic and diastolic blood pressures for all patients. How do the mean and median measures of systolic pressure compare to one another? How do the mean and median measures of diastolic pressure compare to one another? Which of these measures would be best to represent the data?
4. You are reading about a new medication that treats pain, and one of the suspected side effects is nausea. Suppose you have been chosen to design a study to test the impact of the new drug on patients experiencing nausea.
    a) What is the dependent variable, and what is the independent variable for this study?
    b) You have decided to measure nausea by asking patients to rate their nausea on a scale from 1 to 10. What level of measurement is this?
5. You have been asked to present your manager with information about your pharmacy's dispensing of medications used to treat high cholesterol. You know that eight generic and name brand alternatives are stocked at your pharmacy and that two of these medications are rarely, if ever, dispensed.
    a) What level of measurement is being reported when you are asked to list each cholesterol medication kept in stock?
    b) Suppose that your manager has asked to see a histogram that shows how much of each cholesterol medication was dispensed this year. Explain why a histogram is not the best way to represent these data. What type of chart or graph would you propose as an alternative?
    c) If you were reporting the "average" total number of cholesterol medications dispensed per month, would you choose to calculate the mean, median, or mode to best represent these data? Why did you choose that measure?
6. What is the difference between incidence and prevalence?

Use the following scenario for questions 7 and 8.

A research study evaluated the use of computed tomography (CT) in the diagnosis of hamstring injuries. Sixty patients with hamstring injuries confirmed by magnetic resonance imaging (MRI) were evaluated with CT. Forty patients without injuries were also included. The CT results were positive in 40 of the patients with hamstring injuries and in 10 of the patients without hamstring injuries.

7. What is the false positive rate? You may find that constructing a 2 × 2 table similar to what is found in Figure 8-5 helpful.
8. What is the sensitivity of CT for hamstring injury in this study? You may find that constructing a 2 × 2 table similar to what is found in Figure 8-5 helpful.
9. Refer to Figure 8-6. What is the true positive rate at the point labeled "B" on ROC-1?

ONLINE RESOURCES

Diagnostic Test Performance Calculator: http://ilm.medicine.arizona.edu/EBDM/DTPC/calculator.html (Contains a calculator that will compute positive predictive value, negative predictive value, sensitivity, and specificity. Also includes a list of equations commonly employed when evaluating the performance of diagnostic tests.)

EasyCalculation.com: http://easycalculation.com/statistics/statistics.php (Includes step-by-step tutorials for statistical tests and a "calculator" that allows you to input variable values to calculate each of the descriptive statistics discussed in this chapter.)

GCFLearnFree.org: http://www.gcflearnfree.org/excel2010/17.2 (Includes tutorials on how to build charts, tables, and graphs using Microsoft Excel or Google Documents.)

VassarStats Website for Statistical Computation: http://vassarstats.net/ (A useful and user-friendly tool for performing various statistical computations.)

REFERENCES

1. Davidian M, Louis TA. Why statistics? *Science*. 2012;336:10. doi:1126/science.1218685. www.sciencemag.org. Accessed September 27, 2012.
2. Dodge Y. *The Oxford Dictionary of Statistical Terms*. 6th ed. New York, NY: Oxford University Press; 2006.
3. Miles MB, Huberman AM. *Qualitative Data Analysis: An Expanded Sourcebook*. 2nd ed. Thousand Oaks, CA: SAGE Publications; 1994.
4. Rosner B. *Fundamentals of Biostatistics*. 2nd ed. Boston, MA: PWS Publishers; 1986.
5. Kumar CR. *Research Methodology*. New Delhi, India: APH Publishing; 2008.
6. National Vital Statistics System Mortality Data. http://www.cdc.gov/nchs/deaths.htm. Accessed September 23, 2012.
7. Dawson-Saunders B, Trapp RG. *Basic and Clinical Biostatistics*. 2nd ed. Norwalk, CT: Appleton & Lange; 1994.
8. Riegelman RK, Hirsch RP. *Studying a Study and Testing a Test: How to Read the Health Science Literature*. 3rd ed. Boston, MA: Little, Brown; 1996.
9. Wassertheil-Smoller S. *Biostatistics and Epidemiology: A Primer for Health Professionals*. 2nd ed. New York, NY: Springer-Verlag; 1995.
10. The VassarStats Website for Statistical Computation. http://vassarstats.net. Accessed October 4, 2012.
11. Petrie A, Sabin C. *Medical Statistics at a Glance*. Oxford, England: Blackwell Science; 2000.
12. McGee DL. Clinical decision making. In: *The Merck Manual for Health Care Professionals*. http://www.merckmanuals.com/professional/special_subjects/clinical_decision_making/testing.html. Accessed October 4, 2012.
13. Zweig M, Campbell G. Receiver operating characteristic (ROC) plots: a fundamental evaluation tool in clinical medicine. *Clin Chem*. 1993;39:561–577.
14. Okeh UM, Okoro CN. Evaluating measures of indicators of diagnostic test performance: fundamental meanings and formulars. *J Biomet Biostat*. 2012;3:132. doi:10.4172/2155-6180.1000132.

INTERPRETATION AND BASIC STATISTICAL CONCEPTS

Spencer E. Harpe, PharmD, PhD, MPH

CHAPTER OBJECTIVES

▸ Define and differentiate point estimation and interval estimation
▸ Describe important statistical distributions
▸ Explain the role of the central limit theorem in statistical analysis
▸ Explain the basic mechanics of hypothesis testing
▸ Explain how confidence intervals can be used to test hypotheses
▸ Differentiate among various types of hypothesis tests
▸ Define and differentiate statistical significance and clinical significance

KEY TERMINOLOGY

Alternate hypothesis
Central limit theorem
Clinical significance
Confidence intervals
Directional tests
Empirical distribution
Hypotheses
Hypothesis testing
Non-directional tests
Normal distribution

Null hypothesis
Parameters
Point estimate
Population
Power
p-value
Sample
Statistic
Statistical distribution
Statistical estimation

Statistical inference
Statistical significance
Test of difference
Test of equivalence
Test of non-inferiority
Test of superiority
Type I error, or α error
Type II error, or β error

INTRODUCTION

Descriptive statistics provide a useful tool for presenting basic information, such as the central tendency (mean, median, or mode) and spread (standard deviation or interquartile range), of a given sample. While these are useful, the focus is often on taking the findings from a sample used for research and applying them to a target population of interest. For example, in a sample of 200 individuals, half of which received a new medication to reduce LDL cholesterol and the other half received a placebo, the new medication reduced LDL cholesterol by 30 mg/dL. Initially, this finding may seem exciting, but subsequent steps would determine whether the observed reduction was indeed statistically significant (i.e., hypothesis testing) and provide an idea of how large the actual reduction might be in the target population of individuals with high LDL cholesterol (i.e., statistical estimation). Inferential statistics provide the tools to answer these questions.

This chapter begins with a brief discussion of statistical distributions and statistical theory supporting statistical inference. Information about basic principles of point and interval estimation is then presented. The chapter finishes with a discussion of hypothesis testing, which forms the basis for the majority of statistical inference as seen in the biomedical literature.

STATISTICAL DISTRIBUTIONS AND THE CENTRAL LIMIT THEOREM

A variable's distribution is made up of all the possible values and their relative frequency of occurrence. When the values are taken from actual data and the relative frequencies of occurrence are calculated (e.g., the observed lengths of stay for patients in a hospital), this observed distribution is referred to as an **empirical distribution**. A **statistical distribution** is a type of distribution that is defined by some theoretical probability distribution.[1] These statistical distributions are important because they describe the way in which random variables are expected to behave.[2] They also form the basis for statistical testing. While there are many theoretical probability distributions, a few are used commonly in biomedical research.

NORMAL DISTRIBUTION

A **normal distribution** in statistics is what many refer to as a "bell curve" and has some desirable statistical properties. The distribution is symmetrical around the mean. All measures of central tendency are equal (i.e., mean = median = mode). Generally speaking, a normal distribution is any such distribution with a known mean (μ) and standard deviation (σ). Normally distributed variables must be measured at the continuous level (e.g., interval or ratio). From a practical standpoint, two specific distributions can be used when discussing the normal distribution: the z-distribution and the t-distribution.

z-Distribution

The z-distribution is a special type of normal distribution where the data have been transformed to follow the standard normal distribution with a mean of 0 and a standard deviation of 1. While very few, if any, variables actually follow this distribution, it is often approximated by standardizing the data using the following equation:

$$z = \frac{x_i - \bar{x}}{\text{SD}}$$

(1)

This z-score is obtained by dividing the difference between the observed value (x_i) and the mean value ($\bar{x}$) by the standard deviation (SD) of the variable.[a] From a practical standpoint, this translates to the deviation of an observation from the sample mean to the number of "standard units" (or standard deviations) from 0. This translation is useful because it allows probabilities to be attached to the observed values or ranges of values. From the normal distribution, approximately 68% of the values fall within 1 standard deviation above or below the mean (±1 SD), approximately 95% fall within 2 standard deviations (±2 SD), and approximately 99.7% fall within 3 standard deviations (±3 SD). These values become useful in statistical testing.

t-Distribution

The t-distribution, or Student's t-distribution, can be thought of as a modification to the standard normal distribution (or z-distribution) when the sample size is relatively small. From a comparison standpoint, the t-distribution will be very close to the z-distribution as the sample size increases. The t-distribution will become flatter with thicker tails compared to the standard normal curve as the sample size decreases. The amount of difference between the t-distribution and the z-distribution depends on the degrees of freedom[b] available, which is directly related to the sample size. **Figure 9-1** shows the relationship between a standard normal curve (z-distribution)

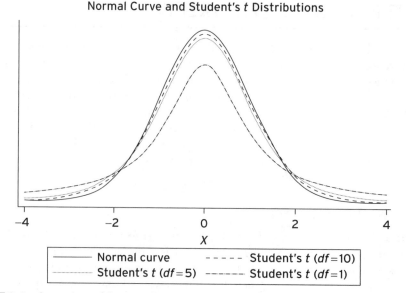

Normal Curve and Student's *t* Distributions

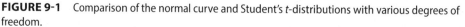

FIGURE 9-1 Comparison of the normal curve and Student's *t*-distributions with various degrees of freedom.

---

[a] Technically, the z-score is calculated by dividing the difference between the sample mean and the hypothesized population mean by the standard error of the mean. This is the approach used in the z-test. More generally, this calculation is used to create scores in terms of standard units and allows the comparison of different measures when the scale of measurement is considerably different.

[b] The degrees of freedom are the number of data points, or observations, that are free to vary when calculating a statistic. Generally speaking, one degree of freedom is lost for each parameter estimated. This is why the equation for calculating the sample standard deviation has $n - 1$ rather than n (the sample size) in the denominator. By calculating the mean, there is one less data point that is free to vary when calculating the standard deviation.

and *t*-distributions for varying degrees of freedom. The *t*-distribution, and the *t*-test based on this distribution, would be used whenever the actual population standard deviation is not known or when a good estimate is not available. In practice, the *t*-test is used more frequently than the *z*-test because the population standard deviation is rarely known.

BINOMIAL DISTRIBUTION

The *z*- and *t*-distributions are useful for continuous variables but do not allow for categorical measurements. The binomial distribution describes a random variable with two possible outcomes, which represents the simplest version of a categorical outcome (e.g., alive vs. dead, treatment success vs. treatment failure, etc.). The binomial distribution describes outcomes in terms of *p* (the probability of success or an outcome of interest) and *q* (the probability of failure or the probability of the outcome of interest not occurring). Using the math of probability, the sum of the probabilities of an event happening (*p*) and the event not happening (*q*) is equal to 1, or $p + q = 1$. For a binary variable, the sampling distribution can be described in terms of the probability of the number of "successes" (or outcomes of interest) for a certain number of trials. Consider flipping a coin. A sampling distribution of possible outcomes could be created for flipping the coin 10 times. The possible outcomes of flipping the coin could be no heads out of 10 flips, 1 head, 2 heads, and so on all the way up to obtaining 10 heads from 10 flips. The probability of obtaining a head on any given coin flip is 0.5 (or 50%). Along the same lines, the approximate number of heads obtained would be about 50% (or one-half) of the number of flips (or trials), which would be 5 out of 10 flips, assuming the coin were "fair." More extreme outcome patterns like flipping 10 heads or 0 heads would be statistically unlikely.

In biomedical research, a "trial" in this situation is not the overall study but the individual patient. If a new medication has an estimated 50% success rate of stopping the growth of a tumor and that drug is given to 50 patients, then there are 50 "trials." In each patient (or trial), there is a 50% chance of success (i.e., stopping tumor growth). The sampling distribution of the outcomes ranges from no successes out of 50 patients to all 50 patients experiencing no tumor growth.

OTHER DISTRIBUTIONS

In addition to the normal distribution and the binomial distribution, there are many other distributions that are used in statistical analyses. Some of these form the basis for specific statistical tests. For example, the chi-square (χ^2) distribution is the basis for the test of the same name, several nonparametric tests, and certain regression analyses, and the *F* distribution is used when conducting analysis of variance (ANOVA) and linear regression analysis. The Poisson distribution is similar to the binomial distribution in that it relates to categorical outcomes. The Poisson distribution is especially useful to describe events when they are relatively rare, such as the number of medication errors per 1,000 patient-days. Holland et al. used Poisson regression when examining the effectiveness of community pharmacist educational visits at reducing hospital readmissions.[3] Another potentially useful distribution is the gamma distribution. Similar to the normal distributions, the gamma distribution is used when the variable of interest is interval or ratio but is very highly skewed. This is often the case when looking at resource utilization or costs, as examined by Wu et al. in a sample of adults with attention-deficit/hyperactivity disorder treated with alternative therapies.[4]

CENTRAL LIMIT THEOREM

Before beginning the discussion of statistical inference, a brief overview of the **central limit theorem** (CLT) is beneficial. This theorem is a fundamental concept providing underlying support for much of the statistical testing seen in the biomedical literature. In statistical theory, a sample is a subset or portion of the population (all observations of interest), and sample size is the number of sampled observations. According to the CLT:

1. The mean of all sample means will equal the population mean.
2. The standard deviation of the sampled means is equal to the standard error of the mean.
3. As the sample size increases, the distribution of the sample means will approach a normal distribution regardless of the underlying distribution of the variable.

Consider trying to determine whether patients spending 24 hours or more in a critical care unit are older than those who spend less than 24 hours in a critical care unit. The CLT suggests that the distribution of the sample mean age difference between the two groups of patients would be normally distributed as long as there is a sufficiently large sample size, regardless of whether the difference in age is actually normally distributed in these patients. One generally accepted rule of thumb is a sample size of at least 30 is sufficiently large as long as there are only moderate departures from the normal distribution. For more severe departures from normality, larger sample sizes become necessary. From a sampling standpoint, samples of various sizes could be obtained: 10 patients (5 in each group), 20 patients (10 in each group), or 500 patients (250 in each group). According to the CLT, the distribution of the sample mean age, or the mean difference in age, to be precise, would approach a normal distribution as the sample size increases.

At a deeper level, the CLT relates to the idea of conducting the same study with different samples. In the critical care unit example, the study could be performed 10 times with different samples of patients from the hospital. From each of these 10 samples, the mean difference in age between the two groups would be calculated. The first tenet of the CLT states that the mean of these differences in mean ages would be equal to, or very close to, the true mean age difference in the underlying population. The second tenet says that the standard deviation of these 10 means (i.e., the standard error of the mean) is equal to, or very close to, the standard deviation of the mean age difference in underlying population. How "close" any given estimate is to the true population parameter depends in part on the number of replicated studies. The estimates may not be very close after repeating the study 10 times. On the other hand, after repeating the study 100 times, or 5,000 times, the differences between the estimates and the true population parameter would become increasingly smaller.

It is important to understand that "sample size" is relevant from two perspectives: the number of subjects in a given study and the number of times a study is repeated. From the first perspective, the distribution of the sampled means will approach a normal distribution as the sample size increases. This is what most people think of when they discuss sample size and the CLT. From the second perspective, the accuracy of the estimates will improve as the number of samples increases. Even though selecting numerous samples is rarely done in practice, this concept relates directly to the idea that the study findings will be correct "in the long run" as discussed later with respect to the interpretation of confidence intervals and errors in hypothesis testing.[c]

---

[c] The idea of being correct "in the long run" is a core principle of the frequentist approach to statistics. This is the approach taken in most statistical analyses used in biomedical research and is characterized by testing a null hypothesis assuming a certain amount of error is acceptable in the long run. The other approach to statistics is called the Bayesian approach.

STATISTICAL INFERENCE

DEFINITION OF STATISTICAL INFERENCE

Because the motivation behind estimation lies to some degree in statistical inference, it may be helpful to define statistical inference in a formal sense before moving into a discussion of estimation. **Statistical inference** is the process of analyzing data from a sample and using those results to infer the related values in the source or target population. The primary characteristic allowing for valid statistical inference is the use of a random sample. Strictly speaking, it is not possible to arrive at valid inferences from a non-random sample; however, non-random samples are used as the basis for inferential statistics in many studies. Researchers frequently use inferential statistics to estimate the "true" effect of an intervention in the larger population through the use of randomized controlled trials, where participation is voluntary and, therefore, a non–random sample. This is not to say that statistically valid inference does not happen in biomedical research. There are various data sets that are collected on random samples of individuals. Many of these data sets, such as the National Ambulatory Medical Care Survey and the Medical Expenditure Panel Survey, are collected and maintained by government agencies (e.g., the National Center for Health Statistics or the Agency for Healthcare Research and Quality) and serve as the basis for a variety of active research endeavors.[5] The growth of electronic medical records can allow for random sampling and valid inference provided the target population of interest is the local institution, which is often the case for quality improvement and program evaluation studies.[6]

POPULATIONS AND SAMPLES

Central to the idea of statistical inference are the concepts of sample and population. The terms are fairly straightforward in that the **population** is the general group of interest in a study while a **sample** is a portion of the population that is selected in order to study some phenomenon in a more efficient manner. Information for these two groups is presented in very specific ways in statistical practice. Quantities related to the population of interest are referred to as **parameters** and are usually represented by Greek letters, while the same quantity from a sample is referred to as a **statistic** and is represented by Latin letters. For example, a mean and standard deviation can be calculated for both a population and a sample. The mean from the population is called a parameter and is represented by μ (the lowercase Greek letter mu). The same measure from a sample is called a statistic and is represented by $\bar{x}$. For the standard deviation, the population parameter is represented by σ (the lowercase Greek letter sigma) and the sample statistic is represented by s or SD. **Table 9-1** shows a comparison of common statistical quantities and their representations for samples and populations.

TABLE 9-1 Statistical Quantities for Samples and Populations		
Quantity	**Sample Statistic**	**Population Parameter**
Mean	$\bar{x}$	μ
Standard Deviation	s or SD	σ
Proportion	p	π
Difference between Two Means	$\bar{x}_1 - \bar{x}_2$	$\mu_1 - \mu_2$
Difference between Two Proportions	$p_1 - p_2$	$\pi_1 - \pi_2$

MECHANISMS OF INFERENCE

Statistical inference can be viewed as happening through two related mechanisms: estimation and hypothesis testing.[7] **Statistical estimation** is a process by which estimates of the population parameters are generated from sample statistics with a focus on generating precise estimates with minimal bias. The second mechanism is through hypothesis testing, where the focus is on making a conclusion about a hypothesized difference or relationship using observations from the sample.

STATISTICAL ESTIMATION

The first approach to statistical inference is the estimation approach whereby a sample statistic is estimated directly using the data obtained from the sample. Calculating the mean, median, and standard deviation are basic examples of estimation. Functions to estimate statistical parameters should be unbiased (i.e., have no systematic error), have minimum variance (i.e., be efficient), be consistent (i.e., theoretically converge at the true population parameter as the sample size increases), and be robust to violations of assumptions.[1,8–9] For example, both the mean and the median are estimates of central tendency. Both should be unbiased estimates of central tendency, but the mean is more efficient than the median because the standard error of the median is considerably larger than that of the mean. On the other hand, the median is a more robust estimate than the mean because a single outlier can drastically affect the mean with little effect, if any, on the median.[1] For more complicated quantities related to relationships between variables or estimating adjusted means and variances, there are often multiple options for estimation functions, so considerable thought must be given to selecting the estimator with the best properties.

POINT ESTIMATION

In point estimation, one single value (i.e., the **point estimate**) is estimated for the statistical quantity of interest. The quantity may be any measure of central tendency or spread, or it could be a measure of association, such as a correlation or regression coefficient. Two examples of point estimates, the arithmetic mean and the proportion, are described further in Chapter 8, "Measurement and Descriptive Analysis." These two measures will be used to illustrate the principals of interval estimation.

INTERVAL ESTIMATION

Point estimates can provide useful information about population parameters, but they provide no information about the precision of the estimate. In order to understand the precision of an estimate, an interval associated with a certain level of acceptable error can be constructed. These intervals are referred to as **confidence intervals**. The general equation for calculating a confidence interval (CI) involves adding and subtracting the product of the error of the estimate and the critical value from the point estimate:

$$\text{Point Estimate} \pm (\text{Critical Value})(\text{Standard Error of the Estimate}) \quad (2)$$

The critical value is selected based on the desired level of confidence. More confidence requires a larger critical value and results in a wider interval. For example, a 99% CI will be wider than a 95% CI for the same point estimate. The standard error of the estimate represents the sampling error associated with a particular estimate. The more error associated with the estimate, the wider the confidence interval will be as long as the confidence level stays constant. Because the standard error is related to the sample size (see equations (3) and (4)), increasing the sample size will decrease error and subsequently reduce the width of the interval. It is important to note that changing the point estimate alone does nothing to the *width* of the interval.

Confidence Interval for a Mean

In order to calculate a CI, the standard error is needed. This is easily calculated from basic descriptive statistics. The standard error of the mean (SE_{Mean}) is obtained by dividing the standard deviation by the square root of the sample size:

$$SE_{Mean} = \frac{SD}{\sqrt{n}} \tag{3}$$

This standard error is then multiplied by the appropriate critical value. Using the two-tailed values from **Table 9–2**, the standard error would be multiplied by 1.96 for a 95% CI. That product would then be added and subtracted from the point estimate to obtain the upper and lower bounds of the CI.[d] **Table 9–3** provides a calculation example.

TABLE 9-2	Approximate Critical Values for Calculating Confidence Intervals and Conducting Hypothesis Tests Using the Standard Normal (z) Distribution	
α **Level**	**One-Tailed Value (upper tail)**	**Two-Tailed Value**
0.10	1.28	1.65
0.05	1.65	1.96
0.01	2.33	2.58

TABLE 9-3	Confidence Interval Calculation
Confidence interval for a mean	**Confidence interval for a proportion**
What is the 95% confidence interval for the mean age of the population given the following sample statistics? Mean: 64.5 years Standard deviation: 10.2 years Sample size: 100 $SE_{Mean} = \frac{SD}{\sqrt{n}} = \frac{10.2}{\sqrt{100}} = \frac{10.2}{10} = 1.02$ Critical value: 1.96 Upper bound: $64.5 + (1.96)(1.02) = 66.5$ Lower bound: $64.5 - (1.96)(1.02) = 62.5$ 95% CI: 62.5 – 66.5	What is the 99% confidence interval for the proportion of adults taking at least one medication given the following sample statistics? Sample proportion: 75% Sample size: 400 $SE_{Prop} = \sqrt{\frac{pq}{n}} = \sqrt{\frac{(0.75)(0.25)}{400}} = 0.022$ Critical value: 2.58 Upper bound: $0.75 + (2.58)(0.022) = 0.807$ Lower bound: $0.75 - (2.58)(0.022) = 0.693$ 99% CI: 69.3% – 80.7%

---

[d] From a technical standpoint, most statistical software packages use the critical values drawn from the *t*-distribution because the standard deviation being used comes from the actual sample rather than from the known population value.

Confidence Interval for a Proportion

Calculating the confidence interval for a proportion is similar to the procedure for a mean. When working with proportions, standard deviations are not provided; however, the variance is calculated as pq, which is simply $p(1 - p)$. The standard error for a proportion (SE_{Prop}) is:

$$SE_{Prop} = \sqrt{\frac{p(1-p)}{n}} = \sqrt{\frac{pq}{n}} \tag{4}$$

Other than that, the steps are the same. Before performing calculations, it is helpful to convert all percentages to proportions before performing the calculations. When finished, they can be converted back to percentages. An example of the calculation is provided in Table 9-3.

Other Types of Confidence Intervals

It is not uncommon to see confidence intervals for many other quantities, such as the difference between two means, the difference between two proportions, odds ratios, or regression coefficients. These intervals are useful complements to traditional hypothesis testing discussed later in this chapter. As with any other confidence interval, they provide a useful way to understand the relative precision of the estimate.

INTERPRETATION AND IMPORTANCE OF THE CONFIDENCE INTERVAL

There are two ways in which CIs may be interpreted. The first way relates to a probabilistic interpretation. In Table 9-3, the 95% CI for age was 62.5 to 66.5 years. The interpretation would be that with 95% confidence, the interval contains the true population mean age (i.e., the parameter). The idea of attaching a probability statement to whether an interval contains the parameter can be related to the earlier discussion of repeating a study on different, repeated samples. In this repeated sampling context, similarly constructed intervals would contain the population parameter at least 95 times if the same study were repeated 100 times using different samples from the same population. Notice how this interpretation has the same motivation of being correct "in the long run."

The second interpretation approach is to say that the estimate of the parameter could be as high as the upper bound or as low as the lower bound (with a certain level of confidence). This interpretation is useful as it emphasizes the range of plausible values that CIs provide. As with the first interpretation, the uncertainty should be placed on the *estimate* of the parameter, not the population parameter itself. Using the age example again, some may say that the estimate of the mean population age was 64.5 years, but that they are 95% confident that true mean age could be as high as 66.5 or as low as 62.5 years. This shifts the uncertainty from the estimate to the parameter, so it is not technically correct; however, it may provide a more straightforward interpretation of the interval.

CIs are a very important part of statistical inference. They provide information about the precision of estimates, which is not provided by an examination of the p-value from a hypothesis test. When looking at estimates of the same quantity (e.g., both estimates of the effect of a drug at lowering LDL cholesterol) and using the same confidence level, narrower intervals indicate more precise estimates. CIs are also important in that they can be used as a method to conduct hypothesis testing while still providing the extra information that a p-value cannot.

HYPOTHESIS TESTING

While estimation provides a form of direct statistical inference, **hypothesis testing** approaches statistical inference in an indirect manner.[8] Hypothesis testing helps guide decisions based on data collected from a study.[7] This second approach to statistical inference, more formally null hypothesis significance testing (NHST), is an older approach than the use of confidence intervals or estimation.

CHARACTERISTICS OF HYPOTHESES

Hypotheses used in statistical testing have several characteristics. A good hypothesis must be a declarative sentence. While the initial idea for a study may be framed as a question, that question must be turned into a statement for hypothesis testing. Second, a hypothesis must describe a relationship between two or more variables. Simply stating that older adults have high blood pressure would not be a good hypothesis. On the other hand, stating that older adults have higher blood pressure than younger adults would be a better hypothesis as it explicitly states a relationship between two variables (age and blood pressure). The final characteristic is that the hypothesis must be testable by empirical means.[10]

TYPES OF HYPOTHESES

In order to test hypotheses to support statistical inference, two types of hypotheses were proposed by Neyman and Pearson: the **null hypothesis** (denoted H_0) and the **alternate hypothesis** (denoted H_A).[11] With a few exceptions noted later, the null hypothesis is generally formulated as stating that there is no relationship or no difference between the variables of interest (e.g., the drug has no effect on the outcome). The alternate hypothesis is usually stated as the opposite of the null hypothesis (e.g., the drug has an effect on the outcome). The NHST process sometimes starts by converting the research question or objective into an alternate hypothesis and then formulating the null, or vice versa. The most important thing to remember, however, is that in hypothesis testing, only the null hypothesis is tested. Based on the principles of NHST, conclusions are only made with respect to the null hypothesis. Furthermore, it is only possible to reject or fail to reject the null hypothesis.[c]

ERRORS IN HYPOTHESIS TESTING

According to Neyman and Pearson, the process of hypothesis testing was prone to two types of errors.[11–12] The errors were originally conceptualized as the probability of committing one of the errors upon repeating the experiment numerous times (i.e., in the long run). Unfortunately, one may never know when these errors are committed because it is rarely, if ever, known whether the null hypothesis is indeed true or false. It is still important to understand their theoretical meaning. **Table 9–4** shows the types of errors in relation to the true state of affairs (i.e., if the null hypothesis is true or false). Both of these errors represent quantities that the researcher sets acceptable levels for when designing the study *before* data are analyzed.

---

[c] Some say that the possible conclusions are to reject or accept the null hypothesis. The idea of "accepting" the null has its philosophical detractors. The important point is that the conclusion is about the null hypothesis, not the alternate hypothesis.

TABLE 9-4 Errors in Hypothesis Testing

		True State of Affairs	
		H_0 is true	H_0 is false
Conclusion from Hypothesis Test	Reject H_0	Type I (α) error	Correct conclusion
	Fail to reject H_0	Correct conclusion	Type II (β) error

Type I Error

The **type I error**, or **α error**, is defined as rejecting the null hypothesis when the null hypothesis is true. This can be thought of as an error of "anxiety" because the conclusion is that there is a difference (or there is something "going on" in the data) when the truth is that there is no difference (i.e., the null hypothesis is true). Consider a study examining the effectiveness of a medication to reduce LDL cholesterol. If the medication is known not to be effective but a study concluded that the medication did reduce LDL cholesterol, a type I error would have been committed as shown in **Table 9-5**. Researchers select an acceptable type I error rate before conducting the study. If the α level is not provided up front, it is impossible to conduct a hypothesis test because the cut-point for rejection of the null hypothesis is not stated. Traditionally, this is set at 5% and may be stated as $\alpha = 0.05$. Other common type I error rates include 1% and 10%.

The acceptable type I error rate is also referred to as the significance level. Authors will sometimes state the acceptable type I error level (or α level) in terms of a p-value, such as "$p \leq 0.05$ was considered statistically significant." This can lead to confusing the true meaning of the p-value with the type I error rate. The **p-value** is the probability of finding the results of the study, assuming the null hypothesis is true.[f] Other common misinterpretations of the p-value include the probability of committing a type I error, the probability that the null hypothesis (H_0) is true, and the probability that the alternate hypothesis (H_A) is true. One useful note about the type I error is its relationship with the confidence level. The level of confidence for a given study is generally related to the type I error rate such that the confidence level is one minus the type I error rate, or $1 - \alpha$. Thus, a type I error rate of 0.05 (or 5%) leads to a 95% confidence level.

Type II Error

The **type II error, or β error**, is defined as failing to reject the null hypothesis when the null hypothesis is false. Some view this as an error of "denial" because they are failing to conclude that there is a difference when, in fact, there is a difference. Using the

TABLE 9-5 Examples of Errors in Hypothesis Testing

		True Efficacy of the Drug	
		Drug does not reduce LDL	Drug reduces LDL
Results of the Study	Conclude the drug reduced LDL	Incorrect conclusion (Type I error)	Correct conclusion
	Conclude the drug did not reduce LDL	Correct conclusion	Incorrect conclusion (Type II error)

---

[f] The complete definition of a p-value is the probability of finding a test statistic as extreme as or more extreme than the observed, or calculated, test statistic given that the null hypothesis is true.

same example of the medication to reduce LDL, a type II error would be committed if the study results suggested that the new medication did not reduce LDL when the medication is known to be effective in reducing LDL (Table 9-5). Statistical **power** is a concept closely related to the type II error rate. Power is the probability of rejecting the null hypothesis given that the null hypothesis is actually false (i.e., finding a difference that actually exists and making a correct conclusion). This value is useful from a research standpoint because it tells us the likelihood of being correct, in the long run, in identifying an effect that actually exists. Typical values for the type II error rate are 20% and 10%, which translate to power levels of 80% and 90%, respectively.

TYPES OF HYPOTHESIS TESTS

When conducting a hypothesis test, the specific type of test being performed must first be determined. The tests can be classified based on whether a direction is being specified in the test. In this situation, the "direction" of a test is defined as whether or not the hypothesis specifies that the difference (or association) will be in a particular direction (e.g., Treatment A is better than Treatment B). Generally speaking, **non-directional tests** (two-sided or two-tailed) are more conservative than **directional tests** (one-sided or one-tailed) because they make it more difficult to reach statistical significance. In a similar fashion, non-directional tests provide more flexibility by allowing researchers to examine differences (or associations) in either a positive or a negative direction rather than locking the analysis into only one direction.

Selecting a directional versus a non-directional test can be likened to crossing the street. If one is unsure of whether traffic on the street is one-way or two-way, then the best option is to look both ways before crossing (i.e., a non-directional test). If there is certainty that the street is one-way, then one only needs to look in that direction before crossing (i.e., a directional test). Obviously, one would only look in a specific direction, or select a directional test, if there is substantial supporting evidence prior to conducting the test. Below are the four types of hypothesis tests that are frequently conducted in research studies. **Table 9-6** presents these hypothesis tests and their appropriate null hypotheses. All of the examples are formulated in terms of comparing the means between two groups. While the underlying calculations would be different for proportions (e.g., the proportion who survive among those receiving Treatment A compared to those receiving Treatment B) or other population parameters, conceptually the tests are the same regardless of the quantity being compared.

Non-Directional Tests

Tests of difference and equivalence are considered non-directional. When these tests are conducted, the focus is not on determining in which direction the difference is. Instead, the focus is on whether there is a difference between the groups or whether the groups are equivalent.

Test of Difference

When conducting a **test of difference**, the null hypothesis is that the difference between two quantities is 0 (i.e., the two quantities are the same or equal). Using gender differences in blood pressure as an example, a test of difference would involve testing whether the mean systolic blood pressure (SBP) in males is different from the mean SBP in females, or H_0: mean SBP_{males} − mean $SBP_{females} = 0$. Testing in this way is non-directional

TABLE 9-6 Types of Hypothesis Tests

Test Type	Conceptual Purpose	Null Hypothesis	Alternate Hypothesis	Assessment
Non-Directional				
Difference	Determine if the means for Group 1 and Group 2 are different	H_0: (Mean$_1$ − Mean$_2$) = 0 *or* H_0: Mean$_1$ = Mean$_2$	H_A: Mean$_1$ − Mean$_2$ ≠ 0 *or* H_A: Mean$_1$ ≠ Mean$_2$	Traditional two-sided test or determine if 0 is contained in the $(1 - \alpha)$ confidence interval for the difference in the means
Equivalence	Determine if the means for Group 1 and Group 2 are practically equivalent (i.e., within an acceptable difference)	H_0: |Mean$_1$ − Mean$_2$| ≥ Δ	H_A: |Mean$_1$ − Mean$_2$| < Δ	Determine if the $(1 - 2\alpha)$ confidence interval for the difference lies completely within the equivalence interval $[-\Delta, +\Delta]$ or conduct two one-sided tests (TOST approach)
Directional				
Superiority	Determine if Group 1's mean is greater than Group 2's mean*	H_0: Mean$_1$ − Mean$_2$ ≤ 0 *or* H_0: Mean$_1$ ≤ Mean$_2$	H_A: Mean$_1$ − Mean$_2$ > 0 *or* H_A: Mean$_1$ > Mean$_2$	Traditional one-sided test or use the one-tailed critical value to calculate the upper bound of the confidence interval to see if the observed value is outside the upper bound
Non-Inferiority	Determine if Group 2's mean is no more than a certain amount lower than Group 1's mean*	H_0: (Mean$_1$ − Mean$_2$) ≥ Δ	H_A: (Mean$_1$ − Mean$_2$) < Δ	Examine the boundary of the confidence interval to see if it crosses the non-inferiority margin

*The relationship between Groups 1 and 2 can be changed as long as the wording and formulation of the hypotheses are rearranged accordingly.

because the direction of the difference is not specified. This test may be performed in the traditional way or through the use of confidence intervals. Because this is a non-directional test, it is important to remember to use the two-tailed critical values. These two-tailed values assign half of the α level to the upper tail and half to the lower tail, effectively maintaining the overall specified α level (e.g., 5%). These two-tailed values would be used regardless of whether the traditional approach or the confidence interval approach is chosen. This is the most commonly seen type of hypothesis test in the biomedical literature and will be illustrated with an example later in this chapter.

Test of Equivalence

In a **test of equivalence**, the objective is to show that two quantities are equivalent (e.g., whether the mean weight loss after exercising three times a week for an hour at a time is equivalent to the mean weight loss after exercising six times a week for 30 minutes at a time). Equivalence cannot be determined by conducting a test of difference and concluding that no significant difference exists when the results are not statistically significant. This conclusion only says that insufficient evidence exists to warrant rejecting the null hypothesis of no difference.[13–14] As Altman and Bland stated, "Absence of evidence is not evidence of absence."[13] Unfortunately, this has happened frequently in the biomedical literature.[15]

In testing for equivalence, remember that the null hypothesis is being tested. This null hypothesis is the opposite of what is trying to be assessed or examined. In the case of equivalence, the purpose is to show that equivalence exists, so the null hypothesis must be constructed appropriately. Equivalence involves identifying a certain amount of difference that is acceptable from a practical standpoint. Selecting an appropriate range of equivalence can be difficult but is crucial to allow for a meaningful conclusion. Although seemingly subjective, the margin of equivalence should be based on prior research or clinical relevance. Using the exercise and weight loss example, one might be inclined to say that the two exercise regimens are equivalent as long as there is less than a 10% difference in weight loss between the two. The null hypothesis must include this range of difference where equivalence would be accepted. Furthermore, because the focus is to determine equivalence, the null and alternative hypotheses must be "reversed" compared to a test of difference.

In the equivalence scenario, the null hypothesis would be that the two quantities differ by some specified amount (Δ) or more, or H_0: $|\text{Mean}_1 - \text{Mean}_2| \geq \Delta$. Using the weight loss example, the null would be stated as H_0: $|\text{Mean weight loss}_{3\text{-day exercise}} - \text{Mean weight loss}_{6\text{-day exercise}}| \geq 10\%$. Although the null hypothesis involves an inequality, the absolute value of the difference between the groups makes the test non-directional. If the absolute value had not been used, then two null hypotheses would be needed: that the difference was greater than or equal to $+\Delta$ and that the difference was less than or equal to $-\Delta$. The absolute value allows a more succinct representation of the null. Given the way the null is specified, rejecting the null allows us to conclude that the two quantities are equivalent (within some specified range).

Performing the test involves using two one-sided statistical tests (or TOST). For example, the researcher may conduct a one-sided (or one-tailed) t-test to look for differences greater than $+\Delta$ and another one-sided t-test to look for differences less than $-\Delta$. Both of these tests need to be conducted to perform the test. A confidence interval approach may be more straightforward and intuitive in the case of a test of equivalence and is equivalent to the TOST approach. To use the confidence interval approach, first construct the appropriate confidence interval for the stated level of statistical significance. Keeping in mind that this approach must reflect the TOST approach, remember that the appropriate confidence interval will actually use twice the stated significance level rather than the traditional ($1 - \alpha$) confidence level. As an example, if $\alpha = 0.05$, then the appropriate confidence interval would be the 90% confidence interval because $2\alpha = 0.10$. Then compare that confidence interval to the equivalence interval, or $[-\Delta, +\Delta]$. If the confidence interval fits completely inside the equivalence interval, then the two groups are said to be equivalent. The determination of bioequivalence during the generic drug approval process is an example of the process of equivalence testing.

DIRECTIONAL TESTS

When conducting directional tests, the focus is on determining whether there is a difference in a pre-specified direction. Tests of superiority and non-inferiority have these directions built into the construction of the hypotheses being tested. Compared to their non-directional counterparts, tests of superiority or non-inferiority will only look in one direction.

Test of Superiority

The **test of superiority** is similar to a test of difference except the focus is to see if one alternative is better than another. Obviously, this would only be performed if there were substantial reason to believe that the effect would only be in one direction. The null hypothesis for a test of superiority would need to include equality and may take the form of H_0: $\text{Mean}_1 - \text{Mean}_2 \leq 0$. Using the blood pressure example from the difference test and assuming that the assumption was that mean SBP in males was higher than in females, the null hypothesis could be stated as H_0: mean $\text{SBP}_{\text{males}} -$ mean $\text{SBP}_{\text{females}} \leq 0$. A traditional one-tailed test could be used to conduct this test using the appropriate one-tailed critical value. A confidence interval approach could also be used to see if the observed value falls outside the upper bound of the confidence interval (again using the one-tailed critical value).

Test of Non-Inferiority

Sometimes the goal of a study is to show that a new treatment is no worse than an existing treatment, which involves a **test of non-inferiority**. Similar to a test of equivalence, the first step involves selecting a margin of non-inferiority based on prior experience, research, or clinical relevance. Also similar to the equivalence test is that the null and alternate hypotheses are "reversed" compared to tests of difference or superiority. Here the null hypothesis is that the comparison treatment (treatment 2) is worse than (i.e., inferior to) the usual treatment (treatment 1) by at least some certain, pre-specified non-inferiority margin (Δ). This might be stated as H_0: $\text{Mean}_2 - \text{Mean}_1 \geq \Delta$. The order of comparisons can be confusing here because the negative direction is being used. Also, one must consider whether lower values are better or worse when constructing the null hypothesis (e.g., lower LDL is better but lower survival rates are worse).

Consider a situation where the objective of the study is to determine the cure rate for a shorter antibiotic course for a respiratory infection. The current recommended course of therapy is 14 days. The new course being examined is 7 days. The outcome is the percent of patients experiencing clinical cure after completing the course of therapy. The defined margin of non-inferiority is 5%, so the percentage with clinical cure in the shorter course group must be less than 5% worse than the standard course to be determined non-inferior. Given this non-inferiority approach, the focus is technically not whether the shorter course is better than the standard course. In this example, the null hypothesis would be that the shorter course is worse than the standard course by at least 5%, or H_0: Mean cure rate$_{\text{14-day}}$ − Mean cure rate$_{\text{7-day}} \geq 5\%$. The alternate hypothesis would be that the difference between the two is less than 5%. Notice how a non-inferiority test could be viewed as taking the alternate hypothesis from a superiority test and including a margin of non-inferiority similar to an equivalence test.

As with the superiority test, a one-sided test or confidence interval could be used to perform the test. Unlike the superiority test, it is not uncommon to see a more stringent confidence level used in non-inferiority tests. Rather than using the one-tailed critical value, the critical value from the two-tailed α level may be used to make the test more conservative.[16] For example, if the desired α level were 0.05, the critical value of 1.96 (the two-tailed critical value for $\alpha = 0.05$) may be used for the non-inferiority test rather than the 1.65 critical value, which would be the usual one-tailed critical value. As with the equivalence test, the focus of the confidence interval approach is to see if the confidence interval includes the non-inferiority margin. If the boundary of the interval crosses the margin, then the null is not rejected and the conclusion is that the new treatment is inferior to the standard treatment. If the boundary of the interval falls completely within the non-inferiority margin, then the null is rejected and the new treatment is said to be non-inferior to the standard. Infectious disease research is a common place where non-inferiority trials are seen. For example, Chastre et al. found that an 8-day course of therapy was non-inferior to a 15-day course of therapy for adults with ventilator-acquired pneumonia.[17]

PROCESS OF PERFORMING A HYPOTHESIS TEST

Two general approaches can be used to perform a hypothesis test. The first is a combination of the original approaches to hypothesis testing set forth by Fisher[18] and Neyman and Pearson.[11–12] The second is an approach that makes use of confidence intervals. Both should produce equivalent conclusions with respect to rejecting or failing to reject the null hypothesis.

To illustrate the process of performing a hypothesis test, consider a scenario to examine whether an automated refill program is effective at improving adherence with chronic medications. The study enrolls 100 people. Half are randomly assigned to the automated refill program. The others are randomly assigned to usual care (i.e., no automated refill). Adherence is measured using the proportion of days covered (PDC) where higher numbers represent greater adherence. For each individual, adherence with chronic medications is measured over a 180-day period after their program enrollment. The goal is to test if mean adherence at the end of the study period is different between the two groups (i.e., a test of difference). The basic findings are presented in **Table 9-7**.

TABLE 9-7 Example of Results from an Adherence Study		
	Automated refill program	**Usual care**
Sample size	50	50
Proportion of days covered (Mean ± SD)	82.5 ± 12.3	75.9 ± 16.7
95% confidence interval*	79.00 – 86.00	71.15 – 80.65
t-statistic		2.250
p-value		0.027
Difference in means (Refill program – Usual care)		6.6
95% confidence interval for the difference between two means		0.78 – 12.42

*The calculation above uses the critical value from the *t*-distribution with *df* = 49, which is 2.01. Using a critical value of 1.96 will result in a CI of [79.09 – 85.91] for the automated refill group and [71.27 – 80.53] for the usual care group.

TRADITIONAL APPROACH

In the traditional approach to hypothesis testing, the researcher follows five steps as explained in the following section. The calculation of the test statistic and the selection of the critical value are usually done by the statistical software being used. Modern computing has allowed for the easy calculation of p-values allowing actual p-values to be presented rather than simply stating that the p-value is greater than or less than the stated significance level (e.g., $p < 0.05$) or simply stating whether the results are statistically significant. The steps to perform a hypothesis test for a difference using the traditional approach are outlined below using the adherence study example and presented in **Table 9-8**.

Step 1. Convert the research question into the appropriate null and alternate hypotheses

Once the desired research question is identified, an appropriate null hypothesis and accompanying alternate hypothesis must be constructed. This is something that must be done with care, as an incorrect hypothesis can drastically alter the conclusions and interpretation. The original research question was to determine if the automated refill program was effective at improving adherence (as measured by PDC). The null hypothesis might be that there is no difference in mean PDC between the automatic refill program (RP) group and the usual care (UC) group. The null hypothesis could be stated as H_0: Mean PDC_{RP} – Mean $PDC_{UC} = 0$ or Mean PDC_{RP} = Mean PDC_{UC}. The alternate would

TABLE 9-8 Example of the Traditional Approach to Hypothesis Testing	
Step	**Example**
1. Convert the research question into an appropriate null and alternate hypothesis	Research question: Is the automatic refill program effective at improving adherence? H_0: Mean PDC among the refill program (RP) patients will be the same as mean PDC among the usual care (UC) patients; or H_0: Mean PDC_{RP} – Mean $PDC_{UC} = 0$. H_A: Mean PDC among the refill program (RP) patients will be different from mean PDC among the usual care (UC) patients; or H_A: Mean PDC_{RP} – Mean $PDC_{UC} \neq 0$.
2. Select the appropriate statistical test	The t-test is selected because it is comparing two independent groups with an assumption that PDC is normally distributed.
3. Select the desired significance level (i.e., α level) and the appropriate critical value for the statistical test	The significance level is set at 5% ($\alpha = 0.05$). The critical value for a two-tailed t-test at the 5% level of significance with 98 degrees of freedom is 1.984.
4. Calculate the test statistic	Based on the provided information, the calculated t-statistic is 2.250 (with 98 degrees of freedom).
5. Compare the test statistic to the critical value and draw conclusions	In comparing the calculated statistic to the critical value, the t-statistic is found to be greater than the critical value. This results in rejecting H_0 and concluding that there is a difference in PDC between the groups. The actual p-value is 0.027.

be that the two groups are different on PDC measurements (H_A: Mean PDC_{RP} – Mean $PDC_{UC} \neq 0$). It is common in statistics textbooks for the population mean for each group to be presented by the Greek letter mu, μ. Thus, the null and alternative hypotheses might also be stated as $H_0: \mu_{PDC_{RP}} - \mu_{PDC_{UC}} = 0$ and $H_A: \mu_{PDC_{RP}} - \mu_{PDC_{UC}} \neq 0$.

Notice that the original research question was actually one-sided, but the null hypothesis was framed as a non-directional null. This is common because two-sided (or non-directional) tests are more conservative than a directional test at the same α level. When reading a research study, look closely to see whether two-sided or one-sided statistical tests were used to determine if the hypothesis testing approach was directional or non-directional because research questions may be stated as directional. This can usually be identified in the statistical analysis section by looking for statements about "two-tailed analyses" or "two-tailed significance levels."

Step 2. Select the appropriate statistical test

In this situation, the comparison is between two independent groups. For the sake of simplicity, assume that PDC (and the difference in PDC) is normally distributed. The appropriate statistical test in this case would be the independent samples t-test. More information about this will be discussed in Chapter 10, "Bivariate Analysis and Comparing Groups."

Step 3. Select the desired significance level (i.e., α level) and the appropriate critical value for the statistical test

The desired significance level must be set up front by the researcher before the data are collected, or at least before data analysis begins. A significance level of 5% (or $\alpha = 0.05$) is selected. Remember that the t-distribution is affected by degrees of freedom. In this situation, there are two groups with 50 subjects each. One degree of freedom is lost in each group in order to estimate the mean, so the total degrees of freedom are 98 ($df = 98$). Because a two-tailed test is being used, the critical t-value for 98 degrees of freedom is 1.984. Notice how this critical value is slightly higher than the similar value for the z-distribution in Table 9-2. This should make sense given that the sample size in the study is moderately large.

Step 4. Calculate the test statistic

Without going into the detailed calculations, based on the information provided in Table 9-7, the calculated t-statistic would be 2.250.

Step 5. Compare the test statistic to the critical value and draw conclusions

The final step in the traditional approach involves comparing the calculated test statistic to the selected critical value. If the absolute value of the test statistic is greater than or equal to the critical value (i.e., |Test statistic| $\geq$ Critical value), then the null hypothesis (H_0) would be rejected. If the critical value is greater (i.e., |Test statistic| < Critical value), then the null would not be rejected (i.e., fail to reject). Remember, the alternate hypothesis is not being tested and is actually not referred to at all during the hypothesis testing process.

As part of this final step, the p-value can be generated. For this example, $p = 0.027$. This means that there is a 2.7% chance of finding a result of this magnitude (or larger) assuming the null hypothesis is true. To put it another way, the chance of finding these results, given that there is no effect of the refill program, is 2.7%. With the computing capabilities available today, it is standard practice to provide the actual p-value rather than stating whether the cut-point for statistical significance is met (e.g., $p < 0.05$ or $p < 0.01$).[19] The p-value can also be conceptualized as the strength of the evidence *against* the null hypothesis. Smaller p-values indicate increasingly strong evidence against the null, so $p = 0.25$ does not suggest strong evidence against the null while $p < 0.001$ would denote strong evidence against the null. Keeping in line with the spirit of hypothesis testing, p-values less than or equal to the α level (or $p \leq \alpha$) denote statistical significance. It is important to remember that the p-value does not represent the strength or size of the finding (i.e., a smaller p-value does not indicate a stronger finding).[9] It only addresses the probability of obtaining a result as large as, or larger than, the observed results assuming the null hypothesis is true.

CONFIDENCE INTERVAL APPROACH

The traditional approach to hypothesis testing has been a source of confusion and misinterpretation.[19–22] CIs have been promoted as a way to overcome some of the problems with interpretations of the p-value and the simple binary conclusions of a hypothesis test.[19,23–24] While these have not completely replaced the traditional approach to hypothesis testing, they have become standard reporting in biomedical research and are included in the *Recommendations for the Conduct, Reporting, Editing, and Publication of Scholarly Work in Medical Journals* promoted by the International Committee of Medical Journal Editors.[25] CIs can also be used to conduct hypothesis tests. The CI approach may actually be more straightforward in some situations like equivalence and non-inferiority than the traditional approach.

The process of conducting a hypothesis test using confidence intervals is similar to the traditional approach in the previous section. The process begins with constructing the appropriate hypotheses. In this approach, there is no statistical test to select, but an α level must still be selected before conducting the study. After stating the α level, the appropriate critical value is chosen to construct the confidence interval. Rather than comparing the test statistic to the critical value, the CI approach involves determining whether the interval contains the value representing the null or a value representing margins for equivalence or non-inferiority. For tests of difference, the null value is usually 0 because the difference between two means would be 0 if they were not different. In certain situations, the ratio of two quantities, such as with odds ratios or relative risks, is being estimated, so the value representing the null is 1 because this reflects the condition where the numerator and denominator in a ratio are equal. If the interval contains the null value of interest, then the null hypothesis is not rejected at a given significance level; if the interval does not contain the null value, the null is rejected at a given significance level.

Using the previous adherence example, the focus is a test of difference between two means; therefore, the null value would be 0. The information provided in Table 9-7 includes the 95% CI for the difference between two means. Looking at this CI, 0 is not included in the interval; thus, the conclusion is that the difference in adherence between the two groups is statistically significant at the 5% level (i.e., the null hypothesis of no difference can be rejected). Note that this is the same conclusion obtained using the traditional approach. From the CI approach, an actual p-value would not be available unless explicitly calculated, but the difference can still be determined to be statistically significant.

In the adherence example, the actual 95% CI for the difference was provided. Sometimes a research article may not provide the CI for the difference. Instead, the point estimates and their CIs, or at least their sample sizes and standard deviations, are provided so each CI could be calculated. In situations where the CI of the difference is not provided, there are methods to construct the CI that involve combining variance estimates of the two groups. This can be difficult if all necessary information is not provided. Some have suggested that an "eyeball test" to check for overlap between the CIs from the two point estimates is an easy way to assess statistical significance in these situations. In the adherence example, the 95% CIs for each group overlap slightly. By using the "eyeball test," the conclusion would be that the PDC for the two programs was not different; however, the formal statistical test and the CI approach using the *difference* in the means suggest that there is a statistically significant difference. This represents the potential drawback to this approach. While one can safely conclude that intervals that do not overlap are statistically significantly different, it is possible for there to be a certain amount of overlap between the CIs of two quantities that are statistically significantly different. Incorrectly concluding that the two means were not significantly different when they were in fact significantly different would result in an incorrect conclusion, but this would make the process more conservative (i.e., more difficult to reject the null) so it may be an acceptable alternative if no other information is available.[26-28]

WHAT "SIGNIFICANT" MEANS

When reading research articles, it is common to see the term "significant" used frequently. Unfortunately, this term may have different meanings in varying contexts and authors may not always be consistent or clear in their use of the term. It is important to recognize the varying meanings of the term "significant" in these different contexts so that statements can be evaluated appropriately. From a statistical analysis standpoint, "significant" has a very specific meaning, which can be quite different from the meaning of the term for applications in practice.

STATISTICAL SIGNIFICANCE

As discussed earlier, one of the final steps in performing a hypothesis test is to determine whether or not the null hypothesis will be rejected. When it is determined that there is sufficient evidence to reject the null hypothesis, then one concludes that the results are statistically significant. One important thing to keep in mind is that **statistical significance** refers to the results of the analysis. On their own, data are neither significant nor non-significant. The differences, associations, or relationships identified in the data while conducting the analysis are determined to be statistically significant.

Because the rules for statistical significance testing do not allow for any gray area in coming to a statistical conclusion, the results of an analysis are either statistically significant or not. Still, some authors use such statements as "marginally statistically significant" or "borderline significant" when the results yield p-values that do not meet the stated level of statistical significance (e.g., $p = 0.06$ when the stated significance level is $\alpha = 0.05$). Stating a "trend toward significance" is problematic when describing the results from one study or one analysis where the p-value is slightly higher than the stated significance level. The term "trend" is not appropriate unless the scenario involves several studies or analyses. Terms like "highly statistically significant" for $p < 0.01$ and "very highly statistically significant" for $p < 0.001$ are also inappropriate and only add to the confusion because the relative size of the p-value is not useful in determining how much more significant a result is.[9,29] Methods have been proposed to incorporate levels of uncertainty regarding making a conclusion after a hypothesis test.[30]

CLINICAL SIGNIFICANCE

Whereas statistical significance relates to whether the null hypothesis is rejected, **clinical significance** speaks to the practical significance or importance of the findings. Statistical significance is strictly related to the statistical analysis. One easy way to conceptualize clinical significance is to consider whether or not the findings will result in a change in practice. It is quite possible for the results of a study to be statistically significant but relatively unimportant from a practice standpoint. Consider a study examining the effectiveness of a new medication in reducing the risk of myocardial infarction (MI) compared to an existing medication that is standard therapy. The researchers may find that the reduction of the 5-year risk of MI is 0.2% compared to the standard therapy with $p = 0.01$. While this result is statistically significant, it is unlikely that this small reduction would prompt clinicians to begin to use this medication in widespread practice instead of the standard therapy. Because p-values and statistical significance can be heavily influenced by sample size, it is important to remember to examine the clinical significance of a result when a very small difference or weak association is determined to be statistically significant and the sample size is large.

It is also important to remember that the absence of a statistically significant finding may be clinically important. For example, consider a new dosing regimen for chemotherapy that has been shown to have an improved side effect profile versus the current standard regimen. When comparing the new dosing regimen to the standard regimen to examine cancer progression and survival, no statistically significant difference was found between the two. This lack of statistical significance could be clinically important and prompt clinicians to change their practice. Admittedly, clinical significance involves a certain level of subjectivity. It is entirely possible that one individual may view the results of a study as clinically significant while another may view them as not clinically significant. Similarly, a difference of the same magnitude may be clinically significant in one therapeutic area but not in another. The use of the number needed to treat (NNT) or the number needed to harm (NNH) can be used when considering clinical significance.[31] While these quantities do not provide absolute cutoffs for clinical significance, they can help provide more concrete values to guide determination of clinical significance. As mentioned earlier, the confidence interval can also help provide an indication of clinical significance, especially when the difference or association is small but statistically significant.

Clinical significance also involves the interpretation of results in the larger context of existing knowledge in an area. While statistical significance is only related to a specific statistical analysis, it is possible to consider the entire study, which may involve multiple analyses, in light of the findings from similar studies when making determinations of clinical significance.

SUMMARY AND CONCLUSIONS

Statistical inference is the process of making a determination about some value or relationship in the target population of interest based on information obtained from a sample. This process is an important part of statistical analysis and draws on basic statistical concepts related to statistical distributions and the central limit theorem. Inference can be conducted directly through estimation or indirectly through hypothesis testing, but both have a useful place in biomedical research. The use of hypothesis testing to generate a p-value and the construction of confidence intervals form the basis for reporting the results of inferential statistics in biomedical research. It is important to understand the general mechanisms behind statistical inference to conduct a research study or to understand and apply the results of other studies in an appropriate manner.

REVIEW QUESTIONS

1. Using the concepts from the central limit theorem, explain why larger samples are viewed as better than smaller samples.
2. For the following research questions, state appropriate null and alternate hypotheses and determine whether the hypothesis test would be directional or non-directional and whether it would be a test of difference, equivalence, superiority, or non-inferiority.
   a) Do students who get at least 8 hours of sleep the night before an exam get different exam grades than those who get less than 8 hours of sleep?
   b) Is the occurrence of vomiting with a higher dose of docetaxel for a shorter duration equivalent to a lower dose of docetaxel for a longer duration? [Note: "Equivalent" here means within 5%.]
3. A study is comparing the difference in the occurrence of abnormalities in serum creatinine associated with a new drug compared to an existing drug. The point estimate for the comparison in creatinine is 0.3 mg/dL with a 95% confidence interval (for the difference) of –0.6 to 1.2. Is this difference statistically significant? Why or why not?
4. A study is testing a new drug that has been developed for improving the understanding of statistics among pharmacy students. Out of a class of 100 students, half are randomly assigned to receive a placebo and half will receive the new drug. The investigators noted that the students in the drug group scored 12 points (SD = 6) higher on the final exam than those in the placebo group. Calculate the 99% confidence interval (two-tailed) for this difference.
5. What is the difference between statistical significance and clinical significance?

ONLINE RESOURCES

Rice Virtual Lab in Statistics: http://onlinestatbook.com/rvls/index.html (Online simulators and calculators for things like confidence intervals, the central limit theorem, sampling distributions, and many others.)

SticiGui: http://www.stat.berkeley.edu/~stark/SticiGui/index.htm (Online introductory statistics "text" that contains calculators and examples of statistics concepts including recorded lectures; developed by Dr. Philip B. Stark at the University of California-Berkeley.)

VassarStats: http://www.vassarstats.net/index.html (Website for statistical computation.)

REFERENCES

1. Dawson B, Trapp RG. *Basic & Clinical Biostatistics*. 4th ed. New York, NY: Lange Medical Books/McGraw-Hill; 2004.
2. Forbes C, Evans M, Hastings N, Peacock B. *Statistical Distributions*. Hoboken, NJ: John Wiley & Sons; 2011.
3. Holland R, Brooksby I, Lenaghan E, et al. Effectiveness of visits from community pharmacists for patients with heart failure: HeartMed randomised controlled trial. *BMJ*. 2007;334(7603):1098.
4. Wu EQ, Birnbaum HG, Zhang HF, Ivanova JI, Yang E, Mallet D. Health care costs of adults treated for attention-deficit/hyperactivity disorder who received alternative drug therapies. *J Manag Care Pharm*. 2007;13(7):561–569.
5. Harpe SE. Using secondary data in pharmacoepidemiology. In: West-Strum D, Yang Y, eds. *Understanding Pharmacoepidemiology*. New York, NY: McGraw-Hill; 2011.
6. Harpe SE. Using secondary data sources for pharmacoepidemiology and outcomes research. *Pharmacotherapy*. 2009;29(2):138–153.
7. Bentley JP. Statistical Analysis. In: Aparasu RR, ed. *Research Methods for Pharmaceutical Policy and Practice*. London, England: Pharmaceutical Press; 2011.
8. Kachigan SK. *Statistical Analysis: An Interdisciplinary Introduction to Univariate & Multivariate Methods*. New York, NY: Radius Press; 1986.
9. Good PI, Hardin JW. *Common Errors in Statistics (and How to Avoid Them)*. Hoboken, NJ: John Wiley & Sons; 2003.

10. Motheral B. Research methodology: hypotheses, measurement, reliability, and validity. *J Manag Care Pharm.* 1998;4(4):382–390.

11. Neyman J, Pearson ES. On the use and interpretation of certain test criteria for purposes of statistical inference. *Biometrika.* 1928;20A(1/2):175–240, 263–294.

12. Neyman J, Pearson ES. On the problem of the most efficient tests of statistical hypotheses. *Philosophical Transactions of the Royal Society of London. Series A, Containing Papers of a Mathematical or Physical Character.* 1933;231:289–337.

13. Altman DG, Bland JM. Absence of evidence is not evidence of absence. *BMJ.* 1995;311(7003):485.

14. Jones B, Jarvis P, Lewis JA, Ebbutt AF. Trials to assess equivalence: the importance of rigorous methods. *BMJ.* 1996;313(7048):36–39.

15. Greene WL, Concato J, Feinstein AR. Claims of equivalence in medical research: are they supported by evidence. *Ann Intern Med.* 2000;132(9):715–722.

16. Lesaffre E. Superiority, equivalence, and non-inferiority trials. *Bull NYU Hosp Jt Dis.* 2008;66(2): 150–154.

17. Chastre J, Wolff M, Fagon J-Y, et al. Comparison of 8 vs 15 days of antibiotic therapy for ventilator-acquired pneumonia in adults: a randomized trial. *JAMA.* 2003;290(19):2588–2598.

18. Fisher RA. *Statistical Methods for Research Workers.* 10th ed. Edinburgh, Scotland: Oliver & Boyd; 1946.

19. Sterne JAC, Davey Smith G. Sifting the evidence—what's wrong with significance tests? *BMJ.* 2001;322(7280):226–231.

20. Glaser DN. The controversy of significance testing: misconceptions and alternatives. *Am J Crit Care.* 1999;8(5):291–296.

21. Weinberg CR. It's time to rehabilitate the P-value. *Epidemiology.* 2001;12(3):288–290.

22. Hubbard R, Bayarri MJ, Berk KN, Carlton MA. Confusion over measures (p's) versus errors (α's) in classical statistical testing. *Am Stat.* 2003;57(3):171–182.

23. Tryon WW. Evaluating statistical difference, equivalence, and indeterminacy using inferential confidence intervals: an integrated alternative method of conducting null hypothesis statistical tests. *Psychol Methods.* 2001;6(4):371–386.

24. Hubbard R, Lindsay RM. Why P values are not a useful measure of evidence in statistical significance testing. *Theory Psychol.* 2008;18(1):69–88.

25. International Committee of Medical Journal Editors. Recommendations for the Conduct, Reporting, Editing, and Publication of Scholarly Work in Medical Journals. http://www.icmje.org/urm_main.html. Accessed December 10, 2013.

26. Schenker N, Gentlemean JF. On judging the significance of differences by examining the overlap between confidence intervals. *Am Stat.* 2001;55(3):182–186.

27. Payton ME, Greenstone, MH, Schenker N. Overlapping confidence intervals or standard error intervals: What do they mean in terms of statistical significance? *J Insect Sci.* 2003;3:Article 34. http://www.insectscience.org/3.34/. Accessed March 28, 2013.

28. Cumming G. Inference by eye: reading the overlap of independent confidence intervals. *Stat Med.* 2009;28(2):205–220.

29. Gehlbach SH. *Interpreting the Medical Literature.* 5th ed. New York, NY: McGraw-Hill, 2006.

30. Schmidt FL, Hunter JE. Eight common but false objections to the discontinuation of significance testing in the analysis of research data. In: Harlow LA, Mulaik SA, Steiger JH, eds. *What if There Were No Significance Tests?* Mahwah, NJ: Erlbaum; 1997.

31. Cordell WH. Number needed to treat (NNT). *Ann Emerg Med.* 1999;33(4):433–436.

BIVARIATE ANALYSIS AND COMPARING GROUPS

MARION K. SLACK, PHD

BISMARK BAIDOO, PHD

CHAPTER OBJECTIVES

▶ Describe statistical tests used to evaluate differences among groups

▶ Define statistically dependent (i.e., dependent or paired observations) samples and state how these affect the choice of a statistical test

▶ Explain how the scale of measurement for the dependent variable influences the choice of a statistical test

▶ Define nonparametric statistical methods and identify common nonparametric tests

▶ Identify statistical tests to evaluate relationships between two continuous variables and between two ordinal variables

KEY TERMINOLOGY

Analysis of variance (ANOVA)
Bivariate analyses
Chi-square test of homogeneity
Independent groups *t*-test
Kruskal–Wallis test
Negative relationship

Nonparametric methods
Paired *t*-test
Parametric methods
Pearson correlation coefficient
Positive relationship
Scatterplot

Sign test
Spearman rank correlation coefficient
Wilcoxon–Mann–Whitney test

INTRODUCTION

The most common research design encountered in biomedicine involves the comparison of outcomes in two groups. Typically one group of patients will receive an experimental treatment and a second group receives a comparison treatment that may be a placebo, a second type of treatment, or usual care. Within pharmacy, the classic two-group study is a study comparing a drug treatment to placebo. The outcomes from each group are compared using a statistical test and conclusions are made regarding the efficacy of treatment based on the results of the statistical test.

The purpose of this chapter is to describe the most commonly used **bivariate analyses**,[a] including those used to compare groups, and to illustrate these techniques using small data sets. The chapter begins by describing the process of statistically comparing averages (or means) and then proportions between two independent groups. The situation of non-independent groups, such as when a group of patients is measured at two different time points, is then discussed. Comparisons of the rank order of responses in two or more groups are also described, as is the calculation of the correlation between two variables. These statistical tests are described in the context of a case scenario. The chapter ends by reviewing the use and assumptions of the described statistical tests for comparing groups as shown with a flowchart.

CASE SCENARIO

Consider the situation of a pharmacist–run community health center where services are provided to a substantial number of patients with type II diabetes. Community health center pharmacists have worked with the local YWCA to provide exercise classes and make gym facilities available to their patients. They know that exercise should have a positive effect on patients with diabetes; that is, exercise increases the impact of diabetes medications on the control of blood sugar in diabetes. They want to gather evidence that the program is effective for their patients, so they have designed a research study. The study will have two groups, a treatment and a comparison group; the patients in the treatment group will participate in the exercise program, while the patients in the comparison group will continue to receive care as it is currently provided, that is, usual care. Eligible patients are assigned to the treatment or comparison group using a random procedure so that the study would be considered a randomized controlled trial (RCT). The primary outcome measure is glycosylated hemoglobin (A1C). A1C indicates the percentage of red blood cells that have become glycated by glucose in the blood and is reported as a percentage; the purpose of the exercise program is to reduce A1C levels to near normal. The next step is to determine what statistical test to use to show that the exercise program produced a statistically significant reduction in A1C compared to the usual care group.

---

[a] *Bivariate analysis* is a term used to denote an analysis with just two variables. Some use the term *univariate analysis* to describe analysis of a single dependent variable, even though there may be multiple independent variables. Using this definition, some of the techniques discussed in this chapter, such as ANOVA and the *t*-test, may also be considered univariate techniques.

CONTINUOUS OUTCOME: COMPARING TWO GROUPS USING THE *t*-TEST

In the case scenario, the exercise program is the independent variable (treatment variable) and has two values: usual care with the exercise program and usual care without the program, making it a discrete variable. The dependent variable is A1C measured as a percentage and treated as a continuous variable. The pharmacists want to show that A1C is reduced in the exercise group compared to the usual care group using a hypothesis test. The process of hypothesis testing was described in Chapter 9, "Interpretation and Basic Statistical Concepts." Using this process, the null hypothesis will be that there is no difference in the mean A1C in the exercise group and the comparison group, or H_0: Mean$_E$ – Mean$_C$ = 0 (this is a non-directional test of difference). It is common in statistics textbooks for the population mean for each group to be presented by the Greek letter mu (μ). Thus, the null hypothesis might also be stated as H_0: $\mu_E - \mu_C = 0$. The A1C data collected after a sufficient period of time for 10 patients in the exercise group and 10 patients in the comparison group are shown in **Table 10-1**. The calculated means are 7.35 for the exercise group and 7.80 for the comparison group (a mean difference of 0.45). Looking at the values, the value is lower for the exercise group, but the difference might be due to random variation. To determine the probability of obtaining these results (or something more extreme) if there were no factors operating but chance (or random variation), a statistical test is needed. The appropriate statistical test in this case is the **independent groups *t*-test**.

TABLE 10-1 Continuous Outcome: Exercise Group vs. Comparison Group*			
Patient ID	**Exercise Group:** **A1C Levels**	**Patient ID**	**Comparison Group:** **A1C Levels**
101	6.8	103	7.6
105	7.3	104	7.9
107	8.1	106	8.1
108	7.1	110	8.4
109	7.7	111	7.8
112	7.3	113	7.5
114	7.6	116	7.7
115	7.2	118	7.2
117	7.5	119	8.2
121	6.9	120	7.6
Mean	7.35		7.80
s^2	0.152		0.129
t-statistic	2.69		
p-value	0.015		

*The A1C levels reported after the exercise program or the comparison (usual care) program are listed in columns 2 and 4, respectively. Total $N = 20$; there are 10 patients in each group ($n_1 = n_2 = 10$).

To obtain the probability of finding an observed mean difference of this magnitude (or larger) assuming the null hypothesis is true (i.e., there were no factors operating but chance; also called a *p*-value), a test statistic is first calculated. After making some assumptions, it is possible to state the distribution of the test statistic when the null hypothesis is true (in this case, the test statistic follows the *t*-distribution). Using this information, a *p*-value can be calculated for the test. The general formula for calculating the test statistic to assess whether the difference between two means is zero (i.e., that the means of two independent groups are the same), called the *t*-statistic, is:

$$t = \frac{\left(\overline{X}_1 - \overline{X}_2\right)}{\sqrt{\frac{s_p^2}{n_1} + \frac{s_p^2}{n_2}}}, \text{ where } s_p^2 = \frac{(n_1 - 1)s_1^2 + (n_2 - 1)s_2^2}{(n_1 + n_2 - 2)}$$

The formula indicates that the calculated value of *t*, the test statistic, depends on the difference between the observed means $\left(\overline{X}_1 - \overline{X}_2\right)$, the variability of the values as represented by the pooled variance estimate (s_p^2), and the square root of the sample size as represented by n_1 and n_2 (the sample sizes for each group).[1] Examination of the equation shows that the value of *t* increases as the difference between the means increases, the pooled variance estimate (variability) decreases, and the sample size increases.

Statistical theory can be used to show that under the null hypothesis of no difference in means, the *t*-statistic is distributed as a *t*-distribution with $n_1 + n_2 - 2$ degrees of freedom. From this knowledge, a *p*-value can be calculated. This *p*-value can then be compared to the acceptable type I error rate that was selected before conducting the study (this acceptable level is called the significance level, or α level). By convention, this generally is set at 5% and may be stated as $\alpha = 0.05$. The general rule of thumb is to reject the null hypothesis if the *p*-value is less than or equal to α and to not reject the null if the *p*-value is greater than α. If it is relatively rare to obtain such results when the null is indeed true (i.e., the data are discrepant with the null hypothesis), the null hypothesis should be rejected. It is important to keep in mind that for the *p*-value derived from the statistical test to accurately reflect the true probability (i.e., be a valid measure), the hypothesis must be stated a priori, that is, before the data are collected and analyzed for a specific study. The standard procedure to ensure validity is to write a proposal in which the hypotheses that will be tested are stated.

The calculated *t*-statistic in Table 10-1 is 2.69 with an associated *p*-value of 0.015. Because the *p*-value is less than the significance level of 0.05, the null hypothesis can be rejected with a conclusion that the two means are not equal (i.e., there was a difference) and those patients in the exercise group, on average, had lower A1C levels than those in the comparison group. There is a statistically significant difference in the mean A1C levels of individuals assigned to the exercise group compared to those in the control group ($p = 0.015$). They, therefore, consider that the exercise program is most likely effective and participating in an exercise program likely will reduce A1C levels. Note that the statistical test did not *prove* that the exercise program is effective; the statistical test provided evidence that if there were no factors operating except for chance, the probability of observing a difference like this is small. Researchers and clinicians need to use their judgment concerning biologic plausibility and other causal criteria including the research design and methods when making assessments of whether a treatment was indeed the cause of any difference.

The primary method of reporting the results of the *t*-test is to report a point estimate of the difference between two means (or the mean for each group) and the *p*-value for the test. Another method of reporting the findings is to report the point estimate and a confidence interval. This approach for a test of difference between two means was discussed in Chapter 9, "Interpretation and Basic Statistical Concepts" (and demonstrated using the *t*-test). This approach can be used for many of the procedures discussed in the current chapter.

ANOVA FOR THREE OR MORE GROUPS

The *t*-test was described for testing the differences in the means of two groups. If more than two groups of patients are included in the study, then different statistical tests are required. The analogous test to the *t*-test for two or more groups is **analysis of variance (ANOVA)**. ANOVA could be used to compare the mean A1C levels for three groups, for example, a placebo group, an exercise group, and a diet counseling group. The means for the three groups are shown in the graph of **Figure 10-1**.

Using an ANOVA requires a two-step analysis process. The first step is to determine if there might be any differences among the means of the three groups by calculating an *F*-statistic and retrieving its associated *p*-value. If the *p*-value is below the stated significance level (α; e.g., 0.05), then a second step is required to determine which groups differ from the others using a modified version of the *t*-test, known as post-hoc tests (examples include Tukey's HSD test and Scheffe's test[2]). In the example, the *p*-value for the comparison between Group 1 (usual care) and Group 2 (exercise) or Group 3 (diet) was less than 0.05, and the null hypothesis of no difference can be rejected for Group 1 versus Group 2 or Group 3. However, the *p*-value for the comparison of Group 2 to Group 3 was greater than 0.05, so the null hypothesis of no difference could not be rejected. Therefore, the findings could be interpreted to indicate that either diet or exercise is better than usual care, but there is no evidence from these data of a difference between the diet and exercise treatments. The *F*-test used in ANOVA can be thought of as an extension of the *t*-test. An ANOVA used to compare two groups would produce the same results as a non-directional *t*-test; the advantage to an ANOVA is its use with three or more independent groups.

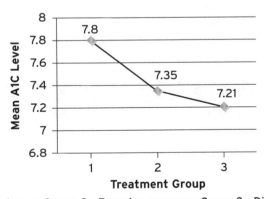

Group 1 = Usual care; Group 2 = Exercise program; Group 3 = Diet counseling

FIGURE 10-1   Graph illustrating findings from an ANOVA.

CATEGORICAL OUTCOME: COMPARING TWO GROUPS USING THE CHI-SQUARE TEST OF HOMOGENEITY

If the goal of the case study is whether a patient is or is not at their goal A1C level, then the researchers could ask whether the proportion (or %) of patients whose A1C levels were at their goal level of 7.5 or less is different in each group; that is, they want to compare the proportion of patients at goal in the exercise group to the proportion of patients at goal in the comparison group. Whether or not a patient is at a treatment goal, a dichotomous variable, represents a different level of measurement than measuring A1C levels. This requires a different statistical test because the type of statistical test used depends on the level of measurement. The appropriate statistical test to assess whether two proportions are equal is the **chi-square test of homogeneity**.

Hypotheses involving categorical outcome variables typically involve proportions. For example, a null hypothesis may be H_0: $P_A = P_B$, where P = population proportion having a given outcome for the A and B groups. The number of patients meeting the criteria for each category of response (e.g., improved and not improved) is counted then expressed as a sample proportion. The null hypothesis is then stated as a comparison of proportions—that there is no difference in the proportion of patients improved in the treatment group and the proportion of patients improved in the comparison group (as with the t-test example, this is a non–directional test of difference).

When comparing two groups on a categorical variable, it is common to present the data in a contingency table. As shown in **Table 10-2**, the proportion of patients who improved in the treatment group is represented as $\dfrac{a}{a+c}$ and the proportion in the comparison group as $\dfrac{b}{b+d}$.

Most introductory statistics books provide formulas for calculating the chi-square test statistic[b] (X^2) from a contingency table (e.g., see Daniel[3]). For a 2×2 contingency table, X^2 can be calculated using this shortcut formula:

$$X^2 = \frac{n(ad - bc)^2}{[(a+b)(c+d)(a+c)(b+d)]}$$

The procedure for interpreting the results is similar to that used for the t-test. Statistical theory reveals that when the null hypothesis of no difference in proportions is true, X^2 is distributed approximately as χ^2 (i.e., a chi-square distribution) with (# rows − 1)(# columns − 1) degrees of freedom (in the case of a 2×2 contingency,

TABLE 10-2 A 2×2 Contingency Table			
	Treatment Group	**Comparison Group**	**Total**
Improved	a	b	$a+b$
Not Improved	c	d	$c+d$
Total	$a+c$	$b+d$	$n = a+b+c+d$

Note: In the table, the two outcomes are "improved" and "not improved." The two comparison groups form the columns and the two outcomes form the rows. This type of table is frequently seen in research reports involving health care. The letters in each cell represent the number of patients improved (or not improved).

---

[b] Also called the Pearson chi–square statistic after its inventor, Karl Pearson.[4]

degrees of freedom = 1). A *p*-value can be then calculated and compared to the significance level, α. The null hypothesis is rejected if the *p*-value is below the value of 0.05 and retained if it is above 0.05.

The data in **Table 10-3** reveal that 70% of the patients in exercise group were at goal, while 20% of the comparison group patients were at goal. The calculated value of X^2 to compare the proportions of patients at goal in these two groups is 5.05, and its associated *p*-value is 0.025. Because the *p*-value is less than 0.05, the null hypothesis can be rejected with a conclusion that there is a statistically significant difference in proportions (if there were no factors operating but chance or random variation, the probability of obtaining these results or something more extreme is small). That is, the proportion of patients at goal in the exercise group is significantly greater than the proportion of patients at goal in the comparison or usual care group.

The chi-square test of homogeneity has some basic sample size requirements. If these requirements are not met, researchers will often use the Fisher exact test to test the null hypothesis of equal proportions in two populations (i.e., $H_0: P_A = P_B$). The test is called an exact test because it calculates the exact probability of obtaining the results or something more extreme (i.e., the *p*-value) rather than relying on an approximation.[3] In the current example, one could argue that the sample size requirements for the chi-square test have not been met and the Fisher exact test should be used. The Fisher exact test for the data in Table 10-3 has a *p*-value of 0.07, suggesting that there is not enough evidence to conclude that the exercise and usual care groups are different in terms of the proportion of patients whose A1C levels were at their goal level. This puts the two pharmacists in the awkward and uncomfortable situation of having an inconclusive answer to their question and nicely highlights the difficulty of working with small samples. In designing and planning their next study, it would be helpful for them to perform a pre-study power analysis to estimate the necessary sample size (see Chapter 13, "Sample Size and Power Analysis" for more information).

The concepts of the odds ratio (OR) and risk ratio (RR) were introduced in Chapter 5, "Cohort and Case-Control Studies." Examples of calculating these measures of association from a 2 × 2 contingency table like that of Table 10-2 were provided. The test of the null hypothesis that two populations have equal proportions on some characteristic of interest (e.g., being at goal) conducted earlier provides valuable information about the RR and OR. If the null hypothesis that there is no difference in proportions is rejected, generally so too will the null hypotheses that the RR = 1 and the OR = 1 be rejected. An RR of 1 and an OR of 1 indicate no association between the two variables of interest. In the present example, it would suggest that when compared to usual care, an exercise program is not effective in increasing the probability of being at goal in terms of A1C. Whether the difference between two proportions (or risks), the RR, or the OR is reported in a given study depends on the type of study design that was employed and the type of statistical technique used to analyze the data. But in the simple case of two nominal variables presented in a 2 × 2 contingency table, the general hypothesis test for whether the difference between two proportions = 0, the RR = 1, and the OR = 1 is the same.

TABLE 10-3	Dichotomous Outcome: Exercise Group vs. Comparison Group		
	Exercise Group	**Comparison Group**	**Total**
At Goal*	7	2	9
Not at Goal	3	8	11
Total	10	10	20

* At goal was defined as having an A1C level of 7.5% or less; the numbers in the "At Goal" row represent the number of patients in the exercise group and the comparison group who were at goal.

As with the case of assessing the difference between two means using the *t*-test, the confidence interval approach can also be used when reporting the difference between two proportions, RR, or OR. Formulas necessary for calculating these confidence intervals from a simple 2 × 2 contingency table are readily available,[5] but can be rather cumbersome. Statistical software packages can easily provide these confidence intervals and the general approach for interpretation and for conducting a hypothesis test using these intervals described in Chapter 9, "Interpretation and Basic Statistical Concepts" apply.

Just like the independent groups *t*-test can be extended to more than two groups by using ANOVA, the chi-square test of homogeneity can be extended and used for the situation of comparing proportions when you have more than two groups (i.e., the contingency table is larger than 2 × 2). It is also possible to use a chi-square test to assess whether two nominal variables of any number of categories are independent (or not associated with each other; again the contingency table is larger than 2 × 2, but now both rows and columns can be greater than 2). This is referred to as the chi-square test of independence, but it is mathematically identical to the chi-square test of homogeneity.[3] Even more tests that use the χ^2 (chi-square) distribution are available if one is able to treat one or more of the classifications as ordinal rather than both as nominal. For more information, see Agresti.[4]

INDEPENDENT VERSUS DEPENDENT GROUPS: THE PAIRED *t*-TEST

Assume that the community health center pharmacists wanted to conduct a study comparing usual care to a combined exercise and diet program. However, developing the combined treatment program would require substantial coordination and development, so they decided to conduct a pilot study first to work out the details related to conducting the study and to determine what type of impact they could expect from the combined treatment program. For the pilot study, they decided to include only 10 patients and that they would measure A1C at the beginning and end of the program. Hence there would be two measures on each patient, one at baseline and one after treatment. The comparison groups would be the baseline group and the post-treatment group, and the same patients would be in both groups.

In general, if the comparison groups used for the statistical comparison involve different groups of patients, then the groups are considered independent. In the first part of the case study, the patients in the exercise group were different patients than those in the usual care group. As shown in Table 10-1, there is one measure of A1C for each patient. If the comparison groups used for the statistical comparison involve more than one measurement on the same patients, then the groups are considered dependent (the sets of observations are said to be paired). The dependence derives from having two measures on the same person and the assumption that the same person will score similarly at both time points.[c] For example, a person who scores high on a baseline measure would be expected to score relatively high on the post-treatment measure. Because the value of

---

[c] In the current example, the same subjects are measured both before and after a treatment—in other words, at two different time points. This is a common scenario giving rise to paired observations. Paired observations can be obtained in a number of different ways. For more information, see Daniel.[3] Also, just as the independent groups *t*-test can be extended to more than two groups by using ANOVA, the paired *t*-test can be extended to the situation where individuals are measured at more than two occasions; this is referred to as repeated-measures ANOVA.

the baseline score correlates to the value of the post-treatment score, the two scores are not independent. In contrast, one person's score should not be correlated to the score of a different person in a second group; that is, their scores are independent and the groups are considered independent. Example data for the study on a combined exercise and diet treatment program using two measures on the same patients are shown in **Table 10-4**.

The null hypothesis for the study can be stated as: There is no difference between the mean A1C level at baseline and post-treatment; H_0: $\text{Mean}_B - \text{Mean}_{PT} = 0$. The test statistic for comparing baseline to post-treatment involves differences in means between dependent groups; therefore, a dependent groups or **paired *t*-test** is used. The *t*-test formula for dependent groups is as follows:

$$ t = \frac{\left(\overline{X}_B - \overline{X}_{PT} \right)}{\sqrt{s_{\overline{X}_B}^2 + s_{\overline{X}_{PT}}^2 - 2rs_{\overline{X}_B}s_{\overline{X}_{PT}}}}, \text{ where } s_{\overline{X}_B}^2 = \frac{s_B^2}{n} \text{ and } s_{\overline{X}_{PT}}^2 = \frac{s_{PT}^2}{n} $$

$$ \left(\begin{array}{l} s_B^2 \text{ and } s_{PT}^2 \text{ are the variances of the scores at baseline and post-treatment;} \\ r = \text{the correlation between the baseline and post-treatment measurements} \end{array} \right) $$

When the null hypothesis of no difference in means is true, this *t*-statistic is distributed as a *t*-distribution with $n - 1$ degrees of freedom. As before, from this knowledge, a *p*-value can be calculated. Notice that the paired *t*-test formula is very similar to that used for a *t*-test for independent groups except that the denominator is reduced by a term allowing for the correlation between the baseline and post-treatment measures.[1] To the extent that the baseline and post-treatment measurements are correlated, the denominator of the test statistic of the scores as represented is reduced and the value of the *t*-statistic is increased. Because of this correlation, the *p*-value for the paired *t*-test will generally be less than the *p*-value for an independent groups *t*-test given the same sample size.

TABLE 10-4	Baseline and Post-Treatment Measures for One Group of Patients	
Patient ID	**Baseline Measure (A1C)**	**Post-Treatment Measure (A1C)**
101	7.6	6.8
102	7.9	7.3
103	8.1	8.1
104	8.4	7.1
105	7.8	7.7
106	7.5	7.3
107	7.7	7.6
108	7.2	7.2
109	8.2	7.5
110	7.6	6.9
Mean	7.80	7.35
s^2	0.129	0.152
t-statistic	3.27	
p-value	0.010	

Example for a dependent groups design where there are 10 patients with two measurements on each patient—a measurement at baseline before the combined diet and exercise treatment and a measurement post-treatment. All patients received the treatment, the combined diet and exercise program. The comparison groups for the statistical test are baseline versus post-treatment. Total $n = 10$; there are 10 patients, each assessed at 2 time points. The *t*-statistic and *p*-value are from a paired *t*-test.

In the case study, the means and variances are the same for both the independent groups *t*-test and dependent groups (or paired) *t*-test (the same data were reformatted to represent the dependent groups version), and the number of patients in the dependent groups example (10) is less than the number in the independent groups example (20). Recall that *p*-value for the independent groups was 0.015; for the paired *t*-test for the data in Table 10-4, $p = 0.010$. The *p*-value is less than 0.05, so the null hypothesis is rejected, and there is some preliminary evidence that the combined exercise and diet program may decrease A1C levels.[d] Because a paired *t*-test is more likely to be statistically significant, a paired *t*-test is said to be more powerful than a *t*-test for independent groups.

ALTERNATIVE APPROACHES FOR COMPARING GROUPS

The Sign Test

Continuing with the pilot study described in the previous section with the data outlined in Table 10-4, because the objective of the study is for the exercise-diet program to decrease A1C, one can tabulate how many patients' A1C levels decreased from baseline to post-treatment. Ideally, all patients' A1C levels would decrease even if the decrease was not adequate to consider them at goal. The null hypothesis would be: The number of patients whose A1C decreased from baseline to post-treatment is equal to the number of patients whose A1C increased from baseline to post-treatment. The **sign test** can be used to test such a hypothesis. This test can be viewed as an alternative to the paired *t*-test when certain assumptions necessary for the paired *t*-test are not met or when the variable of interest cannot be considered continuous.[e]

To obtain the data for the test, the number and direction of changes from baseline to post-treatment are counted. In the example, the desired change is a decrease, so the direction of change is indicated with a negative sign (–). An increase in A1C is indicated by a + sign; no change is indicated by ± and is counted with the + signs. The data for the example study are shown in **Table 10-5**.

The null hypothesis for the sign test is: H_0: N (– signs) = N (+ signs) where N = number of signs. For the example, the null hypothesis will be retained if the number of positive signs is statistically equal to the number of negative signs; if they are not statistically equal, then the null hypothesis will be rejected. The test is conducted by appealing either to the binomial distribution or the normal distribution (an approximation to the binomial distribution) depending on the sample size. A *p*-value can be calculated and compared to a significance level as has been done with the other tests

---

[d] For a variety of reasons, this particular type of design, the pretest-posttest design with no control group, is very limited in providing evidence of a treatment effect; therefore, phrases such as "preliminary evidence" and "may decrease" are used when describing the results.

[e] The Wilcoxon signed ranks test is another alternative to the paired *t*-test. The sign test as described in this section only considers the direction of the change; the Wilcoxon signed ranks test takes into consideration the direction and magnitude of changes.[6] One advantage of the sign test in some situations is that it does not require actual measured values of the variable of interest; one would simply need to determine if the patient increased or decreased (or stayed the same) on the variable between the two time points. Yet another test for paired data, the McNemar test, is used for comparing dependent proportions (e.g., to test the null hypothesis that the proportion of patients at goal at baseline is equal to the proportion at goal post-treatment).

TABLE 10-5	Using Signs to Compare Baseline and Post-Treatment Measurements		
Patient ID	**Baseline Measure (A1C)**	**Post-Treatment Measure (A1C)**	**Sign for Change**
101	7.6	6.8	-
102	7.9	7.3	-
103	8.1	8.1	±
104	8.4	7.1	-
105	7.8	7.7	-
106	7.5	7.3	-
107	7.7	7.6	-
108	7.2	7.2	±
109	8.2	7.5	-
110	7.6	6.9	-

The data are from one group of patients ($n = 10$) tested at baseline and post-treatment. The sign represents the direction of the change in A1C values; a ± indicates no change.

presented in this chapter. Given the data in Table 10-5, eight patients had negative signs and the p-value for the sign test is $p = 0.008$, so the null hypothesis is rejected. Given this information, there is evidence that the patients who took part in the combined exercise and diet program significantly reduced their A1C levels from baseline to post-treatment.

THE WILCOXON–MANN–WHITNEY TEST[f]

Ordinal levels of measurement represent measurements that have an order, for example, from small to large, but do not have equal intervals between the scale values. Ordinal measures are derived by ranking the variable from low to high. For example, the measures of body weight for a group of 10 patients could be ranked from 1 to 10 based on the position of each patient's weight relative to other patients' weights. The data on A1C from the case study presented in Table 10-1 (assuming independent groups) are shown in **Table 10-6** with associated ranks. To obtain the ranks, the data are pooled into one group and numbered from lowest to highest.

When attempting to study differences between two independent groups on a variable that has an ordinal level of measurement (or when that variable is continuous, but heavily skewed with extreme observations), the **Wilcoxon–Mann–Whitney test** can be used. This test can be viewed as a potential alternative to the independent groups t-test under certain conditions. The basic null hypothesis associated with a Wilcoxon–Mann–Whitney test is that there is no difference in the distribution of the scores for

---

[f]Mann and Whitney and Wilcoxon both independently developed equivalent, yet differing versions, of this test; thus, in the literature it goes by the name the Wilcoxon rank-sum test and the Mann–Whitney U test. The Wilcoxon–Mann–Whitney test recognizes each of their contributions.[6] This nomenclature is an important consideration as statistical software may refer to the test by one name or the other. For example, IBM SPSS (New York, NY, USA) refers to the test as the Mann–Whitney U test while SAS (Cary, NC, USA) refers to the test as the Wilcoxon rank-sum test.

TABLE 10-6 Using Rank Order Data to Compare Groups

Patient ID	Exercise Group: A1C Levels	Rank Order:* Exercise Group	Patient ID	Comparison Group: A1C Levels	Rank Order:* Comparison Group
101	6.8	1	103	7.6	11
105	7.3	6.5	104	7.9	16
107	8.1	17.5	106	8.1	17.5
108	7.1	3	110	8.4	20
109	7.7	13.5	111	7.8	15
112	7.3	6.5	113	7.5	8.5
114	7.6	11	116	7.7	13.5
115	7.2	4.5	118	7.2	4.5
117	7.5	8.5	119	8.2	19
121	6.9	2	120	7.6	11
Sum of Ranks		74			136

The data shown are from independent groups—a treatment group and a comparison (usual care group); total $N = 20$; there are 10 patients in each group ($n_1 = n_2 = 10$). The data from both groups are pooled and the ranks assigned for the pooled group.

* Ties are a common problem when assigning ranks to data. A simple method of addressing the issue is to assign each of the tied ranks the mean of the ranks that would be next in the sequence. In the example, patient ID numbers 115 and 118 are tied for the 4th position with an A1C of 7.2; thus each received a rank of 4.5, or $(4+5)/2$. The next scores in rank order are patient ID numbers 105 and 112 with an A1C of 7.3. Because ranks 4 and 5 have already been assigned, these two observations are assigned a rank of 6.5, or $(6+7)/2$.

each group; there is no difference in the sum of the ranks for each group (with some additional assumptions, this procedure can be used to test whether two independent groups have equal medians).[1] For the example using A1C, the hypothesis is that exercise decreases A1C levels; hence, the sum of the ranks for the A1C values for the treatment group are expected to be lower than the sum of the ranks for the comparison group. To calculate a p-value, one can appeal to a specific tabled distribution (which can be found in most nonparametric statistics books[6]), or if the sample is large enough, one can use the normal distribution as an approximation.

Using a standard statistical software package, a p-value of 0.019 was calculated for the data in Table 10-6 using the Wilcoxon–Mann–Whitney test. Therefore, the null hypothesis can be rejected, indicating that the A1C levels for the exercise group are generally lower than those of the comparison group, a finding consistent with the results of the independent groups t-test reported earlier with the same data.

THE KRUSKAL–WALLIS TEST

The **Kruskal–Wallis test** can also be used with ordinal data; it extends the Wilcoxon–Mann–Whitney test to more than two groups when the groups are independent (which is why this test is sometimes referred to as the Kruskal–Wallis one-way analysis of variance by ranks). Again, the scores from both groups are pooled then ranked from lowest to highest and one can test the null hypothesis that the samples come from identical populations with the same median.[6] Thus, the null hypothesis is H_0: $median_A = median_B = median_C$. The formula for the Kruskal–Wallis test statistic is somewhat cumbersome, but p-values can easily be calculated by appealing to a specific tabled distribution or using the χ^2 (chi-square) distribution as an approximation with the degrees of freedom = number of groups − 1.

THE CONCEPT OF CORRELATION

Exercise is the main component of the intervention described in the case scenario to control diabetes and reduce A1C levels. Earlier analyses have shown that A1C values are reduced in the exercise group; however, one cannot determine from these earlier analyses if the response is associated with the amount of exercise—that is, whether the patients who exercised more had lower A1C levels. To answer this question, a bivariate technique to summarize the relationship between two continuous variables called the correlation coefficient can be used.

As a precursor to conducting an analysis of correlation, it is often helpful to display the relationship between the two variables using a **scatterplot**, which is a plot of paired values on each of the variables on a traditional Cartesian coordinate plane (meaning the graph has both X- and Y-axes). Examples of scatterplots can be found in **Figure 10-2**. Graph A demonstrates that as the value of the reference variable on the horizontal axis increases, the value of the second variable shown on the vertical axis also increases. When the value of one variable increases as the value of the second variable increases, the relationship between the two variables is described as a **positive relationship** or association. Graph B illustrates a **negative relationship**; that is, as the value of the reference variable on the horizontal axis increases, the value of the variable on the vertical axis decreases. Both Graphs A and B demonstrate *perfect linear* relationships, meaning all of the data points fall exactly on a straight line. Such perfect relationships will rarely, if ever, occur in practice with real data; real data tend to be messier (i.e., the points do not all fall exactly on a straight line, but rather the points may cluster around it). Chapter 11, "Simple and Multiple Linear Regression," demonstrates how to fit a

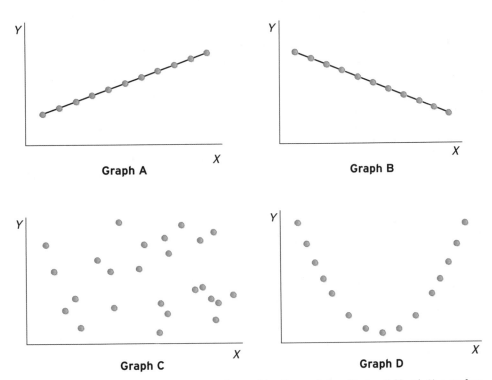

FIGURE 10-2   Scatterplots illustrating a perfect positive linear relationship ($r = 1$) (Graph A), a perfect negative linear relationship ($r = -1$) (Graph B), and no overall linear relationship ($r = 0$) (Graphs C and D).

straight-line equation to a set of such data points. Graph C illustrates a situation where the values of the variable on the horizontal axis do not seem to be linked at all to the values on the vertical axis; in other words, there is no apparent relationship between the X and Y variables. Graph D demonstrates a curved or nonlinear relationship between the values of the X variable and the values of the Y variable; X and Y are negatively related for smaller values of X but positively related for larger values of X.

THE PEARSON CORRELATION COEFFICIENT

If the variables are continuous as illustrated in the graphs in Figure 10-2 statistical procedures can be used to describe the amount of correspondence between the variables using the **Pearson correlation coefficient**, designated as r. The Pearson correlation is a measure of how two variables are *linearly* related.[7] It provides information about the strength and direction of the linear relationship between two continuous variables. The Pearson correlation coefficient varies between +1 and −1. A coefficient of +1 indicates a perfect positive linear relationship between the two variables (Graph A in Figure 10-2). If the correspondence is not perfect—that is many, *but not all*, of the large values of the second variable are paired with large values of the reference variable and many, *but not all*, of the small values of the second variable are paired with small values of the reference variable—the correlation will be positive, but no longer 1 (e.g., 0.8). As fewer and fewer of the values correspond, the value of the Pearson correlation coefficient (r) will decrease; for example, when $r = 0.1$, the linear correspondence between the two variables is small. Keep in mind that what constitutes a small or large correlation is subjectively defined and will vary according to the field of study and the nature of the variables under consideration.[8]

If, as in Graph B in Figure 10-2, the relationship between two variables is negative, the value of the Pearson correlation coefficient will be negative. A coefficient of −1 indicates that there is perfect negative linear correspondence between the two variables. Like positive correlation coefficients, negative coefficients with low values (e.g., −0.15) indicate that there is a small amount of linear correspondence between the values of the two variables. An r of 0 means that there is no overall linear relationship between two variables. Note that this can occur in more than one way. Both Graphs C and D in Figure 10-2 produce Pearson correlation coefficients of 0. Graph C suggests no apparent relationship between the two variables, whereas Graph D suggests a perfect nonlinear relationship. Thus, an $r = 0$ does not mean that two variables are unrelated or independent of each other, only that no linear relationship exists between the two variables. To the extent that the correspondence between the two variables is not linear—for example, represents a curvilinear relationship—the Pearson correlation coefficient will not accurately represent the correspondence between the two variables.

The formula for calculating a Pearson correlation coefficient is shown below.[1] Note that the mean of each variable, X and Y, is used in the calculation; consequently, Pearson's r should be used for data for which a mean can be calculated—that is, continuous data. However, the measurements do not need to be on the same scale; one scale could be height in inches and the other could be weight in pounds.

$$r = \frac{\sum_{i=1}^{n}(X_i - \overline{X})(Y_i - \overline{Y})}{\sqrt{\sum_{i=1}^{n}(X_i - \overline{X})^2 \sum_{i=1}^{n}(Y_i - \overline{Y})^2}}$$

The hypothesis related to correlation, like hypotheses discussed for differences between means or differences in proportions, considers random variation. One could expect that some values of two variables will correspond from random chance even when there is no relationship between the two variables. The hypothesis, then, concerns evaluating the probability of finding the study results or results of greater magnitude, given that there is no truly linear relationship between two variables. The null hypothesis related to a Pearson correlation coefficient could be stated as: The linear correspondence between the variables is zero or H_0: $\rho = 0$ (ρ is the lowercase Greek letter rho and is used by convention to represent the population correlation coefficient).

The test statistic used for the test of the null hypothesis is the t-statistic, shown here (yes, the same t-statistic used for the t-tests discussed above):

$$t = \frac{r\sqrt{n-2}}{\sqrt{1-r^2}}$$

When $\rho = 0$, this test statistic has a t-distribution with $n-2$ degrees of freedom. From this knowledge, a p-value can be calculated and compared to the significance level, α.

Data on the amount of exercise each patient in the study engaged in during the study were collected. The average number of minutes per week is shown for each patient in the right column of **Table 10-7**. The average time engaged in exercise varied from 50 minutes to 210 minutes per week. The post-treatment values for A1C are shown in the second column. As discussed above, correlations can be calculated between two variables, each of which is measured on a different scale. In the current example, one would expect to find a negative correlation, because increased exercise should produce lower A1C values.

The correlation hypothesis for this study could be stated as: There is no correlation between the quantity of exercise and A1C levels at the end of the study, or H_0: $\rho = 0$. As shown in Table 10-7, the calculated value for the Pearson correlation coefficient for this

TABLE 10-7	Data Used to Calculate the Correlation of A1C Levels with Minutes of Exercise	
Patient ID	**Post-Treatment A1C Levels**	**Exercise (average min/wk)**
101	6.8	150
102	7.3	140
103	8.1	50
104	7.1	170
105	7.7	125
106	7.3	150
107	7.6	180
108	7.2	132
109	7.5	90
110	6.9	210
Mean	7.35	139.7
Pearson's r	−0.72	
p-value	0.019	

Total $n = 10$; the correlation involves two different measures on each individual patient: A1C level and average minutes of exercise per week.

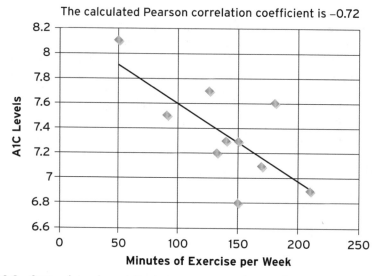

FIGURE 10-3 Scatterplot and correlation between average minutes of exercise per week and A1C levels.

group of 10 patients is $r = -0.72$. A graphic representation of the correlation between amount of exercise and blood sugar levels as represented by A1C levels is shown in **Figure 10–3**.

The graph clearly shows that the correlation is negative; that is, the more time patients engaged in exercise, the lower their A1C levels. The p-value associated with an r of -0.72 with $n = 10$ is 0.019, which is less than 0.05. Therefore, the null hypothesis of no linear correspondence between A1C and minutes of exercise can be rejected with a conclusion that there is evidence of a negative linear relationship between the amount of exercise and A1C levels.

THE SPEARMAN RANK CORRELATION COEFFICIENT

The **Spearman rank correlation coefficient**, r_s (note that the subscript s is used to differentiate the Spearman rank correlation coefficient from the Pearson correlation coefficient), is very similar to r; it measures the degree to which the values on a reference variable increase or decrease relative to the values on the second variable. Unlike r, though, r_s does not account for the amount of difference between the values; it only considers whether the rank of the second variable is higher or lower than the rank of the reference variable.[1] Because r_s is for ranked data (ordinal data), it can be used when the data on the two variables are not measured on an interval or ratio scale. If one variable is measured on a ratio or interval scale and the other variable is measured on an ordinal scale, then the variable measured on the ratio or interval scale must be transformed into ranks before calculating r_s.

A reasonable hypothesis is that the amount of exercise is negatively correlated with frequency of visits to the pharmacy; the more a patient exercises, the less often they visit the pharmacy. The two pharmacists in our case scenario have no objective data on frequency of pharmacy visits, but they both know the patients and know which patients visit the pharmacy most, and which least. Therefore, they rank patients based on the frequency of visits where 1 = the most visits and 10 = the least visits. The data are shown in **Table 10–8**.

Patient ID	Exercise (average min/wk)	Rank for Average Exercise	Rank for Frequency of Visits to Pharmacy	Difference (*d*) between Ranks	*d²*
101	150	6.5	4	2.5	6.25
102	140	5	9	−4	16
103	50	1	10	−9	81
104	170	8	7	1	1
105	125	3	8	−5	25
106	150	6.5	5	1.5	2.25
107	180	9	3	6	36
108	132	4	2	2	4
109	90	2	6	−4	16
110	210	10	1	9	81
Spearman r_s			−0.63		268.5

TABLE 10-8 Rank Data for Calculating r_s

The data are for 10 patients and there are two measurements on each patient: the average number of minutes of exercise per week and their rank for relative number of pharmacy visits. The data for average minutes of exercise per week is converted to ranks for calculation of r_s. The difference is calculated for each pair of ranks, then squared to calculate r_s.

When there are no tied ranks, the formula for r_s is:

$$r_s = 1 - \frac{6 \sum_{i=1}^{n} d_i^2}{n(n^2 - 1)},$$

where d_i is the difference between a pair of ranks

and n is the number of pairs of ranks.

There is correction to this formula when there are ties; however, one can simply calculate the Pearson r on the ranks (rather than raw data) even when there are ties and this approach will produce the Spearman rank correlation, r_s.[6] Like r, the value of r_s varies between −1 and +1; a negative correlation indicates that as one variable increases, the other decreases. Again, like r, values close to 0 indicate that there is little or no correspondence between the ranks of one variable and the second variable while values close to either −1 or +1 indicate a close correspondence between the ranks. The calculated r_s for the example is −0.63, indicating that there is a moderate negative correspondence between the average amount of exercise and the number of visits to the pharmacy—the number of pharmacy visits was negatively associated with amount of exercise.

As indicated above, r_s and r are very similar. The calculation of both measures of association is also readily available in standard statistical software packages. However, r_s can be used in situations when interval or ratio data are not available. In the example, the pharmacists had no data on frequency of visits but could rank the patients based on their knowledge of who visited the pharmacy most often, least often, and so on. Thus r_s allows one to statistically test a relationship when limited data are available. As demonstrated above, r_s can be used with interval and ratio data after transformation into ranks. Its use with this type of data is preferred when the variables of interest have skewed distributions because r_s is less sensitive to extreme values compared to r.

A FINAL NOTE ON CORRELATION

Establishing the relationship between independent and dependent variables of interest is an important step in the research process, but these relationships should be interpreted with caution. The methods for describing relationships in this section may indicate that the variables are correlated, but this relationship may not necessarily be causal. Correlation simply indicates that the independent and dependent variables are related to each other, whereas causality further asserts that the independent variable is the "cause" or explanation for the values of the dependent variable. Correlation (or association) is but one piece of evidence for a causal relationship; although necessary, correlation itself does not provide sufficient evidence to establish causality.

USING A FLOWCHART TO IDENTIFY THE APPROPRIATE STATISTICAL TEST FOR COMPARING GROUPS

The primary topic of this chapter has been calculating a test statistic and obtaining its corresponding p-value to test the null hypothesis of no difference between study groups. Several procedures can be used to test the null hypothesis of no difference, including independent groups t-test, paired t-test, ANOVA, chi-square test, sign test, Wilcoxon–Mann–Whitney test, and Kruskal–Wallis test. All of these statistical tests are included in the group of statistical tests used to make inferences concerning location or central tendency. The types of statistical tests included in this group are summarized in **Figure 10–4**.

The primary factors used to determine which statistical test to use are the

- independence or dependence of the groups (samples)
- level of measurement of the dependent (outcome) variable
- assumptions on which specific statistical tests are based

Groups are independent if the values on the measure in one group are in no way influenced by the values on the measure in the other group. If there are different people in each group, blood pressure readings in one group generally would not influence the blood pressure readings in the second group. In contrast, if the groups are dependent—for example, the same people are in both groups—then blood pressure levels in the second group will be influenced by the blood pressure levels in the first group.

The second factor that determines which statistical test to use is the level of measurement on the dependent or outcome variable. If the outcome variable is continuous, the mean or average for each group can be calculated, and a statistical test, i.e., a t-test or ANOVA, can be used to determine a p-value. If the outcome variable is categorical (or nominal), then a chi-square test can be used to calculate a p-value and test the null hypothesis.

The third factor that determines which statistical test to use is the assumptions on which the statistical tests are based. In general, there are two groups of statistical methods, **parametric methods** and **nonparametric methods**,[g] and each group has different assumptions. Although not always clear-cut, parametric tests are analysis methods

---

[g] Note that "parametric" and "nonparametric" are used to refer to analysis methods. The statistical test is nonparametric or parametric; one should not describe data as being parametric or nonparametric. Thus, the phrase "nonparametric data" should not be used.

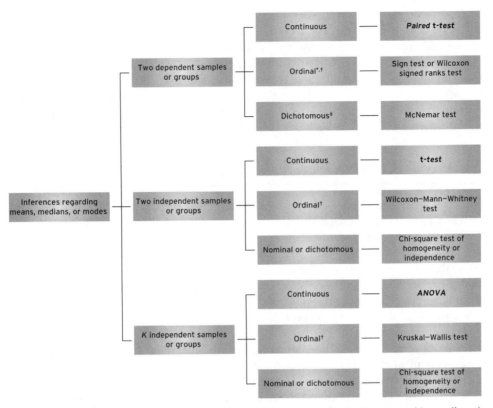

To use the flowchart, identify the study design (e.g., dependent samples or groups) and the level of measurement (e.g., continuous), and then identify the type of statistical test to use (e.g., paired *t*-test). Parametric tests make certain assumptions, such as the data are normally distributed and homogeneity of variance (e.g., the variances of the scores are equal in all comparison groups), and are identified in **bold and italicized** lettering.

*The data for the sign test can also be dichotomous, but there must be some order implied by the dichotomy (e.g., increased or decreased).

†The scale of measurement of the dependent variable can be ordinal or continuous (interval or ratio) and assumptions of an alternative parametric test, such as normality, are not reasonable.

‡The McNemar test is used when the outcome variable is dichotomous and the interest is in comparing two dependent proportions.

FIGURE 10-4 Flowchart for identifying appropriate statistical tests for comparing groups.

that attempt to test hypotheses that contain statements about population parameters (e.g., about populations means) and/or rely on assumptions about the specific nature of the sampled population (e.g., the variable on which the groups are being compared is normally distributed in each population). The parametric statistical methods are shown in **bold and italics** in Figure 10-4 and include the paired *t*-test, *t*-test, and ANOVA. In contrast, nonparametric statistical methods make few if any assumptions about the populations that generated the samples and/or focus on testing hypotheses that are not about specific population parameters. Hence, if the assumptions required for parametric tests cannot be met, one alternative is to use a nonparametric test. Nonparametric tests shown in Figure 10-4 include the McNemar test, sign test, Wilcoxon signed ranks test, chi-square test, Wilcoxon–Mann–Whitney test, and Kruskal–Wallis test.

The upper arm of the diagram displays the tests for paired samples or dependent groups when the dependent variable is measured at the nominal, ordinal, and continuous levels. For example, if investigators have a hypothesis of no difference between the means at baseline and post-treatment, they would follow the track in the paired samples arm through continuous measures to a paired *t*-test.

The center arm of the flowchart displays the statistical tests to use with two independent samples (groups) when the dependent variable is measured at the nominal, ordinal, or continuous levels. For example, if the null hypothesis stated that there were no differences in the means between the two groups, the track through the continuous level of measurement to the t-test would be followed.

The lower arm of the flowchart illustrates selection of a statistical test for more than two (K) independent samples. For continuous variables when the hypothesis is no difference between three or more means, the statistical test would be an ANOVA. The corresponding test for ordinal level data, or with continuous data when the assumption of normality is not tenable, such as a skewed distribution, is the Kruskal–Wallis test.

SUMMARY AND CONCLUSIONS

Bivariate analysis is used to describe methods for analyzing just two variables, such as when testing hypotheses when an experimental treatment is compared with a placebo or a comparison treatment to determine if the differences between the groups can be deemed to be statistically significant. Such analyses also include assessing the association between two variables, such as the Pearson correlation or the Spearman rank correlation. Although not comprehensive in nature, this chapter has attempted to introduce the reader to common bivariate analyses and illustrate these statistical methods with small data sets based on the questions from two pharmacists working in a community health center. The importance of considering study design issues, such as whether observations should be considered to be dependent or paired and the level of measurement of the outcome variable, in selecting an appropriate statistical test was demonstrated. Two general types of statistical methods were identified: parametric and nonparametric. The use of these tests to evaluate whether statements can be made concerning statistical significance of results by comparing a p-value to a stated significance level (α) was highlighted.

REVIEW QUESTIONS

1. Example dependent variables and study designs are listed in columns 1 and 2 in the table below. Identify the level of measurement for the dependent variable in column 3 and the appropriate statistical test in column 4.

Example Dependent Variable/Outcome	Study Design	Level of Measurement	Statistical Test
Difference in mean blood pressure level in two groups (e.g., 120 vs. 125 mmHg)	Independent groups (2)		
Difference in mean blood pressure level before and after an intervention (e.g., 120 vs. 125 mmHg)	Dependent groups (baseline vs. post-treatment)		
Difference in mean blood pressure level in three groups (e.g., 120 vs. 125 vs. 130)	Independent groups (3)		
Proportion at blood pressure goal in two groups (e.g., 10/20 vs. 3/20)	Independent groups (2)		

Example Dependent Variable/Outcome	Study Design	Level of Measurement	Statistical Test
The number of patients in a single group with increased/decreased BMI when comparing two time points	Dependent groups (baseline vs. post-treatment)		
Rank order of task completion in two groups	Independent groups (2)		

2. The formula for calculating the *t*-statistic from the independent groups *t*-test is presented below. Based on the formula, complete each statement below using the appropriate term: *increases* or *decreases*.

$$t = \frac{\left(\overline{X}_1 - \overline{X}_2\right)}{\sqrt{\dfrac{s_p^2}{n_1} + \dfrac{s_p^2}{n_2}}},$$

a) As the difference between the treatment mean ($\overline{X}_1$) and placebo mean ($\overline{X}_2$) increases, the value of the *t*-statistic _____ (increases or decreases) and the associated *p*-value _____ (increases or decreases).

b) As the standard deviation increases, the value of the *t*-statistic _____ (increases or decreases) and the associated *p*-value _____ (increases or decreases).

c) As the number of subjects in the sample increases, the value of the *t*-statistic _____ (increases or decreases) and the associated *p*-value _____ (increases or decreases).

3. If the difference between two proportions is 0, show why the risk ratio is 1.

ONLINE RESOURCES

quantpsy.org: http://www.quantpsy.org/chisq/chisq.htm (A user-friendly website for calculating chi-square tests without having to use the raw data.)

VassarStats: http://www.vassarstats.net/index.html (Another useful website.)

REFERENCES

1. Minium EW. *Statistical Reasoning in Psychology and Education*. 2nd ed. New York, NY: John Wiley & Sons; 1978.
2. Huck SW, Cormier WH, Bounds WG Jr. *Reading Statistics and Research*. New York, NY: Harper & Row; 1974.
3. Daniel WW. *Biostatistics: A Foundation for Analysis in the Health Sciences*. 8th ed. Hoboken, NJ: John Wiley & Sons; 2005.
4. Agresti A. *An Introduction to Categorical Data Analysis*. 2nd ed. Hoboken, NJ: John Wiley & Sons; 2007.
5. Rothman KJ. *Epidemiology: An Introduction*. New York, NY: Oxford University Press; 2002.
6. Siegel S, Castellan NJ. *Nonparametric Statistics for the Behavioral Sciences*. 2nd ed. New York, NY: McGraw-Hill; 1988.
7. Last JM. *A Dictionary of Epidemiology*. 4th ed. New York, NY: Oxford University Press; 2001.
8. Wassertheil-Smoller S. *Biostatistics and Epidemiology: A Primer for Health Professionals*. 2nd ed. New York, NY: Springer-Verlag; 1995.

11

SIMPLE AND MULTIPLE LINEAR REGRESSION

DAN FRIESNER, PhD

JOHN P. BENTLEY, PhD

CHAPTER OBJECTIVES

▸ Identify and describe situations where a research design is not amenable to bivariate statistical analysis

▸ Define and describe the causes (i.e., confounders, omitted variables, mediators, effect modifiers) and consequences (i.e., bias or inefficiency) of inappropriately using bivariate statistical analysis

▸ Explain how linear regression is commonly used in the drug literature to account for these causes and consequences

▸ Describe and appropriately interpret the coefficient estimates and predictions produced by linear regression

▸ Describe how the coefficient estimates and predictions produced by linear regression, when properly interpreted, can be used to evaluate a research hypothesis

KEY TERMINOLOGY

Biased
Bivariate linear regression
Coefficient estimates
Confounder
Confounding effect
Dummy variables
Effect modification
Effect modifier

Inefficient
Interaction
Linear regression
Mediating effect
Mediator
Moderator
Moderator effect
Multiple linear regression

Omitted variable
Ordinary least squares (OLS)
Residual
R-squared (R^2)
Simple linear regression

INTRODUCTION

In an ideal experimental setting, a researcher has complete control over study design and implementation. This complete control over the experiment allows the researcher to anticipate and account for potential sources of bias that might affect the outcome of the experiment. Once all major sources of bias have been identified and accounted for, the remaining sources of error can be adjusted for in a traditional randomized controlled trial (RCT). These can include minor variability in laboratory methods and measurement errors in the resulting data. Random sampling methodologies, as well as the random assignment of patients to treatment and control groups, are sufficient to ensure that these minor differences "average out" across the groups and do not bias or otherwise influence the results of the experiment. As a result, experimental data can be used to statistically test the researcher's null hypothesis in a fairly straightforward manner.

Unfortunately, in many practical settings, the researcher does not have full control over the design of a study. For example, many types of observational studies use secondary data like administrative claims previously collected by third-party payers for non-research purposes.[1] Similarly, in certain types of clinical studies, ethical considerations prohibit researchers from employing randomization or conducting experiments.[2] Third, some research must be collected through survey techniques, where study participants may not be willing or able to respond to all questions posed by a researcher.[3] Without the ability to control the study design to adjust for possible biases inherent in these designs, it is difficult to argue that the results add anything substantial to the current states of knowledge and clinical practice. This is problematic, given the wide array of topics and issues in clinical and administrative pharmacy practice that can *only* be investigated using observational study designs.

The approach used by most clinical and academic researchers in these instances is to apply more sophisticated methods of statistical analysis to data that are derived from partially controllable or non-controllable experiments. Statisticians also refer to these types of experiments as *natural experiments*, because the researcher must take some or all of the experimental design as given, or as a "state of nature."[4,5] The logic behind the analysis of natural experiments is to attempt to identify all possible sources of bias that might occur in the study. One subsequently collects data on both the performance of the control and test groups (although the independent variable of interest does not have to be a nominal grouping variable—it can be a continuous variable), as well as these possible sources of bias. The potential sources of bias are included in the statistical analysis and used to adjust for (or hold constant) any unwanted effects. Thus, any potential sources of bias are removed statistically, or "averaged out" in much the same manner that randomization accounts for minor sources of bias in an RCT. The common methods of statistical analysis that are used to account for these sources of bias are generally known as "regression analysis." This chapter provides an introduction to regression analysis, and more specifically **linear regression** analysis, as it is used in clinical research. It provides a brief discussion of bias and inefficiency that may result from bivariate analyses and introduces simple linear regression. The chapter concludes with a discussion of multiple linear regression with a demonstration of how this statistical method can be used to account for some of the potential problems associated with bivariate analyses.

CASE SCENARIO

Consider the study analyzed by Willems and Saunders[6] (as well as a related study by Schorling and colleagues[7]), who used interview and community-based participatory research methods to examine the prevalence of type II diabetes (hereafter, diabetes) and cardiovascular disease (CVD) among African Americans in two rural Virginia (Buckingham and Louisa) counties. The research team interviewed 1,046 subjects and successfully screened 403 individuals for diabetes and CVD. The raw data are available at http://biostat.mc.vanderbilt.edu/wiki/Main/DataSets. After eliminating observations with missing values,[a] the data set contains 366 observations. This reduced sample will be used in the chapter as a simple context in which to explore regression analysis. Diabetes is typically diagnosed using glycosylated hemoglobin (A1C), with higher levels indicating the onset of diabetes.[6] It is also generally hypothesized that obesity, as measured by the ratio of the waist (in inches) to the hip (in inches), is an accurate predictor of diabetes.[6] As discussed in Chapter 10, "Bivariate Analysis and Comparing Groups," it is possible to examine the magnitude and the statistical significance of the Pearson correlation coefficient between the two variables of interest, which in this case is 0.2157 (p-value <0.0001). This relationship can also be expressed graphically via a two-dimensional scatter plot, as shown in **Figure 11-1A**.

Clearly, the relationship between the two variables is positive. Assuming that the researcher has performed the calculations correctly, there is nothing inherently invalid about Figure 11-1A from a *purely statistical* perspective. The problem of bias occurs when the researcher attempts to *interpret* the statistical result *within the context of her/his own discipline or practice setting*. For example, many clinical and health services researchers would argue that the relationship expressed in Figure 11-1A is misleading because it attempts to express a relationship between obesity and the onset of diabetes in an oversimplified manner. Examples of this oversimplification include, but are not limited to, the following:

1. There are other, alternative methods to measure obesity. For example, one could use the body mass index (or BMI) as a measure of obesity.
2. Waist and hip circumferences depend on body frames. People who are naturally larger in stature will exhibit fundamentally different waist-hip ratios and if body

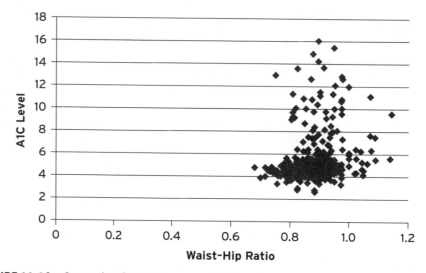

FIGURE 11-1A   Scatterplot of A1C level versus waist-hip ratio.

---

[a] There is substantial literature dealing with missing data, including missing data mechanisms and methods for addressing the presence of missing data (for more information, see Enders[8]). To simplify the case scenario used in this chapter, the relatively simple approach known as a complete-case analysis was used.

3. Males tend to be larger in stature than females, so if stature matters, gender might also matter in explaining A1C levels.
4. The study examines African Americans in two rural counties in Virginia. The relationship between A1C levels and waist–hip ratio may be fundamentally different in other geographic areas (i.e., urban areas or other rural areas of the United States) or among different socioeconomic structures (i.e., among Hispanic or Asian populations).

frame is also related to A1C, then failing to account for it in an analysis may give the wrong impression about the waist–hip ratio and A1C relationship.

OMITTED VARIABLES, CONFOUNDERS, BIAS, AND EFFICIENCY

These four items help illustrate several terms that researchers typically use to critique studies involving observational studies. The first and most general terms are **confounder** and **omitted variable**. In its global usage, a confounder is any factor that prevents the researcher from directly and appropriately interpreting a statistical result within the practical context of the study.[9] An omitted variable is a specific and observable factor, but is omitted from the analysis.[4,5] Note that the term *confounder* is a broader term than an omitted variable, since a confounder could be an omitted variable, but it could also reflect a flaw in the study's design. The decision to study patients in two rural Virginia counties could represent lack of generalizability, without necessarily being construed as an omitted variable. On the other hand, a failure to account for a participant's gender would be both an omitted variable and a confounder.

The presence of a confounder (whether an omitted variable or otherwise) in a study typically causes the study to provide results that may differ in direction, magnitude, and practical interpretation from an otherwise similar study that has accounted for the confounding effect. For example, if the researcher omits the variable from the analysis, the study will generate an estimate that on average is fundamentally different than the population parameter that one is trying to estimate. In the language of statistics, such sample estimates are said to be **biased**.[4,5] On the other hand, if the researcher adjusts for the confounder statistically, the sample estimates should be very similar to the population parameter being estimated; in such cases, the estimate is said to be unbiased. The difference between the average confounded sample estimate and the non-confounded population parameter is an estimate of the *magnitude of the bias*. Henceforth, all references to the term "bias" refer to the statistical definition, rather than the vernacular use of the term.

If adjusting for the confounder leads to changes in any estimate of variation (usually a reduction in the standard deviation or standard error), then any results obtained without adjusting for confounding (usually exhibiting higher levels of variation) are said to be **inefficient**.[4,5] The *amount of inefficiency* is essentially the difference between the two measures of variation with and without adjusting for confounder effects.

Researchers are often interested in the relationship between two variables, a primary independent variable and a dependent variable. The consideration of other variables may alter the interpretation and meaning of the relationship between these two variables. Failure to appropriately handle these other variables in the analysis may impact or otherwise generate biased or inefficient results. In many instances, there are three common explanations. The first is generally known as a **confounding effect**, and the variable that produces the effect is known as a confounder. Thus, the term *confounder* has both a global meaning, as described earlier, and a more specific connotation, as used here. A confounder is a variable that when accounted for in an analysis leads to a meaningfully different interpretation of the relationship between the primary independent variable and the dependent variable compared to when the confounding variable is ignored in or excluded from the analysis.[10] In the present example, consider a variable indicating the person's stature as a potential confounder. Confounding would be present if the estimate of the relationship between A1C and waist–hip ratio is substantially different depending on whether or not stature is considered as a predictor of A1C together with waist–hip ratio. Thus, if a researcher can account for how large the person is naturally, it is possible to interpret the relationship between A1C and the waist–hip ratio more appropriately. More information on the concept of confounding can be found in Chapter 5, "Cohort and Case-Control Studies."

The second explanation is known as **effect modification**, and any variable that produces a modifying effect is known as an **effect modifier**.[11] In other areas of research, effect modification is known as a **moderator effect** and the variable that produces the effect is called a **moderator**.[12] An effect modifier alters the strength and/or direction of the relationship between the independent variable and the dependent variable.[13] Thus, the relationship between the independent variable of interest and the dependent variable depends on the values of a third variable, the effect modifier. An example of an effect modifier is when different subgroups respond differently to a treatment. In the present example, consider the county of residence of the participants. There may be fundamentally different sociocultural and economic factors across the two counties in this study. If diets, lifestyles, and genetic predispositions are fundamentally different across the two counties, one might expect to see corresponding differences in the A1C and waist–hip ratio relationship between the two counties (e.g., the relationship may be stronger in one county compared to the other). In clinical trials, effect modifiers typically occur when people in different age groups like the elderly respond fundamentally differently to a drug than other age groups like young adults.

The third explanation is known as a **mediating effect**, and the variable that produces the effect is known as a **mediator**.[13] A mediator is similar to a confounder in that, if you can account for the mediator in the analysis, it is possible to interpret the relationship between the independent variable of interest and the dependent variable more appropriately. The difference between a confounder and a mediator is that a confounder is not an intermediate variable in a causal pathway, whereas a mediator attempts to link the primary independent variable and the dependent variable.[12] In other words, a mediation model can be used to assess whether a primary independent variable leads to changes on another variable (mediator), which in turn causes changes on the main dependent (outcome) variable. Consider the potential role of systolic blood pressure (SBP) in the relationship between measures of obesity (waist–hip ratios and BMI) and the occurrence of cardiovascular disease (CVD). Obesity (as signified by higher waist–hip ratios and greater BMI) leads to higher SBP, which in turn leads to greater CVD risk. Such a finding suggests that obesity increases CVD risk partly through its effect on other risk factors, such as SBP. Accounting for this mediating effect affects the accuracy and precision of any empirical results because doing so provides more information about the causal nature of the relationship between the variables being analyzed.

It is important to note that in any single analysis, any combination or permutation of these potential sources of error may be present. Confounders, effect modifiers, and mediators may exist independently or simultaneously. One may have confounders, moderators, mediators, all, or none. While there are statistical methods available to test for the presence of each of these, there is no substitute for using common and clinical sense for appropriately adjusting and accounting for these effects. Each of these effects arises not in the application of statistical methods, but in the interpretation of the results within a practical context. It is therefore important for researchers and clinicians to have a solid understanding of clinical practice, identify errors of omission and commission, and adjust for them accordingly. At the very least, such issues should be discussed as limitations in the resulting manuscript. For clinicians, the ability to identify the presence of these effects can be valuable in determining whether the study findings can be applied to practice.

The confounding effect will be discussed and demonstrated after considering some basic principles of linear regression. The moderator effect (effect modification) and the concept of statistical interaction also will be briefly explored, building on the multiple regression model. However, the analysis of mediating effects is not discussed in this chapter; for more information on statistical mediation, see MacKinnon.[12]

SIMPLE LINEAR REGRESSION

An examination of Figure 11-1A provides a simple and straightforward means to introduce regression analysis, specifically linear[b] regression analysis with a single independent variable, referred to as **simple linear regression** (also called **bivariate linear regression**). Suppose for simplicity that obesity, as measured by the waist–hip ratio, causes elevated A1C levels, and thus drives the onset of diabetes. Thus, waist–hip ratio is the independent variable (sometimes called a predictor variable or regressor) and A1C is the dependent variable (sometimes called the response variable or outcome variable). In this case, it is appropriate to place the waist–hip ratio on the horizontal axis of Figure 11-1A and A1C levels on the vertical axis. Suppose now that one is interested in identifying how small changes in the average patient's level of obesity increase the likelihood of developing diabetes. Empirically, how does a slight increase (or decrease) in waist–hip ratio, on average, increase (decrease) patient A1C levels?

The most straightforward means to characterize this relationship is to draw a linear trend or regression line through the middle of the data in the scatterplot, as shown in **Figure 11-1B**. Like all linear trend or regression lines, the equation for the line can be characterized using a slope and an intercept; that is, $Y = b_0 + b_1 X$, where Y indicates the dependent variable on the Y-axis, X indicates the independent variable on the X-axis, b_0 is (an estimate of) the equation's intercept and b_1 is (an estimate of) the slope. The slope of the line is especially interesting to the researcher because it characterizes the relationship (or *marginal effect*)[4,5,14] of waist–hip ratio (X) on A1C levels (Y). The relationship between

---

[b] *Linear* refers to the fact that the resulting equation is linear in the regression coefficients (i.e., the *b* coefficients as defined later in the chapter). This means that the independent variables are multiplied by the regression coefficients and then these products are summed to calculate a predicted score on the dependent variable. There are no restrictions on how the independent variables and the dependent variable are defined. Linear regression can be used to capture nonlinear (e.g., curvilinear) relationships between variables using a special case of linear regression called polynomial regression or by transforming the independent and/or dependent variables prior to analysis (e.g., taking the natural log of the variables). For more information see Wooldridge,[4] Stock and Watson,[5] and Kleinbaum et al.[10]

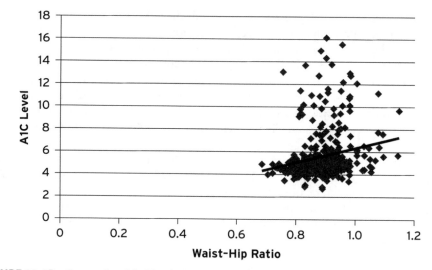

FIGURE 11-1B   Scatterplot of A1C level versus waist-hip ratio.

each individual observation and the trend line, or the measure of how far above or below the trend line each participant in the study is, can be measured by the vertical distance between each data point and the trend line. This is known as the (estimated) *error term*, or **residual**. Individuals whose data points lie above the trend line have positive (estimated) errors, while those below the trend line have negative (estimated) errors. Since regression produces estimates that reflect mean values, the sum of all residuals in the data set will automatically be zero. Mathematically, the equation governing the scatterplot is given by the following:[14]

$$Y_i = b_0 + b_1 X_i + u_i \tag{1}$$

where $i = 1, \ldots, n$ indexes each of the n observations (in this case, people) in the sample of data; Y represents each patient's A1C reading; X represents each patient's waist-hip ratio; and u is the error term. As noted earlier, the first part of the equation ($Y_i = b_0 + b_1 X_i$) essentially gives an estimate of the equation for the trend line, while the u_i depicts how each individual observation in the data set relates to the trend line. Because the trend line reflects the mean value in the data set, it also implies that $\sum_{i=1}^{n} u_i = 0$; that is, all positive values for u will offset the negative values.

Regression analysis is the process of specifying and estimating these trend lines. **Ordinary least squares (OLS)** is the simplest form of estimation for regression analysis, in that it assumes that the variable on the Y-axis of the scatterplot is a continuous variable. To estimate b_0 and b_1 (the **coefficient estimates**), it is necessary to solve a calculus problem.[14] More specifically, OLS seeks to choose the value of b_0 and b_1 to make the sum of the squared values of the residual u_i as small as possible.

$$\text{minimize}_{b_0, b_1} \sum_{i=1}^{n} (u_i)^2$$

$$\text{or} \tag{2}$$

$$\text{minimize}_{b_0, b_1} \sum_{i=1}^{n} (Y_i - b_0 - b_1 X_i)^2$$

In other words, OLS chooses the values for the slope and the intercept to ensure that the trend line is set as close to the middle of the data in the scatterplot as possible without overestimating or underestimating the equation of the line. In the case of a single variable on the X-axis (i.e., a single independent variable, or a single regressor), OLS estimates the intercept and slopes via the following equations:

$$b_1 = \frac{\sum_{i=1}^{n}\left[\left(X_i - \overline{X}\right)\left(Y_i - \overline{Y}\right)\right]}{\sum_{i=1}^{n}\left(X_i - \overline{X}\right)^2} \tag{3}$$

$$b_0 = \overline{Y} - b_1 \overline{X} \tag{4}$$

where $\overline{X}$ represents the sample mean for the independent variable (in this case, the waist–hip ratio) and $\overline{Y}$ represents the sample mean for the dependent variable (in this case, the A1C level). Although researchers generally rely on statistical software to perform these calculations rather than using these formulas, an appreciation of the complexity of these calculations, and the computing power necessary to produce them, is warranted. **Table 11–1** displays the results of the regression equation estimated using Microsoft Excel's Analysis Tool Pack (Microsoft Corporation, Redmond, WA). The estimated intercept of the line is −0.1011 while the estimated slope is 6.4774.

TABLE 11-1 Simple Linear Regression Results

SUMMARY OUTPUT

Regression Statistics						
Multiple *R*	0.2157					
R-Squared	0.0465					
Adjusted *R*-Squared	0.0439					
Standard Error	2.1815					
Observations	366					

ANOVA						
	df	*SS*	*MS*	*F*	p-*value*	
Regression	1	84.5280	84.5280	17.7612	<0.0001	
Residual	364	1732.3296	4.7591			
Total	365	1816.8576				

	Coefficients	*Standard Error*	*t-statistic*	p-*value*	*95% Confidence Limits*	
Intercept	−0.1011	1.3593	−0.0744	0.9407	−2.7742	2.5719
whratio	6.4774	1.5370	4.2144	<0.0001	3.4550	9.4999

whratio = waist-hip ratio

Examining Table 11-1 yields several additional features of linear regression with OLS estimation. First, because both the slope and intercept estimates are based on a sample of data, there is inherently some measure of variation attached to each estimate. OLS estimates these measures as standard errors. Second, assuming (1) that the data has been collected appropriately as a random sample; (2) that the distribution for the error term can be approximated by a normal distribution; and (3) that the equation is properly specified, the distribution for each parameter estimate can also be shown to be closely approximated by a normal distribution (and exactly specified by Student's *t*-distribution). This allows the researcher to apply simple *t*-tests to the slope and intercept to test hypotheses of interest to the study.[14] The formula for the test statistic is given by:

$$t = \frac{b - \beta_{H_0}}{SE_b} \tag{5}$$

where b represents the regression coefficient estimate produced by OLS (either b_0 or b_1); SE_b is the estimated standard error produced by OLS for b; and β_{H_0} is the statement about the value of the corresponding population parameter specified under the null hypothesis. The degrees of freedom for the test is $n - k$, where n is the number of observations in the data set and k (in this case, 2) is the number of slope and intercept parameter estimates. From this knowledge, a *p*-value can be calculated for the test. The most common hypothesis test applied in any regression analysis is:

$$H_0 : \beta = 0$$
$$H_A : \beta \neq 0 \tag{6}$$

Under this hypothesis test, the value for β_{H_0} in equation (5) is zero. Intuitively, a value for zero as specified under the null hypothesis, and applied to the slope estimate b_1, suggests that there *is no linear relationship* between the variables X and Y. In practical terms, this null hypothesis implies that *there is no causal link between obesity (as measured by the waist-hip ratio) and the presence of diabetes (as measured by A1C levels)*. A rejection of this null hypothesis in favor of the alternative suggests (with a significance level previously specified by the researcher, such as $\alpha = 0.05$) that there is a linear relationship between these two variables. Examining Table 11-1, the large *t*-statistic value (4.2144) and correspondingly small *p*-value (less than $\alpha = 0.05$) indicate that the null hypothesis for the slope estimate b_1 can be rejected.

Once the coefficient's statistical significance has been established, the magnitude of the slope, 6.4774, can be interpreted in a practical, clinical context. In linear regression, coefficient estimates are interpreted as marginal effects.[4,5,14] This implies that for every small, one-unit change in the waist-hip ratio, the mean A1C level increases or decreases by 6.4774 units. Thus, if the waist-hip ratio increases by 0.001, the A1C level increases by 0.0064774 units (or 0.001*6.4774).

Another feature of linear regression with OLS estimation is that it provides several very simple and intuitive links to basic descriptive statistics. For example, suppose that the true population value for b_1 (or β_1) is exactly equal to zero. According to equation (4), $b_0 = \overline{Y} + 0\overline{X} = \overline{Y}$. That is, when there are no independent variables included in the regression (or when they are all statistically no different from zero, and do not predict the dependent variable), OLS provides an intercept estimate that is equal to the sample mean of the dependent variable (A1C levels). In addition, if the researcher applies the basic hypothesis test specified in equation (6) to the slope estimate (b_1) and the null hypothesis is rejected, this implies that the linear regression model provides valuable information over and above simple descriptive statistics and hypothesis tests conducted using those descriptive statistics.[14]

A final feature of linear regression is that it attempts to explain the amount of variation in the dependent variable, Y. In OLS estimation, the error term can be used to measure the relative degree with which the regression model predicts changes in the dependent variable (A1C levels). This is also known as "assessing the OLS model's fit." If the regression provides valuable information over and above simple descriptive statistics, then the regression model should account for a large portion of the total variation in the dependent variable. Using the example, variation in waist-hip ratios should explain a large portion of the variation in A1C levels. Mathematically, this relationship can be expressed as **R-squared (R^2)**. The measure of R^2 must take values between 0 and 1. As R^2 approaches 0, the regression explains very little variation in the dependent variable (Y). If the regression explains the dependent variable well, then the R^2 approaches 1.

R^2 is a useful measure of overall model fit for several reasons. First, it is intuitive. It is simply the proportion of total variation that the OLS linear regression model explains, with higher values indicating that OLS does a better job of predicting the dependent variable, and lower values indicating that OLS does a worse job of explaining the dependent variable. Second, OLS can be interpreted within the context of descriptive statistics. One can actually demonstrate that (in the case of a single independent variable, X) the R^2 is simply the square of the bivariate (Pearson) correlation coefficient; that is, $R^2 = (r_{XY})^2$.[14] Third, the R^2 measure can be interpreted within the context of the scatterplot depicted in Figure 11-1A. When OLS produces a regression with a high R^2 value, all of the data points are very tightly clustered around the trend or regression line. At the extreme case where $R^2 = 1$, all data points lie *exactly on* the trend line. This makes the values for the residual (the u_i's) very close to zero, both individually and collectively, and the R^2 close to one. When the R^2 is closer to zero, most of the data are scattered across the plot far away from the trend line, which makes the u_i's very large. Some might ask how large should R^2 be when evaluating model fit? Unfortunately, there is not an easy answer to this question. Rather, it depends on the application. Some suggest that regressions are considered excellent model fits when the R^2 value is in excess of 0.66, moderate fits for R^2 values between 0.33 and 0.66, and poor fits for R^2 values below 0.33 (i.e., explains less than one-third of the variation in the dependent variable). However, there are situations where an R^2 less than 0.33 can be considered acceptable. Note that the R^2 value produced by the regression in Table 11-1 is 0.0465, which implies that the regression model exhibits relatively poor fit.

MULTIPLE LINEAR REGRESSION

GENERAL FEATURES

The use of regression analysis provides researchers analyzing observational data with a simple and straightforward means to address possible confounders. Consider first those confounders that can be addressed by collecting information on one or more omitted variables. As an example in the Willems diabetes study,[6] suppose that the researcher collected data on the body frames of each study participant (variable Z). If the variable Z

can somehow be incorporated into the regression model, then any statistical bias or inefficiency that results from failing to include Z would be eliminated, since the researcher has adjusted, or controlled, for this variable in the empirical analysis. As such, variables such as Z are frequently referred to as *control variables*.[14,15]

Mathematically, control variables are added to the model through the error term or residual. In equation (1), the residuals (u_i's) effectively incorporate all sources of variation in the dependent variable (Y, or A1C levels) that are not captured by the primary regressor(s) (X, or the waist-hip ratio). Hence, any omitted variable is automatically included in the residuals. But if data are collected on the omitted variable Z, the effect of the variable Z can be separated from the residual by incorporating the variable in the equation for the trend or regression line. Specifically, let

$$u_i = b_2 Z_i + \varepsilon_i \tag{7}$$

where b_2 is a coefficient estimate and ε is another residual with characteristics that are similar to those of u. All other notation remains the same. Also note that, since the sum (and mean) of all of the u_i's is zero, there is no need to specify an intercept for this equation. Substituting equation (7) into equation (1), it follows that:

$$Y_i = b_0 + b_1 X_i + u_i$$

$$\text{or} \tag{8}$$

$$Y_i = b_0 + b_1 X_i + b_2 Z_i + \varepsilon_i$$

This incorporation of the effects of the variable Z in equation (8) is known as a **multiple linear regression** equation, since the right-hand side of the equation contains more than one regressor. Multiple regression is also called multivariable analysis, multivariable adjustment, or multivariable modeling.[16] With only two regressors, X and Z, equation (8) could be represented as a three-dimensional scatterplot, and the trend line $Y_i = b_0 + b_1 X_i + b_2 Z_i$ becomes a plane instead of a line.[14,15]

The frame variable (Z) is described as a confounder, in that understanding the body frames of the study participants can help to more appropriately interpret the relationship between the waist-hip ratio and A1C levels. If the estimates from equation (8) inclusive of (Z) are compared with the estimates in equation (1), then the coefficient estimate and standard error for the waist-hip ratio changes. This is because we have held constant, or controlled for, the effects of the confounding variable, and the interpretation of the regression coefficient for waist-hip variable takes that into account. In equation (1), the estimate b_1 reflects the marginal impact of a small change in the waist-hip ratio (X) on A1C levels. In equation (8), the estimate b_1 reflects the marginal impact of a small change in the waist-hip ratio (X) on A1C levels, *holding constant, or controlling for, the specified confounding variables*. Assuming there is some theoretical and/or clinical rationale for the variable Z to be included as a control variable, the difference in magnitude between the two measures provides an approximation of the magnitude of the bias that occurs due to the omission of a confounder.

Generally, a regression equation contains many potential omitted variables that must be accounted for to produce unbiased estimates. Hence, it may be necessary to separate the effects of many control variables in equation (7):

$$u_i = b_2 Z_i + b_3 W_i + \ldots + b_k V_i + \varepsilon_i \tag{7b}$$

where b_2, b_3, . . . ,b_k depict additional slope (or regression coefficient) estimates for each control variable; Z, W, . . . , V represent the required control variables; and the remaining terminology is as described previously. This, in turn, leads to a more complicated (but theoretically and/or clinically appropriate) specification of equation (8):

$$Y_i = b_0 + b_1 X_i + b_2 Z_i + b_3 W_i + \ldots + b_k V_i + \varepsilon_i \tag{8b}$$

As the specification of (8) becomes more complicated, it is important to understand the consequences of the new specification on OLS parameter estimates. First, it is difficult (and visually unappealing) to present scatterplots that have more than three dimensions. Hence, in multiple regression, trend lines and other empirical results are commonly presented as equations and tables of parameter estimates, rather than scatter plots. Second, while the interpretation of each slope estimate can be interpreted as a marginal effect, one must note that the effect is based on holding constant all other control variables in the model. Hence, the interpretation of b_1 would be *the marginal impact of a one-unit change in the waist-hip ratio* (X) *on A1C levels* (Y), *holding all other specified regressors (predictors) in the model constant.* Third, the mechanics underlying the calculation of the slope and intercept estimates becomes more complicated. As a result, the solutions for each b estimate become much more complicated than what is expressed in equations (3) and (4). Standard computer packages (including SPSS, SAS, and Microsoft Excel's Analysis ToolPak feature) can easily conduct multiple regression analyses with nearly as much speed as a simple regression, and report the results in an identical fashion, including estimated standard errors for each slope/intercept estimate. Fourth, individual t-tests can be applied to specific parameter estimates in a manner that is identical to the simpler form of linear regression discussed previously.

Multiple regression also requires the researcher to develop two new metrics to assess the overall "fit" of the regression equation. The first is an adaptation of the R^2 measure. In multiple regression, the R^2 becomes less useful as a measure of model fit for two reasons. One is that, with the addition of more than one control variable, the R^2 is no longer the simple square of the Pearson correlation coefficient between Y and X. Second, the R^2 is a limited measure in that anytime a new control variable is added to the equation, the R^2 will *always* increase, whether or not the variable is clinically or practically meaningful. In the diabetes example, one would expect the model to predict A1C levels more accurately if a variable such as participant's body mass index (BMI) were included in the model, and thus the R^2 should increase by a considerable amount if BMI were added as a control variable. On the other hand, the R^2 would increase (albeit by a smaller amount) if an irrelevant variable were added to the model, for example, the distance in miles from the participant's home to the nearest U.S. Post Office.

To account for these limitations, researchers have developed what is known as the adjusted R^2, or $\overline{R}^2$.[14–17] This measure adapts the R^2 formula by adding a penalty for each extra parameter that is added to the model. Thus, the $\overline{R}^2$ measure forces a trade-off between the complexity of the model (as measured by the number of regressors) and the gain in model fit (R^2) that those regressors provide. Adding regressors will always increase the R^2, and the R^2 will always be at least as large as the $\overline{R}^2$. A large difference in magnitude between the R^2 and $\overline{R}^2$ may indicate the presence of one or more superfluous regressors in the model. Smaller differences indicate that each regressor in the model contributes some useful amount of statistical information to the model.

Table 11-2 uses the diabetes data to estimate an example of a multiple regression model using a variety of additional regressors, including the patient's total cholesterol level (*chol*), county of residence (*Buckingham*), age (*age*), gender (*female*), BMI (*bmi*), body frames (*small* and *large*, respectively), systolic blood pressure (*bp.1s*), and diastolic blood pressure (*bp.1d*). Note several interesting changes in the model as these additional regressors were added to the regression. First, the R^2 increased from 0.0465 to 0.1798. Additionally, the $\overline{R}^2$ takes a value of 0.1567, which is very close in magnitude to the R^2.

TABLE 11-2 Multiple Linear Regression Results

SUMMARY OUTPUT

Regression Statistics	
Multiple R	0.4240
R-Squared	0.1798
Adjusted R-Squared	0.1567
Standard Error	2.0488
Observations	366

ANOVA

	df	SS	MS	F	p-value
Regression	10	326.6894	32.6689	7.7827	<0.0001
Residual	355	1490.1682	4.1977		
Total	365	1816.8576			

Variable	Coefficients	Standard Error	t-statistic	p-value	95% Confidence Limits	
Intercept	−1.3633	1.6473	−0.8276	0.4085	−4.6030	1.8764
whratio	2.5881	1.6978	1.5244	0.1283	−0.7509	5.9271
chol	0.0099	0.0026	3.8129	0.0002	0.0048	0.0150
Buckingham	0.2699	0.2224	1.2136	0.2257	−0.1675	0.7074
age	0.0318	0.0082	3.8815	0.0001	0.0157	0.0480
Female	−0.2104	0.2603	−0.8083	0.4195	−0.7224	0.3016
bmi	0.0405	0.0200	2.0190	0.0442	0.0010	0.0799
small	−0.0551	0.2791	−0.1976	0.8435	−0.6040	0.4937
large	−0.1125	0.2956	−0.3805	0.7038	−0.6938	0.4688
bp.1s	0.0065	0.0069	0.9485	0.3435	−0.0070	0.0201
bp.1d	−0.0104	0.0107	−0.9729	0.3313	−0.0315	0.0106

whratio = waist-hip ratio; chol = total cholesterol level; Buckingham = county of residence; female = gender; bmi = body mass index; small and large refer to dummy variables representing the discrete variable, body frame; bp.1s = systolic blood pressure; bp.1d = diastolic blood pressure

While overall model fit is still somewhat poor, the implication is that adding these regressors to the model does significantly increase the model's ability to explain A1C levels among the study's participants. Three regressors exhibit significant t-statistics: patient total cholesterol, patient age, and patient BMI. The coefficient estimate for the patient's cholesterol is 0.0099, indicating that a small, one-unit increase in the typical patient's total cholesterol increases A1C levels by 0.0099 units, holding the other regressors constant. Similarly, a one-unit increase in the patient's age increases A1C levels by 0.0318 units while holding the other regressors in the model constant. Lastly, a one-unit increase in the patient's BMI increases A1C levels by 0.0405 units, holding the other specified regressors constant. All three results make sense clinically, as older patients, patients with cardiovascular disease, and more obese patients are all more prone to the onset of type II diabetes. Interestingly, once other patient characteristics are controlled for, the waist–hip ratio measure's *t*-statistic and *p*-value indicate that this regressor is no longer a significant determinant of A1C levels. This suggests the presence of confounding with respect to the relationship between waist–hip ratio and A1C. However, it is important to recognize that in certain cases, adding additional regressors does not remove the source of the bias. Whether adding regressors reduces the bias is as much a function of clinical and theoretical knowledge as it is the application of statistics.

Another extension commonly used in multiple regression is the need to test hypotheses about more than one parameter (i.e., *joint tests* of model parameters). As with the *t*-statistic and *t*-test, most computer packages automatically calculate *F*-statistics and perform *F*-tests under one or more standard null and alternative hypotheses. Under the null hypothesis, the *F*-statistic is distributed as an *F*-distribution, allowing for the calculation of a *p*-value. The most common null hypothesis is

$$H_0 : \beta_1 = \beta_2 = \ldots = \beta_k = 0$$
$$H_A : \text{Not } H_0$$

(9)

Under this null hypothesis, all of the population values for slope coefficients are jointly equal to zero, which implies that none of the regressors have any joint impact on the dependent variable. Thus, the regression does not add anything over and above simply computing mean A1C levels. Rejecting the null implies that the regressors, when considered collectively, do explain a significant amount of variation (or significantly predict) A1C levels. The second panel in Table 11-2 contains the results of this test. The *F*-statistic's value is 7.7827, and the corresponding *p*-value is less than 0.05, indicating that we reject the null hypothesis at the 0.05 level of significance. That is, it was "worth it" to run the regression.

DUMMY VARIABLES

Notice that several regressors used in the multiple regression reported in Table 11-2 are discrete variables (i.e., county of residence, gender, body frames). It is possible to include such variables in regression analysis in general, and in linear regression analysis in particular. To include discrete variables in regression analysis, **dummy variables** can be used to represent the categories of a discrete variable.[14,17] Dummy variables are specific types of control variables that are binary in nature. Perhaps the most commonly used dummy variable coding scheme is reference cell coding, which uses $a - 1$ dummy variables, with a being the number of categories of a discrete variable, and each dummy variable can have a value of 0 or 1, indicating membership in a category (1 if a member of a group and 0 otherwise).[10]

Consider the case of a binary regressor, such as whether the study participant resides in Buckingham County or Louisa County. Perhaps there might be differences across the two counties that should be controlled for in the analysis; thus it is included as a predictor variable in the analysis. Since the county of residence variable has two categories, one dummy variable is needed. In the analysis reported in Table 11-2, the variable Buckingham takes on a value of 1 if the study participant resides in Buckingham County and a value of 0 otherwise (i.e., the participant resides in Louisa County).

When the dummy variable is included as a regressor and the regression equation is estimated, a coefficient estimate will be produced for the dummy variable. The question is how to interpret this coefficient estimate, since the dummy variable is binary, and therefore cannot represent a marginal effect in the truest sense. In such cases, the coefficient estimates for dummy variables indicate *the mean change (increase or decrease) in the dependent variable (Y) that occurs due to membership in the category where the dummy variable takes a value of 1 (relative to a value of 0), holding the other specified regressors constant*. In the case of our diabetes regression, the dummy variable's coefficient estimate represents the mean increase in A1C levels experienced by residents of Buckingham County (over and above residents of Louisa County), holding the other specified regressors constant. That is, at the mean, how much better or worse are A1C levels in Buckingham County than in Louisa County, after we have controlled for all other determinants of A1C levels in the model? In the present example, this difference is not statistically significant ($p = 0.2257$).

Also note that dummy variables are always interpreted in a relative context (the ones relative to the zeros). As a result, the use of one dummy variable provides information on both groups, and it is unnecessary to include a second dummy variable to identify the Louisa County residents with a value of 1. Similarly, in some cases there will be a series of mutually exclusive and collective exhaustive dummy variables to measure multiple categories. An example might be a series of variables that measure race or ethnicity. Suppose that we have five categories: Caucasian, African American, Asian, Hispanic, and all other races/ethnicities. In such cases, the researcher would choose four dummy variables to represent the five categories, and these four dummy variables would be included in the regression. All dummy variables would be measured relative to the omitted category (called the reference category). Note that if you include all five dummy variables in the equation, OLS will generally crash! This is a phenomenon known as *perfect multicollinearity*, which occurs when the researcher includes a series of variables that contain *exactly* the same quantity of information, but the information is included twice.[14] In the case of the five dummy variables, the combination of the first four dummy variables tells you exactly the same thing that the fifth dummy variable does (i.e., through process of elimination, if you aren't in the first four dummy variables you must be included in the fifth one). The choice of which $a - 1$ dummy variables are included in the regression is generally left to the researcher, as any combination of $a - 1$ variables will contain the same amount of statistical information. However, it is generally good practice to use the dummy variable that exhibits the highest number of ones (and the lowest number of zeros) as the omitted dummy variable.

EFFECT MODIFICATION

Suppose county of residence is added as a regressor variable in a linear regression equation examining the relationship between A1C (the dependent variable) and waist–hip ratio. In the process of conducting the analysis, a researcher asks whether the relationship between waist–hip ratio and A1C is significantly different between participants who reside in Buckingham County and those who reside in Louisa County. As described earlier, this is a question of effect modification or moderation, and county of residence would be called an effect modifier or moderator. Effect modification is present when there is a statistical **interaction** between two independent variables; thus, a typical way to test for effect modification is to include an interaction term as an additional independent variable in the regression equation. This term is the product of the two variables in question; in the present case, this term would equal *waist–hip × county of residence*. If the null hypothesis that the regression coefficient for the interaction term is zero is rejected, then this is evidence of effect modification.

A moderated regression analysis (not shown) revealed no evidence in the Willems' study data[6] that there is an interaction between waist–hip ratio and county of residence in the prediction of A1C ($p = 0.4826$). The decision to include interaction terms in a regression equation should not be based solely on statistical evidence. Researchers should also provide clinical and/or theoretical considerations for their inclusion.

MULTIPLE LINEAR REGRESSION EXAMPLE FROM THE LITERATURE

Figure 11-2 is from a study exploring the relationship between mental health stigma, mental health literacy, and the willingness of pharmacists to provide services for patients with schizophrenia.[18] The figure contains an annotated table from the original study that demonstrates one approach for displaying the results from a multiple linear regression analysis, namely, a listing of independent variables and a statement of the estimated regression coefficients for each independent variable (denoted as β in the table), along with 95% confidence intervals and *p*-values. The findings from this table suggest that higher schizophrenia literacy is associated with a greater willingness to provide medication counseling, while higher social distance scores (indicating higher levels of stigma) are associated with less willingness to provide medication counseling (after controlling for the other variables in the model). Both of the dependent variables (i.e., willingness to provide medication counseling and identify drug-related problems) and the primary independent variables of interest (i.e., mental health literacy and mental health stigma) studied by O'Reilly and colleagues[18] are derived from multi-item, self-reported measurements and are treated as continuous variables in the analysis. Because the measurement scales for these variables are somewhat arbitrary, some researchers will report standardized estimates to aid interpretation rather than what is presented in Figure 11-2.

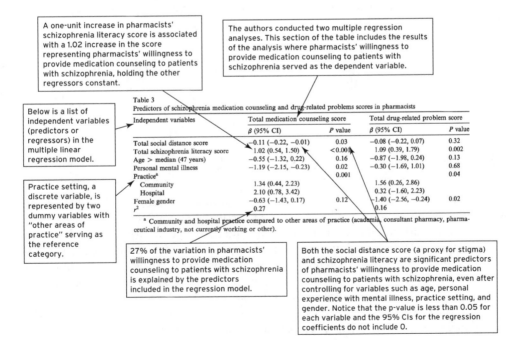

FIGURE 11-2   Results from multiple linear regression analysis exploring predictors of pharmacists' willingness to provide services to patients with schizophrenia.

Reproduced from O'Reilly C, Bell J, Kelly P, Chen T. Exploring the relationship between mental health stigma, knowledge and provision of pharmacy services for consumers with schizophrenia. *Res Social Adm Pharm.* 2013 Apr 27. doi:pii: S1551-7411(13)00057-0. 10.1016/j.sapharm.2013.04.006. [Epub ahead of print]

CASE STUDY 11-1	Linear Regression with Diabetes Data

The specification of any regression model is based on the experience of the researcher, an evaluation of the literature, and theory-based prior expectations. Please use your clinical knowledge, prior expectations, and theoretical knowledge to answer the following question.

What is the appropriate specification for the regression depicted in Table 11-2? In specifying this regression, what variables in the current data set should be included, and what additional variables should the researchers have collected data on to include in the regression?

HINT: If the current regression explains less than 20 percent of the variation in A1C levels, there is more than 80 percent left to be explained. This implies that a number of variables are missing!

CASE STUDY 11-2	Literature Evaluation with Linear Regression

Andreassen and colleagues conduct a multiple linear regression to explain the serum concentration of oxycodone among 439 cancer patients. Regressors include the total daily dose of oxycodone, gender, time from the last oxycodone dose to the blood sample, the presence of a CYP3A4 inducer, and the presence of a CYP3A4 inhibitor. Please read the article and answer the following questions.

1. Evaluate the authors' regression specification and their results. Does the regression model display good fit? Which variables are significant? Do the empirical results coincide with prior expectations? Are there any omitted variables?
2. The authors conduct two additional regressions to predict (1) the ratio of oxymorphone/oxycodone and (2) the ratio of noroxycodone/oxycodone. Repeat the evaluation conducted in question 1 for each of these additional regressions.

Data from Andreassen T, Klepstad P, Davies A, et al. Influences on the pharmacokinetics of oxycodone: a multicenter cross-sectional study in 439 adult cancer patients. *Eur J Clin Pharmacol.* 2011;67:493–506.

SUMMARY AND CONCLUSIONS

Linear regression analysis is one of the most common statistical techniques in clinical research and is used when the dependent variable is continuous and there is a need to adjust for variables that cannot be accounted for by manipulating a study's design. Under the appropriate circumstances, linear regression models can be highly successful in accounting for many potential confounders and for assessing effect modification. A regression analysis will produce accurate and precise results when (1) the assumptions underlying the model are consistent with the data being analyzed and (2) sufficient data and explanatory variables (or regressors) are available to control for each and every relevant confounder. If these criteria are not met, then the statistical technique will not provide results that are useful to clinicians. Also, the results will not inform clinical practice if important data and/or regressors are omitted or included inappropriately. At the same time, clinicians should approach this issue with a certain degree of understanding about the research process. The simple fact is that no study is perfect; however, not all flaws in a research project are necessarily fatal. It is important for clinicians and researchers to recognize that such flaws may exist. The goal of the researcher is to ensure that every attempt has been made to minimize the impact of those flaws, and be very transparent in the manuscript about the presence of any limitations or flaws that may be unaccounted for in the study. Similarly, clinicians should always ask whether accounting for such flaws would fundamentally alter the study's major conclusions. In general, clinicians and researchers must use theory, common sense, and practical experience to make such assessments.

REVIEW QUESTIONS

1. Explain the concept of effect modification *in your own words* and give an example of an effect modifier.
2. What is the difference between a confounder and a mediator? Give an example of each from the clinical literature.
3. Using a statistical definition, what does it mean for an estimate to be biased? Inefficient?
4. Explain why testing the null hypothesis that all of the slope coefficients in a regression are equal to zero is equivalent to evaluating the use of linear regression versus descriptive statistics for the dependent variable.
5. Can a regression's R^2 ever be less than its adjusted R^2? Explain.

ONLINE RESOURCES

UCLA Statistical Consulting Group: http://www.ats.ucla.edu/stat/ (A useful website complete with answers to frequently asked questions, tutorials, and various worked examples, including some with annotated output. It also includes webpages developed for many textbooks, including some devoted to the topics covered in this chapter, showing how to work the examples in these books using various statistical software packages.)

REFERENCES

1. Pizzi L, Lofland J. *Economic Evaluation in U.S. Health Care*. Boston, MA: Jones & Bartlett; 2006.
2. Chow S-C, Liu J-P. *Design and Analysis of Clinical Trials: Concepts and Methodologies*. Hoboken, NJ: Wiley-Interscience; 2004.
3. Dillman D. *Mail and Internet Surveys: The Tailored Design Method*. 2nd ed. New York, NY: John Wiley & Sons; 2000.
4. Wooldridge J. *Introductory Econometrics: A Modern Approach*. Cincinnati, OH: South-Western; 2000.
5. Stock J, Watson M. *Introduction to Econometrics*. Boston, MA: Pearson; 2007.
6. Willems J, Saunders J, Hunt D, Schorling J. Prevalence of coronary heart disease risk factors among rural blacks: a community-based study. *Southern Med J*. 1997;90(8):814–820.
7. Schorling J, Roach J, Siegel M, et al. A trial of church-based smoking cessation interventions for rural African Americans. *Prev Med*. 1997;26:92–101.
8. Enders C. *Applied Missing Data Analysis*. New York, NY: Guilford Press; 2010.
9. Keppel G, Wickens T. *Design and Analysis: A Researcher's Handbook*. 4th ed. Upper Saddle River, NJ: Pearson/Prentice Hall; 2004.
10. Kleinbaum D, Kupper L, Nizam A, Muller K. *Applied Regression Analysis and Other Multivariable Techniques*. 4th ed. Belmont, CA: Duxbury Press; 2008.
11. Piantadosi S. *Clinical Trials: A Methodological Perspective*. Hoboken, NJ: John Wiley & Sons; 2005.
12. MacKinnon D. *Introduction to Statistical Mediation Analysis*. New York, NY: Lawrence Erlbaum and Associates; 2008.
13. Baron R, Kenny D. The moderator-mediator variable distinction in social psychological research: conceptual, strategic, and statistical considerations. *J Personality Soc Psych*. 1986;51:1173–1182.

14. Studenmund A. *Using Econometrics: A Practical Guide*. 5th ed. Boston, MA: Pearson/Addison Wesley; 2006.

15. Daniel W. *Biostatistics: A Foundation for Analysis in the Health Sciences*. 8th ed. New York, NY: John Wiley & Sons; 2005.

16. Katz M. Multivariable analysis: a primer for readers of medical research. *Ann Intern Med*. 2003;138:644–650.

17. Gujarati D. *Basic Econometrics*. 4th ed. Boston, MA: McGraw-Hill; 2003.

18. O'Reilly C, Bell J, Kelly P, Chen T. Exploring the relationship between mental health stigma, knowledge and provision of pharmacy services for consumers with schizophrenia. *Res Social Adm Pharm*. April 27, 2013. doi:pii: S1551-7411(13)00057-0. 10.1016/j.sapharm.2013.04.006. [Epub ahead of print]

LOGISTIC REGRESSION AND SURVIVAL ANALYSIS

JOHN P. BENTLEY, PhD

DAN FRIESNER, PhD

CHAPTER OBJECTIVES

▸ Describe how binary logistic regression and Cox regression are commonly used in the drug literature

▸ Distinguish the nature of the outcome variable for logistic regression and Cox regression compared to linear regression

▸ Describe and appropriately interpret the coefficient estimates and predictions produced by binary logistic regression and Cox regression

▸ Describe how the coefficient estimates and predictions produced by binary logistic regression and Cox regression can be used to evaluate a research hypothesis

▸ Interpret an estimated survival curve

▸ Evaluate a Kaplan–Meier plot comparing the survival curves of two different groups

KEY TERMINOLOGY

Binary logistic regression
Censoring
Cox proportional hazards
   regression model
Hazard
Hazard function
Hazard ratio (HR)

Kaplan–Meier
   method
Logit
Log-rank test
Maximum likelihood
   estimation (MLE)
Odds ratio (OR)

Survival analysis
Survival curve
Survival function

INTRODUCTION

In general, the linear regression model is used when the dependent variable or outcome variable of interest is a continuous variable, such as glycosylated hemoglobin (A1C) or systolic blood pressure. However, in clinical research, many outcome variables of interest cannot be conceptualized as being continuous. In some cases, the outcome variable may be categorical (e.g., a dichotomous or binary variable, such as whether or not one has a disease), while in many other situations the outcome variable may be the time until an event occurs and it is possible that the researcher may not know when (or whether) the event occurs for everyone in the study.

The purpose of this chapter is to discuss additional methods of regression analysis that are appropriate for such situations. The chapter begins with a discussion of the methodology behind, and appropriate use of, logistic regression for the analysis of an outcome variable that is binary (or dichotomous). The second part of the chapter provides an overview of two different techniques that fall under the general umbrella of survival analysis, the Kaplan–Meier procedure and Cox regression. Both are widely used in the clinical literature when the outcome variable is the time until the occurrence of an event.

BINARY LOGISTIC REGRESSION

In Chapter 11, "Simple and Multiple Linear Regression," the case scenario involved the prediction of patient A1C levels, a continuous variable (see http://biostat.mc.vanderbilt .edu/wiki/Main/DataSets).[1,2] From a clinical perspective, the linear regression model using ordinary least squares (OLS) estimation has a limitation. Although higher A1C levels do indicate a more pronounced onset of diabetes, when diagnosing patients there must be some practical cutoff, above which a patient "has" diabetes, and below which the patient "does not have" diabetes. Most pharmacotherapy guidelines use an A1C level of 7 as this cutoff point.[3] It is conceivable to characterize this discrete decision by creating a new variable in the diabetes data set that takes a value of 1 for patients whose A1C levels exceed or equal 7 and a value of 0 otherwise. Clinical researchers often encounter such binary outcome variables, where the variable can only take on two values. Although such variables can consist of continuous variables with a meaningful cutoff point (like A1C), many times the binary variable is a true discrete variable (e.g., dead or alive, experienced an adverse event or did not, case or control). When an outcome variable consists of only two categories, **binary logistic regression** is an appropriate statistical method. There are generalizations of logistic regression for situations when the response variable has more than two nominal categories or when the response variable is a set of ordered categories. Binary logistic regression is an oft-used statistical method in the biomedical literature.

To correctly predict a variable that takes only two possible values, one must attempt to predict the *probability* or *chance* that the dependent variable takes a value of 0 or a value of 1. That is:

$$P(Y_i = 1) = b_0 + b_1 X_i + b_2 Z_i + b_3 W_i + \ldots + b_k V_i \tag{1}$$

where $P(Y_i = 1)$ denotes an estimated probability that the dependent variable (Y) takes on the value of 1 (i.e., has the event or outcome of interest).[a] One of the many

---

[a] Since the dependent variable is mutually exclusive and collectively exhaustive, and since the probability that *some* value for Y must occur with certainty (a probability of 1), we can immediately deduce the probability that $Y_i = 0$ once we have estimated the probability that $Y_i = 1$.

problems[b] associated with using linear regression with OLS estimation for equation (1) is that probabilities must range between 0 and 1, inclusive, but predicted values (i.e., estimated probabilities) from equation (1) using linear regression with OLS estimation may be less than 0 or greater than 1. To ensure that the probabilities are appropriately constrained to be between 0 and 1 and to subsequently estimate these probabilities, we must identify a function for $P(Y_i = 1)$. A common choice is to assume that $P(Y_i = 1)$ follows a logistic distribution. The logistic distribution is similar to the normal distribution, except that the tails of the distribution are slightly thicker.[4,5] For cumulative probabilities, the logistic distribution is:

$$P(Y_i = 1) = \frac{e^{b_0 + b_1 X_i + b_2 Z_i + b_3 W_i + \ldots + b_k V_i}}{1 + e^{b_0 + b_1 X_i + b_2 Z_i + b_3 W_i + \ldots + b_k V_i}} \tag{2}$$

where e^x is the exponential function evaluated at x (sometimes expressed as exp(x)). This function is the antilog (or inverse) of the natural logarithm (base e exponentiation).

Equation (2) can be rearranged to arrive at the following:

$$\ln\left(\frac{P(Y_i = 1)}{1 - P(Y_i = 1)}\right) = b_0 + b_1 X_i + b_2 Z_i + b_3 W_i + \ldots + b_k V_i \tag{3}$$

Equation (3) is the called the binary logistic regression model. Notice that the right-hand side of the equation is virtually identical to the linear regression model in equation (8b) in Chapter 11, "Simple and Multiple Linear Regression." However, the left-hand side of the model is quite different. This expression is called the **logit** (or log-odds) and it is the natural log of the odds of success for Y_i (i.e., the odds of having the event of interest). Note that $\left(\frac{P(Y_i = 1)}{1 - P(Y_i = 1)}\right)$ is the odds that $Y_i = 1$. The transformation of P to $\ln\left(\frac{P(Y_i = 1)}{1 - P(Y_i = 1)}\right)$ is called the logit transformation, which is why logistic regression models are also called logit models.

To estimate the parameters, one must use a different method than OLS to account for the binary nature of the dependent variable. The estimation method most commonly used for logistic regression is known as **maximum likelihood estimation (MLE)**.[4-6] As the names suggest, the difference between OLS and MLE is that OLS focuses on identifying the equation of a trend line that *minimizes* the residuals that relate each data point to the trend line. MLE focuses on maximizing the *predictive* capabilities of the regression, rather than minimizing its residuals.

Table 12-1 contains results from a binary logistic regression analysis. Since Microsoft Excel does not include logistic regression in its Analysis ToolPak feature, the results were produced using SAS Version 9.3 (SAS Corporation, Cary, NC). For simplicity, the same set of explanatory variables from Table 11-2 in Chapter 11, "Simple and Multiple Linear Regression," was used in the logistic regression model. As with linear regression, the logistic regression model provides a list of coefficient estimates for the slopes and intercept. It also provides a standard error estimate for each estimate. However, there are some notable differences in Table 12-1 compared to the previous results generated by linear regression. First, because it is inappropriate to use an OLS trend line to estimate the regression model, it is also inappropriate to use the standard R^2 measure of model fit (there are R^2 analogs for use in logistic regression, but they do not have the same proportion-of-total-variation interpretation). Also, the

---

[b] There are others; see Menard.[7]

TABLE 12-1	Binary Logistic Regression Analysis						
Dependent Variable: Diabetes (Binary Variable Identifying A1C Scores above 7)							
Variable	**Coeff.**	**Standard Error**	**Chi-Square Statistic**	**p-value**	**Odds Ratio**	**95% Confidence Limits for Odds Ratio**	
intercept	−11.3118	2.4607	21.1324	<.0001			
whratio	3.1805	2.3976	1.7597	0.1847	24.0590	0.2190	>999.999
chol	0.0090	0.0034	6.8211	0.0090	1.0090	1.0020	1.0160
Buckingham	0.1238	0.3315	0.1395	0.7088	1.1320	0.5910	2.1670
age	0.0418	0.0124	11.4317	0.0007	1.0430	1.0180	1.0680
female	−0.2570	0.4035	0.4054	0.5243	0.7730	0.3510	1.7060
bmi	0.0714	0.0286	6.2401	0.0125	1.0740	1.0160	1.1360
small	0.1012	0.4600	0.0484	0.8259	1.1060	0.4490	2.7260
large	−0.0474	0.4026	0.0139	0.9062	0.9540	0.4330	2.0990
bp.1s	0.0069	0.0091	0.5756	0.4480	1.0070	0.9890	1.0250
bp.1d	−0.0043	0.0162	0.0700	0.7914	0.9960	0.9650	1.0280
Chi-square test statistic value			51.3355	<0.0001			
Degrees of freedom			10				
Number of observations			366				

whratio = waist-hip ratio; chol = total cholesterol level; Buckingham = county of residence; female = gender; bmi = body mass index; small and large refer to dummy variables representing the discrete variable, body frame; bp.1s = systolic blood pressure; bp.1d = diastolic blood pressure

test of the overall model (i.e., the test of the null hypothesis that all population values for the coefficients are jointly equal to zero—see equation (9) in Chapter 11, "Simple and Multiple Linear Regression") is not performed using an F-statistic, but rather a chi-square statistic. The question asked by this test in logistic regression is the same basic question as in linear regression, but the nature of the dependent variable is different. Thus, it asks, taken collectively, does the *entire set* of independent variables contribute significantly to the prediction of the binary dependent variable? The bottom of Table 12-1 contains this test (test statistic = 51.3355) and its associated p-value (<0.0001), which indicates a rejection of the null hypothesis; so one can conclude that the predictors, taken collectively, do allow better predictions of $P(Y_i = 1)$ than could be made without them.

Similarly, t-statistics are not used to test the significance of individual predictors in logistic regression. The standard null hypothesis for such a test is given by:

$$H_0 : \beta_k = 0 \tag{4}$$
$$H_A : \text{Not } H_0, \text{ or } \beta_k \neq 0$$

There are several ways of constructing this significance test, but the most commonly reported by statistical software (and what appears in Table 12-1) is known as the Wald test. Under the null hypothesis stated in equation (4), the test statistic is simply $\left(\dfrac{b_k}{SE_{b_k}}\right)^2$, where b_k indicates a specific coefficient estimate and SE_{b_k} is the estimated standard error for b_k. Under the null hypothesis, this test statistic has an approximately χ^2 (chi-square) distribution with degrees of freedom = 1. For the clinician, there is little difference in the interpretation of the results compared to linear regression. *p*-values less than conventional levels (usually 0.05) indicate a rejection of the null hypothesis. Similar to Table 11-2 in Chapter 11, "Simple and Multiple Linear Regression," three regressors in Table 12-1 exhibit significant chi-square statistics: total cholesterol, age, and BMI.

A final difference of note between binary logistic regression and linear regression is in the interpretation of the coefficient estimates. The logistic regression coefficients as stated in equation (3) represent the change in the log-odds of success for Y_i for a one-unit increase in the regressor of interest, holding the other regressors constant. The concept of log-odds is not intuitive. To interpret the magnitude of the relationship between a regressor and the dependent variable, it is common to calculate an **odds ratio (OR)** for each parameter estimate.[6] The idea behind an odds ratio in the context of logistic regression is the same as the odds ratio concept that was introduced in Chapter 5, "Cohort and Case-Control Studies." Using equation (3) together with an understanding of the difference between probability and odds and some knowledge of the laws of exponents, it can be shown that the natural antilogarithm (base *e* exponentiation) of the estimated logistic regression coefficient (e^b) is an estimated odds ratio.[8] Thus, consider a predictor *x*. The odds ratio compares the odds of success at $x + 1$ to the odds of success at *x*, holding constant the other regressors. The estimated odds of success at $x + 1$ equal the estimated odds of success at *x* multiplied by the odds ratio, e^b. If a marginal change in the value of a regressor does not noticeably impact a model, it will not allow the model to distinguish between observations where $Y_i = 1$ and $Y_i = 0$. If that is the case, $\beta = 0$ and the odds ratio would equal 1 ($e^0 = 1$). On the other hand, if a small change in a regressor is informative, it will help the model better distinguish between cases where $Y_i = 1$ and $Y_i = 0$, and the corresponding odds ratio would move away from a value of 1 and $\beta \neq 0$.

Just like with the coefficient estimates, it is possible to build confidence intervals (usually 95% confidence intervals) around odds ratio estimates and conduct hypothesis tests. If the confidence interval for an odds ratio includes 1, this implies that the variable does not play any statistical role in explaining the dependent variable. This is equivalent to single parameter hypothesis tests discussed in equation (4), where the null hypothesis identifies a case where a population parameter is set equal to 0. If the value of 1 falls outside of the confidence interval, we reject the null hypothesis that the odds ratio for the population equals 1. This implies that the regressor in question plays a statistical role in explaining the dependent variable.

Despite the differences in the mathematical mechanics between linear regression and binary logistic regression, the practical interpretation of the results remains highly consistent between the two models. Examining Table 12-1, note that the chi-square tests indicate that the overall model is statistically significant, just as the *F*-tests indicated in Table 11-2 in Chapter 11, "Simple and Multiple Linear Regression". Additionally, only three regressors have statistically significant coefficient estimates: total cholesterol, age, and BMI. All three coefficient estimates are positive in sign and have odds ratio estimates (i) that are greater than 1 and (ii) whose 95% confidence interval estimates do not include the value of 1. Thus, higher values for any one of these variables (holding constant the other specified regressors) lead to a greater likelihood of developing diabetes. For example, the interpretation of the results for the age variable is: After adjusting for the other predictors, the estimated odds of having an A1C equal to or exceeding 7 multiply by 1.043 for each one-year increase in age.

Thus, holding constant the other predictors, the estimated odds of having an A1C equal to or exceeding 7 for a 51-year-old are 1.043 times the estimated odds for a 50-year-old (or 4.3% higher). Rather than a single year, it may be more interesting to examine the odds ratio associated with a decade change in years. This is easily accomplished by multiplying the logistic regression coefficient by 10 before exponentiating. Thus, we have $e^{(10*0.0418)} = \left(e^{(0.0418)}\right)^{10} = OR^{10} = 1.519$, which means that the estimated odds of having an A1C equal to or exceeding 7 for a 60-year-old are 1.519 times the estimated odds for a 50-year-old (or 51.9% higher), holding the other predictors in the model constant.

Similarly, the potential for various confounding effects remains the same across both methods (linear regression and logistic regression). Notice that it is also possible to use dummy variables to represent categories of a discrete variable in logistic regression just like in linear regression (odds ratios give a comparison of the odds of having the event for one group relative to another). The presence of confounders and effect modifiers may create bias and inefficiency in the resulting estimates through different statistical mechanisms, but the fact that these effects occur remains the same. Hence, clinicians and academic researchers should always exercise care to ensure that the underlying study and data collection processes, as well as the specification of the regression model, are constructed and implemented appropriately and in accordance with theory and clinical practice.

To further illustrate the practical interpretation of the results from a logistic regression analysis, consider **Figure 12–1**, which is from a study that examined whether certain demographic and clinical factors were significantly associated with experiencing

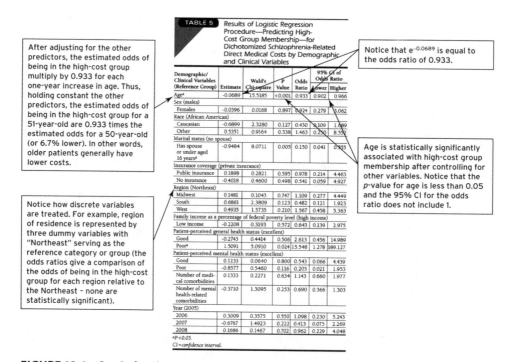

FIGURE 12-1 Results from logistic regression analysis exploring predictors of high-cost group membership in patients with schizophrenia.

Reproduced from Desai P, Lawson K, Barner J, Rascati K. Identifying patient characteristics associated with high schizophrenia-related direct medical costs in community-dwelling patients. *J Manag Care Pharm.* 2013;19(6):468–477.

high schizophrenia–related direct medical costs in a group of patients with schizophrenia living in the community setting using data from the Medical Expenditure Panel Survey (MEPS).[9] The figure contains an annotated table from the original study that demonstrates one approach for displaying the results from a logistic regression analysis. The table contains a list of independent variables, the estimated logistic regression coefficients for each independent variable, the Wald test statistic and *p*-value for each independent variable, and the value of the odds ratio that corresponds to the logistic regression coefficient for each predictor, along with 95% confidence intervals for the odds ratio. The dependent variable used in the analysis presented in Figure 12-1 was a dichotomous variable indicating whether the respondent was in a high-cost group (annual expenditures ≥$16,000) or a low-cost group (annual expenditures <$16,000). The significant predictors of group membership in the multivariable model included age, marital status, and perceived general health status.

CASE STUDY 12-1   Logistic Regression with Diabetes Data

Because the same data set is used to estimate the binary logistic and linear regressions (see Table 11-2 in Chapter 11, "Simple and Multiple Linear Regression"), it is possible to make some basic comparisons across both models. Answer the following questions:

1. Suppose you are the researcher who has the choice to estimate either a linear model (using the A1C reading) or a binary logistic model (using a binary cutoff of 7.0) to explain and predict the onset of type II diabetes. Holding the number and types of regressors constant across both models, which estimation approach is most appropriate from a clinical perspective? Please explain your answer.
2. The binary logistic regression model discussed above uses an A1C level of 7.0 as a cutoff point for the onset of type II diabetes. While this cutoff point is consistent with guidelines, it is not set in stone.[3] Is there a different cutoff point that should be used? Please explain your answer.

HINT: Some clinicians focus on specific types of diabetes; for example, prediabetes and unmanaged diabetes. How does your answer change depending on the type of diabetes you are attempting to predict?

CASE STUDY 12-2   Literature Evaluation with Binary Logistic Regression

Brannstrom and colleagues conduct a series of four binary logistic regressions (see Table IV in their paper) to explain the use of various diuretics among 467 elderly participants in northern Sweden. Regressors include factors such as age, gender, a diagnosis of heart failure, a diagnosis of hypertension, and the presence of dementia. Please read the article and answer the following questions.

1. Evaluate the authors' regression specification and its results. Which variables are significant? Do the empirical results coincide with prior expectations? Are there any omitted variables?
2. The authors appear to use the same model specification (i.e., the same set of regressors) for each type of diuretic. From a clinical perspective, does this make sense? Please explain your reasoning.
3. The authors conduct an additional regression to predict the use of short-acting nitroglycerin (see their Table V). Repeat the analysis you conducted in questions 1 and 2 for this regression.

Data from Brannstrom J, Hamberg K, Molander L, Lovheim H, Gustafson Y. Gender disparities in the pharmacological treatment of cardiovascular disease and diabetes mellitus in the very old: an epidemiological, cross-sectional survey. *Drugs Aging*. 2011;28(12):993–1005.

SURVIVAL ANALYSIS

GENERAL FEATURES

In certain types of studies, the question of interest is not simply *whether* something occurs, but *how long* something will last.[c] Once again, consider the diabetes data described previously. A related research question may be the following. Suppose these same study participants were followed over a number of years. During the follow-up period, the participant provides samples for routine testing. Can we predict how long it will take for the average person in the study to develop nephropathy? And more specifically, does being diagnosed with diabetes reduce the length of time before the onset of nephropathy? A second example commonly occurs in clinical trials of experimental medicines, particularly for various types of cancer. Suppose the researcher identifies and collects a sample of participants, all of whom have the same late-stage cancer. Half are randomly assigned to receive the traditional treatment protocols (if the condition is terminal, perhaps it is simply pain management) and half receive the experimental treatment in addition to pain management. Questions that one may ask include: What is the median survival time in both groups? What is the survival probability at different points in time (e.g., 6-month, 1-year, 5-year survival rates)? and Is there any evidence that the survival experience of patients is different between the groups?

When the outcome of interest in a study concerns the *occurrence* and the *timing* of an *event* (i.e., a time-to-event outcome), the statistical methods commonly employed are called **survival analysis**. There are actually a collection of survival analysis methods, and the two most common in the biomedical literature are the **Kaplan–Meier method** and the **Cox proportional hazards regression model**. Before discussing these methods, it is first necessary to describe the concepts of **censoring** and censored data. When evaluating a time-to-event outcome, it quite possible that researchers will encounter some censoring of data. Censoring occurs when the time to the event occurrence is not known exactly; thus, there is some information about survival time, but not complete information. Censoring may occur for a number of reasons, for example, because participants drop out of the study before its conclusion. Additionally, some participants may not experience the event over the time frame of the study. Survival analysis methods, including the Kaplan–Meier method and Cox regression, are capable of handling censored data. Without appropriately accounting for censored data, other methods of estimating survival (e.g., calculating the mean survival time) will lead to potential biases.

THE KAPLAN–MEIER METHOD

A common product of the Kaplan–Meier method are estimates of something called the **survival function** (also referred to as the **survival curve**—although in practice with real data, they look more like step functions than smooth curves). The Kaplan–Meier survival curve summarizes the probability of survival over time estimated from a sample. Examples of Kaplan–Meier survival curves can be found in Figures 12-2A and 12-2B. Both figures are from a study reporting the results of an RCT comparing radiotherapy

---

[c] The same question is often asked following a randomized controlled trial; thus, the approaches discussed in this section are commonly used to compare groups following an RCT. The techniques described here used in such situations can be considered bivariate analyses with a response variable that is a time-to-event variable, possibly with censoring.

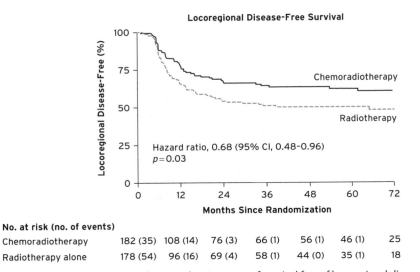

Locoregional Disease-Free Survival

No. at risk (no. of events)

Chemoradiotherapy	182 (35)	108 (14)	76 (3)	66 (1)	56 (1)	46 (1)	25
Radiotherapy alone	178 (54)	96 (16)	69 (4)	58 (1)	44 (0)	35 (1)	18

FIGURE 12-2A Kaplan-Meier survival curves showing rates of survival free of locoregional disease during 72 months of follow-up. The *p*-value is from the log-rank test and the hazard ratio is from a Cox proportional hazards model.

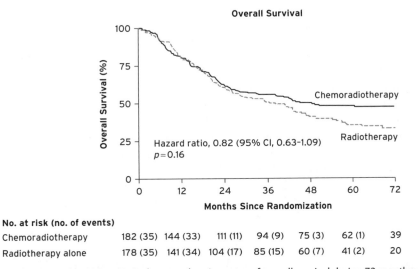

Overall Survival

No. at risk (no. of events)

Chemoradiotherapy	182 (35)	144 (33)	111 (11)	94 (9)	75 (3)	62 (1)	39
Radiotherapy alone	178 (35)	141 (34)	104 (17)	85 (15)	60 (7)	41 (2)	20

FIGURE 12-2B Kaplan-Meier survival curves showing rates of overall survival during 72 months of follow-up. The *p*-value is from the log-rank test and the hazard ratio is from a Cox proportional hazards model.

Reproduced from James N, Hussain S, Hall E, Jenkins P, Tremlett J, Rawlings C, Crundwell M, Sizer B, Sreenivasan T, Hendron C, Lewis R, Waters R, Huddart R, for the BC2001 Investigators. Radiotherapy with or without chemotherapy in muscle-invasive bladder cancer. *N Engl J Med.* 2012;366:1477–88. © Massachusetts Medical Society. Reprinted with permission from Massachusetts Medical Society.

alone versus radiotherapy concurrent with chemotherapy consisting of fluorouracil and mitomycin C (chemoradiotherapy) in the treatment of muscle-invasive bladder cancer.[10] The results for the primary study endpoint, locoregional disease-free survival, are found in **Figure 12-2A**, while the results for one of the tertiary study outcomes, overall survival, can be found in **Figure 12-2B**.

To compare the overall survival experience of both groups with respect to the study outcomes (i.e., to test the null hypothesis that the two curves are equivalent), the **log-rank test** was used by the authors. The results of these tests are also displayed in the figures. For the primary study endpoint, the test was statistically significant ($p = 0.03$), while there is no evidence in the data that the two treatments are different with respect to overall survival ($p = 0.16$). In examining Figure 12-2A, the survival curve for the chemoradiotherapy group is always higher than the survival curve for the radiotherapy group, suggesting that the chemoradiotherapy group has longer times to locoregional disease recurrence (defined as recurrence in pelvic nodes or bladder). The authors also report a 2-year recurrence-free rate of 67% in the chemoradiotherapy group and 54% in the radiotherapy group, providing further evidence that the use of fluorouracil and mitomycin C combined with radiotherapy improved locoregional control of bladder cancer when compared to radiotherapy alone.

The Cox Proportional Hazards Regression Model

Although Kaplan–Meier survival curves are relatively simple and intuitive to understand, they are limited if one wants to adjust for predictors when the dependent variable consists of possibly censored time-until-event data. Furthermore, such procedures do not allow one to quantify the effect of a predictor variable on survival time (i.e., no parameter estimates are provided). Regression analysis techniques that can be used to control for additional characteristics of participants were previously introduced for the cases of a continuous outcome variable (linear regression) and a binary outcome variable (logistic regression). There are other regression techniques that can be used when the outcome variable is the occurrence and the timing of an event, with the possibility of censored data. These methods can be used to address the typical multivariable problems addressed by multiple linear and logistic regression (e.g., confounding, effect modification, dummy variables). Thus, it is possible to place survival analysis in a regression-based context. The most commonly used method in the biomedical literature to accomplish this goal is known as the Cox proportional hazards regression model.[6,7,11]

To understand the Cox model, it is helpful to understand the concepts of **hazard** and the **hazard function**. The hazard of an event at any point t can be thought of as the risk of event occurrence at time t.[12] Technically, the hazard is a rate and takes the form of the number of events per interval of time. The collection of an individual's hazard for an event over time is called his or her hazard function, or $h_i(t)$. The hazard function can be modeled as a function of a set of predictors:[12]

$$h_i(t) = h_0(t) \exp(\beta_1 X_i + \beta_2 Z_i + \beta_3 W_i + \ldots + \beta_k V_i) \tag{5}$$

Equation (5) is called the proportional hazards model and is the basic model for Cox regression. This says that the hazard for person i at time t is the product of two factors:

- $h_0(t)$: a baseline hazard function (which is generally of little importance in Cox regression because it does not even have to be estimated to make any inferences of the effects of the predictors)
- A set of predictor variables—like regressors in multiple regression

Taking the natural logarithm of both sides of equation (5), the model can be rewritten as:

$$\ln h_i(t) = \ln h_0(t) + \beta_1 X_i + \beta_2 Z_i + \beta_3 W_i + \ldots + \beta_k V_i \tag{6}$$

The right-hand side of equation (6) looks strikingly similar to that of linear and logistic regression (with the exception that population regression parameters, βs, are used rather than sample estimates, bs). The βs describe the way that the hazard (and also survival time) is affected by the predictor. Thus, when $\beta = 0$, there is no effect, and when:

- $\beta > 0$: an increase in the predictor leads to an increase in the hazard or a decrease in survival
- $\beta < 0$: an increase in the predictor leads to a decrease in the hazard or an increase in survival

The β coefficients are estimated using a method similar to that used in logistic regression, called maximum partial likelihood estimation. As in the other regression models, it is possible to generate standard errors for each parameter estimate, thereby facilitating hypothesis tests and confidence interval construction. These coefficients represent the impact of a small (one-unit) change in the regressor on the natural logarithm of the hazard rate, holding the other specified regressors constant. With a little math, it can be shown that the natural antilogarithm of a parameter (e^{β}) from Cox regression is a **hazard ratio (HR)**, a very useful property of the model that aids in interpretation of the results. An HR is conceptually identical to a rate ratio (a ratio of two rates), and the interpretation of the HR is similar to that of an odds ratio. Thus, HR = 1 ($e^{0} = 1$) suggests no relationship between the predictor and the timing of event occurrence. For example, Figures 12-2A and 12-2B provide the HR estimated from a Cox model comparing chemoradiotherapy to radiotherapy only, with radiotherapy only as the reference group. For the primary outcome, locoregional disease-free survival, the point estimate of the HR is 0.68, with a 95% CI of 0.48–0.96, indicating statistically significant treatment effect (the 95% CI does not include 1). This point estimate says that at any point in time the hazard of recurrence of locoregional disease for the chemoradiotherapy group is 0.68 times (or "68% of" or "32% less than") the hazard for the radiotherapy group.

As with linear regression and logistic regression, additional predictor variables can be added to address the possibility of confounding or effect modification. For example, James and colleagues[10] evaluated the hazard ratio for the primary endpoint of locoregional disease-free survival, adjusting for variables such as age, tumor stage, performance status, and tumor grade. They found basically the same results, namely that there was a statistically significant benefit associated with chemoradiotherapy.

A final note on Cox regression concerns the meaning and assessment of proportional hazards assumption. This is a basic assumption of the model (although the model can be generalized to allow for non-proportional hazards). Basically, this assumption means that the ratio of hazards is constant over time. Practically speaking, this implies that the effect of each predictor (at least those that are not time-varying) is the same at all time points. There are a number of methods for checking this assumption and authors will often discuss how this assumption was assessed and the subsequent findings. For example, James et al.[10] note: "The proportional hazards assumption of the Cox model, which was tested with the use of Schoenfeld residuals, held for the primary endpoint and two secondary endpoints (disease-free survival and time to invasive locoregional recurrence) but did not hold for the time to cystectomy, and there were slight departures for overall, bladder-cancer-specific, and metastasis-free survival." Additional discussion of the assumption and potential solutions to violations can be found in Allison.[12]

CASE STUDY 12-3	**Literature Evaluation with the Cox Proportional Hazards Model**

Butler and colleagues estimate a Cox proportional hazards regression model (see their Table 3) to explain the rate at which Maricopa County, Arizona, Medicaid patients visit the emergency department. The study includes 127,916 individuals. Age and medication non-adherence are included as the primary regressors. Separate regressions are conducted for a variety of disease states, including hypertension, COPD, congestive heart disease, diabetes, and high cholesterol. Please read the article and answer the following questions.

1. Evaluate the authors' regression specifications and their results. Which variables are significant? Do the empirical results coincide with prior expectations? Are there any omitted variables?
2. The authors appear to use the same model specification (i.e., the same set of regressors) for each chronic condition. From a clinical perspective, does this make sense? Please explain your reasoning.

Data from Butler R, Davis T, Johnson W, Gardner H. Effects of nonadherence with prescription drugs among older adults. *Am J Manage Care*. 2011;17(2):153–160.

CASE STUDY 12-4	**Literature Evaluation with the Cox Proportional Hazards Model**

Wu and colleagues estimate a Cox proportional hazards regression model (see their Table 2) to explain the rate at which patients enrolled in selected managed care programs and who are currently being treated for major depressive disorder using either escitalopram or citalopram switch to a different antidepressant. Please read the article and answer the following question.

The authors find that "[T]he rate of discontinuation with switching to another second-generation antidepressant was also lower in the escitalopram group (24.7% vs 29.3%; $P < .001$)." From a pharmacotherapy perspective, does this result make sense?

Data from Wu E, Greenberg P, Ben-Hamadi R, Yu A, Yang E, Erder M. Comparing treatment persistence, healthcare resource utilization, and costs in adult patients with major depressive disorder treated with escitalopram or citalopram. *Am Health Drug Benefits*. 2011;4(2):78–87.

SUMMARY AND CONCLUSIONS

Logistic and Cox regression methods are valuable statistical tools to analyze binary and time-to-event outcomes, respectively. Notable differences among linear regression, logistic regression, and Cox regression include how the dependent variable is measured, the approach to parameter estimation, and how coefficient estimates are interpreted. However, these regression methods are used to address typical multivariable problems, such as confounding, effect modification, and the use of dummy variables. In addition, the basic principles of confidence interval construction and the conduct of hypothesis tests apply to all three regression models. Because the tools are extensions of the linear regression model, the limitations of these tools are similar to those found in linear regression. Consequently, the primary detriment of binary logistic regression and Cox proportional hazards regression models is not in their use, but in their *appropriate* use. Whether the tool actually produces a result that is useful depends on how the researcher uses the tool. Thus, clinicians must always evaluate analyses to understand the practical and clinical implications of variables that are missing, mismeasured, or inappropriately used by researchers. Clinicians and researchers have important and complementary roles to advance the practice based on evidence derived on theory, common sense, and practical experience.

REVIEW QUESTIONS

1. Compare and contrast linear regression, logistic regression, and Cox regression. Specifically, how do they differ in terms of the nature of the outcome variable and the interpretation of the coefficient estimates?
2. Explain why testing the null hypothesis that $\beta = 0$ in logistic regression and Cox regression is the same thing as testing the null hypothesis that the odds ratio = 1 in logistic regression and that the hazard ratio = 1 in Cox regression.
3. Can an odds ratio be negative (i.e., less than zero)? Explain.
4. Using a practical, clinical example, please explain why the vast majority of survival models contain some form of censoring.

ONLINE RESOURCES

UCLA Statistical Consulting Group: http://www.ats.ucla.edu/stat/ (A useful website complete with answers to frequently asked questions, tutorials, and various worked examples, including some with annotated output. It also includes webpages developed for many textbooks, including some devoted to the topics covered in this chapter, showing how to work the examples in these books using various statistical software packages.)

REFERENCES

1. Willems J, Saunders J, Hunt D, Schorling J. Prevalence of coronary heart disease risk factors among rural blacks: a community-based study. *Southern Med J*. 1997;90(8):814–820.
2. Schorling J, Roach J, Siegel M, et al. A trial of church-based smoking cessation interventions for rural African Americans. *Prev Med*. 1997;26:92–101.
3. DiPiro J, Talbert R, Yee G, Matzke G, Wells B, Posey L. *Pharmacotherapy: A Pathophysiologic Approach*. 6th ed. New York, NY: McGraw-Hill; 2005.
4. Studenmund A. *Using Econometrics: A Practical Guide*. 5th ed. Boston, MA: Pearson/Addison Wesley; 2006.
5. Greene W. *Econometric Analysis*. 4th ed. Upper Saddle River, NJ: Prentice Hall; 2000.
6. Lachin J. *Biostatistical Methods*. 2nd ed. Hoboken, NJ: John Wiley & Sons; 2011.
7. Menard S. *Applied Logistic Regression Analysis*. 2nd ed. Thousand Oaks, CA: Sage Publications; 2002.
8. Agresti A. *An Introduction to Categorical Data Analysis*. 2nd ed. Hoboken, NJ: John Wiley & Sons; 2007.
9. Desai P, Lawson K, Barner J, Rascati K. Identifying patient characteristics associated with high schizophrenia-related direct medical costs in community-dwelling patients. *J Manag Care Pharm*. 2013;19(6):468–477.
10. James N, Hussain S, Hall E, et al, for the BC2001 Investigators. Radiotherapy with or without chemotherapy in muscle-invasive bladder cancer. *N Engl J Med*. 2012;366:1477–1488.
11. MacKinnon G III. *Understanding Health Outcomes and Pharmacoeconomics*. Burlington, MA: Jones & Bartlett Learning; 2013.
12. Allison P. *Survival Analysis Using SAS: A Practical Guide*. 2nd ed. Cary, NC: SAS Institute; 2010.

SAMPLE SIZE AND POWER ANALYSIS

JOHN P. BENTLEY, PhD

CHAPTER OBJECTIVES

▸ Explain the basic information needed to calculate sample size

▸ Describe additional considerations that may need to be addressed before calculating a sample size

▸ Identify examples of available software for power and sample size calculation

▸ Demonstrate how to calculate sample size requirements for basic study designs

▸ Differentiate between sample size calculations based on precision analysis and power analysis

▸ Explain the limitations associated with retrospective power analysis

KEY TERMINOLOGY

α

β

Cohen's d

Effect size

One-sided test

Power

Power analysis

Precision analysis

Retrospective power analysis

Standardized effect size

Two-sided test

Type I error

Type II error

INTRODUCTION

In the conduct of research, resources are often limited. Furthermore, ethical standards with respect to research with human subjects require that researchers minimize the number of individuals who are exposed to a research protocol to the number that is needed to accomplish a particular purpose. On the other hand, studies that are smaller than necessary run the risk of generating invalid scientific knowledge while exposing subjects to risks and burdens, which is also considered unethical.[1] Thus, it is imperative for researchers to consider sample size needs when planning a project: studies that are too large waste resources and may unnecessarily expose subjects to risks, inconveniences, and burdens with limited additional societal benefit,[2] while studies that are too small are underpowered, leading to findings that may be invalid, misinterpreted, or never disseminated.

The basic principles of statistics can be used to calculate a justifiable sample size for a study. In addition to obtaining an appropriate and defensible estimate of the number of subjects needed, this process is important for several reasons. It requires researchers, often in collaboration with a statistician, to consider the availability of existing information, the data analysis plan, and the magnitude of the treatment effect considered to be important. Although the final sample size for a study is often affected by the availability of subjects, financial resources, and ethical considerations, sample size calculation is a necessary first step to balance statistical needs with issues of feasibility.

The purpose of this chapter is to introduce the statistical principles underlying sample size calculation. It begins with a few examples of such calculations from the biomedical literature that will be used to subsequently illustrate certain concepts. General principles necessary for understanding sample size estimation are then reviewed, followed by a discussion of needed information when using the method of sample size determination referred to as power analysis. After a brief review of some available software, a few worked examples from basic designs are conducted using a free software program. The chapter concludes with a discussion of some other considerations when estimating sample size for a study.

CASES FROM THE LITERATURE

Many articles in the biomedical literature include information justifying the sample size used in the study. This section is usually, but not always, found in the "Statistical Analysis" section of an article. Below are excerpts from four manuscripts from the biomedical literature where the authors have provided such information. These examples are used to illustrate some commonly used terminology and also to set the stage for a more detailed discussion of several points. As concepts regarding sample size calculation and power analysis are introduced later in the chapter, references will be made back to these four cases.

Bentley and Thacker attempted to assess the effects of risk and payment on subjects' willingness to participate in research using a set of hypothetical scenarios together with a 3 (level of risk) × 3 (level of monetary payment), randomized, between-subjects, factorial design.[3] Here is their statement of the number of participants needed for the study:

> Power analysis indicated that 23 cases per treatment group ($n = 207$) were necessary to have power of 0.80 to detect medium main and interaction effects with a significance level of 0.05.

Using a randomized controlled trial (RCT), Poldermans and colleagues studied whether beta-receptor blockade (using bisoprolol) immediately before vascular surgery and then 30 days postoperatively in high-risk patients was able to reduce the risk of adverse cardiovascular outcomes when compared to standard perioperative care.[4] They report the following information about the number of patients initially thought necessary for their study:

> The calculation of sample size was based on a previous study in which we noted a 28 percent incidence of serious perioperative cardiac events in patients who had clinical risk factors as well as positive results on dobutamine echocardiography. We calculated that the inclusion of 266 patients would allow us to detect a reduction in the incidence of the primary end point from 30 percent to 15 percent with an alpha level of 0.05 and a statistical power of 0.80.*

James et al. report the results of an RCT comparing radiotherapy alone versus radiotherapy concurrent with chemotherapy consisting of fluorouracil and mitomycin C (chemoradiotherapy) in the treatment of muscle-invasive bladder cancer.[5] The following is from their "Statistical Analysis" section:

> We originally determined that an enrollment of 460 patients (194 events) would provide a power of 90% to detect an improvement of 15 percentage points (from 50% to 65%) in the primary end point in the chemoradiotherapy group, as compared with the radiotherapy group, at 2 years (hazard ratio, 0.62) with a two-sided alpha level of 0.05. In 2005, with the support of the independent trial steering committee, we reduced the power to 80% because of slow recruitment. The revised target sample size was 350 patients (140 events).[†]

And finally, Murdoch et al. describe the results of an RCT designed to evaluate whether vitamin D supplementation can prevent upper respiratory tract infections.[6] Their assumptions and sample size calculation included the following:

> On the assumption that participants would have an average of 1.6 URTIs per year and follow-up of 18 months and that the intervention would need to reduce the mean number of infections by 20% to have clinical relevance, we calculated that a sample of 240 participants would be required to observe this effect with a power of 80% at the .05 level of significance. This number was increased to 320 to compensate for the potential influence of influenza vaccination and loss to follow-up.[‡]

GENERAL CONCEPTS

In general, sample size calculations are typically based on type I and/or type II errors. These errors were defined and discussed in Chapter 9, "Interpretation and Basic Statistical Concepts," and are illustrated in **Table 13-1**. Probabilities are assigned to these errors. Thus, α refers to the probability of a **type I error** (sometimes called the level of significance or the significance level) or the probability of rejecting the null hypothesis

TABLE 13-1 Errors in Hypothesis Testing			
		True State of Affairs	
		H_0 is true	H_0 is false
Conclusion from Hypothesis Test	Reject H_0	Type I (α) error	Correct conclusion
	Fail to reject H_0	Correct conclusion	Type II (β) error

---

*Reproduced from Poldermans D, Boersma E, van Urk H, et al. The effect of bisoprolol on perioperative mortality and myocardial infarction in high-risk patients undergoing vascular surgery. Dutch Echocardiographic Cardiac Risk Evaluation Applying Stress Echocardiography Study Group. *The New England Journal of Medicine.* 1999;341(24):1789–1794.

†Reproduced from James N, Hussain S, Huddart R, et al. Radiotherapy with or without chemotherapy in muscle-invasive bladder cancer. *The New England Journal of Medicine.* 2012;366(16):1477–1488.

‡ Reproduced from Murdoch D, Slow S, Scragg R, et al. Effect of vitamin D3 supplementation on upper respiratory tract infections in healthy adults: the VIDARIS randomized controlled trial. *JAMA.* 2012;308(13):1333–1339.

when it is true. Likewise, α refers to the probability of a **type II error**, or the probability of failing to reject the null hypothesis when it is false. Subtracting β from 1 provides another probability that plays a critical role in sample size calculation. **Power**, or $(1 - \beta)$, is defined as the probability of correctly rejecting the null hypothesis when it is false.

A commonly used approach for sample size calculation for hypothesis-testing studies attempts to minimize the probabilities of type I and type II errors (alternatively, minimize α and maximize power), or least minimize them at some acceptable level. In essence, a researcher uses a predetermined α and attempts to achieve a desired level of β (or, conversely, power) by choosing a sample size to detect some clinically or scientifically meaningful effect. This general approach to sample size determination is referred to as **power analysis**[7] and is the primary method discussed in this chapter. Another approach to sample size calculation referred to as precision analysis will be briefly discussed later.

Before the conduct of a study, investigators may choose to calculate a necessary sample size for achieving a specified power. This is referred to as sample size estimation. However, it is also possible to use the principles of power analysis to justify a given sample size, which may be limited due to budgetary or other constraints. Thus, it is possible to calculate power when given a specific sample size or even to calculate how big an effect can be detected given a specific sample size. Thus, one might ask, given the number of subjects we have access to, is the size of the effect that can detected even realistic? If not, one might reconsider the study. This type of power analysis is referred to as sample size justification. The focus of this chapter is on sample size estimation, but the basic principles are the same for both types of power analysis.

Before discussing the mechanics associated with power analysis, it is worth mentioning the importance of assuring consistency of sample size estimation and the data analysis plan. Thus, it is critical for the research team to carefully consider their study design, the measurement of their primary endpoint, and their proposed data analysis plan before attempting a power analysis. If the research team proposes to use a Wilcoxon–Mann–Whitney test to assess the main study hypothesis, then the power analysis to determine the required sample size should *not* be based on the assumption that a *t*-test will be used. As an example of an appropriate way to handle the situation where the measurement of the primary study outcome is changed before analysis, necessitating a change in the sample size calculation, consider the study reported by Kripalani et al., who evaluated the effect of a pharmacist intervention on the rate of clinically important medication errors.[8] The initial data analysis plan called for comparing the proportion of patients in each treatment group experiencing at least one clinically important medication error (i.e., a dichotomous outcome), most likely using a chi-square test of homogeneity. This planned data analysis was used to calculate an initial sample size estimate. The primary outcome was changed prior to study initiation to reflect the number of clinically important medication errors per patient (i.e., a count variable), still a categorical outcome, but one necessitating a different and more complex analysis strategy (negative binomial regression was used by Kripalani and colleagues). The authors proceed to describe how big an effect they were able to detect in terms of their new outcome measure given their initial sample size estimate.

INFORMATION NECESSARY TO COMPUTE SAMPLE SIZE USING POWER ANALYSIS

To calculate a required sample size based on a power analysis, several pieces of information are needed. The most critical information includes the following: knowledge of how the primary endpoint is measured (type of data), the type of hypothesis test proposed, a measure of variance or precision, a specification of the magnitude of effect one wishes to detect, the stated level of significance (α), and the target level of power ($1 - \beta$). Each of these is discussed, while other considerations that may need to be addressed before calculating a sample size will be discussed later in the chapter.

TYPE OF DATA

The measurement of the primary outcome of the study (i.e., the dependent variable) drives the selection of the statistical method used to analyze the data, knowledge of which is necessary when conducting a power analysis. There must be consistency between a power analysis and the data analysis plan. In general, there are three broad categories for type of data that one must consider: (1) discrete responses, with the most common example being dichotomous or binary responses (e.g., dead or alive), (2) continuous responses (e.g., cholesterol levels), and (3) time-to-event responses (i.e., time until the occurrence of an event). Examples for the first two outcome types will be provided later in this chapter. Power analysis for time-to-event responses are somewhat more complicated, and examples will not be provided. However, it is worth noting a few issues that researchers should consider when performing sample size calculations for a time-to-event response. When comparing groups in terms of survival (see Chapter 12, "Logistic Regression and Survival Analysis" for more details), the key is that there needs to be a reasonable *number of events* during the study period. So this is the initial concern rather than total number of observations. Thus, sample size calculation for comparing the survival experience of two groups consists first of calculating the required number of events and *then* calculating the required number of patients one eventually needs for the study (see Chow et al.[7] for more details and the case above from James et al.[5] for an example).

TYPE OF HYPOTHESIS TEST

The four different types of hypothesis tests (i.e., test for difference—also called test for equality, test for superiority, test for equivalence, and test for non-inferiority) were described in Chapter 9, "Interpretation and Basic Statistical Concepts" and comprise the second piece of information necessary when calculating a required sample size. Furthermore, these tests are associated with certain trials of the same name, as introduced in Chapter 4, "Randomized Controlled Trials." Thus, a non-inferiority test is associated with a non-inferiority trial designed to show whether a new therapy is *no worse* than a standard, and a superiority test is associated with a superiority trial designed to show whether a new therapy is more effective than a standard. Researchers must clearly state the hypothesis of interest when performing a sample size calculation. Which type of hypothesis test is selected will have an effect on the required sample size needed for a study.

Recall that the tests for difference and test for equivalence are two-sided (non-directional), whereas tests for superiority and non-inferiority are one-sided (directional) tests. The use of **one-sided tests** versus **two-sided tests** is still a somewhat controversial matter, especially in the clinical trials literature, and especially with respect to tests of superiority versus tests for difference.[7,9,10] That being said, two-sided tests are generally preferred and used in the biomedical literature for a variety of reasons (unless there is a strong justification for using a one-sided test). Indeed, even when investigators and statisticians say superiority test, oftentimes they are referring to a two-sided test.[11] These days, non-inferiority trials (and also equivalence trials) are becoming increasingly common, largely because of an increased emphasis on comparative effectiveness research.[12] The examples used in this chapter will consist of tests for differences, although a sample size calculation for a non-inferiority trial considering a binary outcome will also be demonstrated.

Measure of Precision (or Variance)

In general, a more precise method of measurement (i.e., smaller variance) will permit detection of any given treatment effect with a smaller sample size. Thus, as statistical variability increases, the sample size needed to detect a given effect size increases. Studies with large levels of variability coupled with small sample sizes will show statistically significant differences only if there is a large difference between the two groups. With continuous outcomes, this parameter is usually represented by the population standard deviation (σ), while with dichotomous outcomes, it depends on the proportion of those with the event in the control group and the increase (or decrease) in the proportion having a given outcome in the treatment group. Although researchers generally do not have control over the population variance in practice, they often have some level of control over the selection of measures used in their studies to assess outcomes. Thus, measures with psychometric unreliability should be avoided as they generally lead to increased variance (decreased precision), requiring larger samples to detect a given effect.[13] Similarly, repeating the measurement (i.e., administering a pretest) and then using that information in the analysis either as a covariate or by using a difference score (i.e., posttest score − pretest score) as the outcome variable can be shown to increase precision (reduce variance) under many conditions, thus reducing the required sample size.[7,14–16]

Magnitude of Effect

This is also called the **effect size** and reflects a clinically (or scientifically) relevant treatment effect that the study should be able to detect. It may be the difference between two population means or proportions in the case of a two-group problem. The choice of the detectable effect size can have a significant effect on sample size requirements. All other things being equal, the necessary sample size for a study increases as the size of the treatment effect decreases. Thus, if the effect size of interest is small, a large sample size will be required. Choosing this parameter should be based on clinical judgment, experience, expertise, and a firm understanding of the content area, *not* statistical considerations. The detectable effect size should reflect effects that are clinically important, thus power analysis for sample size planning attempts to ensure both statistical and clinical significance.

Readers of the biomedical literature are likely to encounter **standardized effect sizes**. One way to think of a standardized effect size is the effect size adjusted for standard deviation[7] such that the effect size is expressed in "standard" units rather than the original measurement units of the dependent variable. Thus, a standardized effect size combines the effect size and the measure of variance into a single metric. For most standardized effect measures, there are also guidelines suggesting what to consider as a small, medium, or large effect. Consider the comparison of the means from two independent groups. **Cohen's *d*** is a standardized effect size that is calculated by dividing the difference between the two means by an estimate of the population standard deviation (e.g., the pooled standard deviation for the two groups).[13] Thus, a Cohen's *d* of 0.2 reflects a difference between two groups of two-tenths of a standard deviation (or the two groups differ by 0.2 SDs), a small effect according to conventional standards.[13] This approach to effect size estimation when conducting a pre-study power analysis is often used when the measurement scale for the dependent variable is arbitrary; see the case above from Bentley and Thacker[3] for an example. It is also used when there is limited information available before a study about the raw (unstandardized) effect size of interest or the measure of variance.

There are critics of standardized effect sizes,[17,18] especially when the measurement units of the dependent variable have meaning. The primary criticism is that standardized effect sizes ignore other important considerations such as the reliability of measurement instruments for the response variable or the degree of heterogeneity in the population under study. As long as the ratio of the raw effect size to the standard deviation remains the same, the sample size estimate does not change. Thus, the specification of a medium effect size for a power analysis will lead to the same sample size estimate, even if there are noticeable differences in the reliability of available measurement instruments. But an instrument with a higher reliability, and hence a smaller standard deviation, should be able to detect a smaller absolute (or raw) effect size, all other things being equal. Standardized effect sizes essentially ignore this.

Specified Significance Level

The significance level, or α, is chosen by researchers early in the study planning period. Conventionally, it is set at $\alpha = 0.05$, although other values are possible (such as 0.01 and 0.10). All other things being equal, the required sample size for a study increases as the probability of a type I error decreases. Stated differently, one way to increase the power of a statistical test would be to increase the probability of a type I error one is willing to accept.

Target Level of Power

As with α, power is also set in advance by researchers. Its conventional level is 0.80, although people who run clinical trials and statisticians are increasingly suggesting a power of 0.90,[19] as studies using 90% power provide more "wiggle room" in terms of the impact of potentially flawed assumptions in other design parameters when performing the calculations than studies designed with 80% power. Power curves (e.g., plotting power on the Y-axis and different potential samples sizes on the X-axis) can help to demonstrate the impact of small changes in design parameters on power. Such a plot will be demonstrated later and will be used to show why a power of 0.90 is generally preferred over a power of 0.80. All other things equal, sample size requirements increase with increasing target levels of power.

SOME AVAILABLE SOFTWARE

There are a multitude of resources available for performing sample size calculations based on power analysis. These include commercial software, free software, as well as a number of websites. Some commercial software is stand-alone (expressly designed for power analysis and sample size calculation), while others are modules available as part of multipurpose statistical software (see **Table 13–2**).

There are some free stand-alone power analysis programs and a number of excellent websites that allow the user to conduct sample size estimations. See **Table 13–3** for selected resources.

TABLE 13-2 Selected Commercial Software for Sample Size Calculation and Power Analysis

Package	Program/Procedure	Type
SAS (SAS Institute, Cary, NC, USA)	PROC POWER PROC GLMPOWER	Multipurpose
Stata (StataCorp LP, College Station, TX, USA)	SAMPSI	Multipurpose
PASS (NCSS, LLC, Kaysville, UT, USA)	Not Applicable	Stand-alone
SamplePower (IBM SPSS, New York, NY, USA)	Not Applicable	Stand-alone
nQuery Advisor (Statistical Solutions, Saugus, MA, USA)	Not Applicable	Stand-alone

TABLE 13-3 Selected Free Programs and Internet Sites for Sample Size Calculation and Power Analysis

Site	Comment	Link
Russell Lenth's power and sample size website	Includes a number of applets and software that can be run stand alone	http://homepage.stat.uiowa.edu/~rlenth/Power/index.html
PS: Power and sample size calculation	Stand-alone program	http://biostat.mc.vanderbilt.edu/PowerSampleSize
G*Power[20,21]	Stand-alone program	http://www.gpower.hhu.de

WORKED EXAMPLES

The following examples use G*Power to estimate the required sample sizes for a few basic designs and also attempt to demonstrate some of the basic precepts discussed previously. In all cases, the assumption is made that a parallel design is being used (i.e., a trial design in which patients receive only one of two or more concurrently administered treatments, such that two or more *separate* groups are being compared).

COMPARING TWO GROUPS—CONTINUOUS RESPONSE

Suppose a research team wishes to compare cholesterol levels in group of patients receiving care through a medication therapy management (MTM) program compared to a control group receiving usual care. Based on past literature, a difference in cholesterol level of 15 mg/dL is considered clinically meaningful. The team is attempting to estimate the sample size necessary to detect this difference in cholesterol level with 90% power. The standard deviation, estimated from previous data, is assumed to be 50 mg/dL. The team plans to conduct a two-sided hypothesis test (test for equality) at the 5% significance level. The following hypotheses are thus considered, and an independent-groups *t*-test will be used to analyze the data:

$$H_0 : \mu_{\mathrm{MTM}} = \mu_{\mathrm{UC}}$$
$$H_A : \mu_{\mathrm{MTM}} \neq \mu_{\mathrm{UC}}$$

(1)

Figure 13-1 shows a screenshot from G*Power that illustrates this calculation while **Figure 13-2** provides an example of a power curve with power on the *Y*-axis and total sample size on the *X*-axis. Given these parameters, the results shows that a total sample

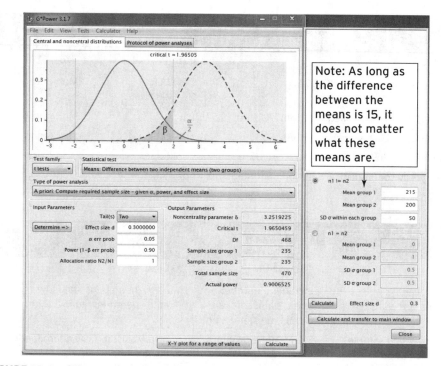

FIGURE 13-1   G*Power calculation of the required sample size for independent-groups *t*-test.
Courtesy of G*Power.

size of 470 (or 235 per treatment group) is needed. Notice in Figure 13-2 that if 80% power was used rather than 90% (total required sample size of 352), the results would be closer to the "shoulder" of the curve, such that small changes in the sample size actually achieved would have a greater effect on power. In terms of variance, if the estimate of the standard deviation was increased to 60 mg/dL, a total sample size of 676 (or 338 per treatment group) would now be required with 90% power, a fairly substantial increase.

Comparing Two Groups—Dichotomous Response

Consider the case example described from the study conducted by Poldermans and colleagues.[4] The essential sample size calculation question is this: Estimate the sample size necessary to detect a 15% decrease in the incidence of the primary endpoint (death from cardiac causes or nonfatal myocardial infarction during the perioperative period) associated with beta-blockade using bisoprolol with 80% power. Assume that standard perioperative care leads to an event rate of 30% and that the investigators want to conduct a two-sided hypothesis test (test for equality) at the 5% significance level.

The following hypotheses are considered and the authors state in the statistical analysis section that differences between the groups in terms of the proportion experiencing the primary endpoint were evaluated using Fisher's exact test:

$$H_0:P_B = P_{SC}$$
$$H_A:P_B \neq P_{SC}$$
(2)

Figure 13-3 shows a screenshot from G*Power that illustrates this calculation. Given these parameters, the results show that a total sample size of 262 (or 131 per treatment group) is needed (slightly different than the estimate of 266 in the original

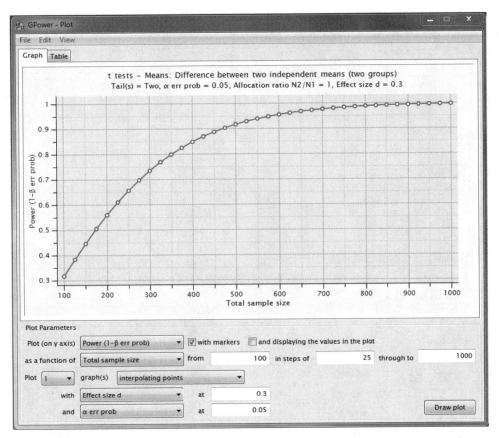

FIGURE 13-2   Power curve with sample size on the *X*-axis for independent-groups *t*-test example.
Courtesy of G*Power.

study, most likely due to subtle differences in the algorithms in the programs used to perform the calculations or possibly rounding error). The hypothesis for this study also could have been tested using a chi-square test of homogeneity. Given this test, and keeping all other parameters the same, results in a total sample size estimate of 242 (or 121 per treatment group), which is slightly less than the requirement assuming that the analysis would be conducted using Fisher's exact test. Although this finding is not always true, it is generally true that the use of Fisher's exact test will lead to a larger sample size estimate than the use of the chi-square test of homogeneity.

As mentioned earlier, for a dichotomous response, the measure of variance depends on the proportion of those with the event in the control or reference group. In general, the variance is largest when $P = 0.5$ and smallest when P is near 0 or 1. Therefore, larger sample sizes are required to detect a change in the difference in two proportions when the two proportions are closer to 0.5. In the present example, assume that standard perioperative care leads to an event rate of 45% rather than 30%. Assuming everything else is the same, the total required sample size to detect a 15% decrease in the incidence of the primary endpoint would be 348 (or 174 per treatment group).

TEST FOR NON-INFERIORITY: COMPARING TWO GROUPS ON A DICHOTOMOUS RESPONSE

As discussed in the Chapter 9, "Interpretation and Basic Statistical Concepts," the goal of a study may be to show that a new treatment is no worse than an existing treatment, necessitating a test of non-inferiority. Consider the case of a non-inferiority test when

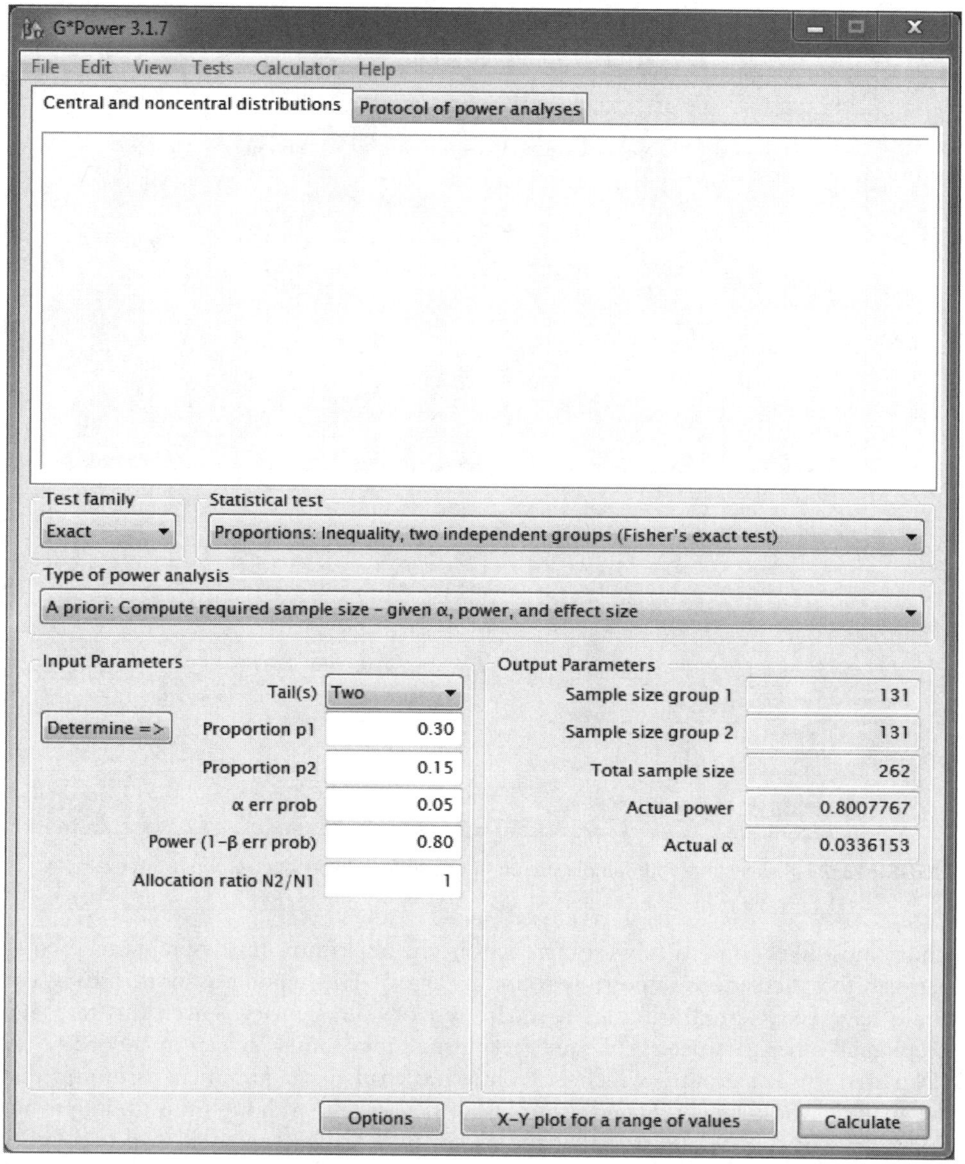

FIGURE 13-3   G*Power calculation of the required sample size for Fisher's exact test.
Courtesy of G*Power.

comparing two groups on a binary outcome (assuming a good outcome, such as survival or cure). The null and alternative hypotheses for this situation are:

$$H_0 : P_{NT} - P_S \leq -\delta$$
$$H_A : P_{NT} - P_S > -\delta \tag{3}$$

where P_{NT} and P_S refer to the probabilities of the outcome (or the proportions experiencing the outcome) in the new treatment group and the standard treatment group, respectively. Understanding these hypotheses involves somewhat reversed thinking when compared to tests for superiority or difference. Thus, the null hypothesis is stating that there is a difference between the groups. In other words, the proportion of successes in the new treatment group is at least an amount δ (called the non-inferiority margin) worse than the proportion of successes in the standard treatment group. The alternative hypothesis, what we want to demonstrate, is stating that there is no real difference between the groups. In other words, the proportion of successes in the new treatment group is no worse than δ lower than the proportion of successes in the standard treatment group (the new treatment is non-inferior to the standard treatment). Assume that δ is 0.035 and the groups are two different antibiotics for the treatment of an infection. Given this, the new treatment would be non-inferior to the standard therapy if probability of a cure is no more than 3.5% lower with the new treatment than with the standard treatment.

To conduct a power analysis with non-inferiority testing, one needs to consider the non-inferiority margin (δ) and the true difference in proportions, which is usually assumed to be 0.[22] Assume that a non-inferiority trial was being conducted to compare two antibiotics for the treatment of an infection. The standard treatment has a cure rate of 90%, and any difference between the two treatments of less than 3.5% is considered to have no clinical relevance ($\delta = 0.035$). Given this information, and assuming equal group sizes, power of 0.80, and $\alpha = 0.05$, how many subjects are needed in each treatment group? G*Power cannot be used to perform this calculation. However, PROC POWER in SAS can. To accomplish this, the following command statements can be used in SAS:

```
Proc Power;
TwoSampleFreq
Test = PChi
Sides = U
Alpha = 0.05
NullProportionDiff = -0.035
ProportionDiff = 0.00
RefProportion = 0.90
Power = 0.80
Npergroup = .
;
Run;
```

Given these parameters, the results are that a total sample size of 1,818 (or 909 per treatment group) is needed. The choice of non-inferiority margin (δ) is critical and sometimes can be quite controversial. Holding everything else constant and decreasing δ to 0.03 leads to a substantial increase in the required number of subjects (now 1,237 per group or 2,474 total).

COMPARING THREE OR MORE GROUPS— CONTINUOUS RESPONSE

Now consider the case of comparing three groups on a continuous outcome, perhaps a new method to improve adherence with chronic medications versus an automated refill program (an active control) and usual care (i.e., a three-arm trial). Assume that the primary endpoint is continuous, such as scale scores generated from patients' responses to a newly developed self-reported non-adherence measurement instrument. Given the lack of information concerning the clinical significance and meaning of differences along the new measurement scale, investigators decided to use a standardized effect before performing a power analysis. The specification of α, power, and a standardized effect completely determines the sample size.[17] Thus, one might ask: How many subjects would be required to have power = 0.90 to detect a medium-sized effect, assuming $\alpha = 0.05$ and a 3-group design? The following hypotheses are considered and ANOVA will be used to perform the omnibus test of whether there are differences among the means:

$$H_0 : \mu_1 = \mu_2 = \mu_3$$
$$H_A : \text{The three population means are not all equal} \tag{4}$$

The results from G*Power are shown in **Figure 13-4**. Notice that the analyst directly enters the stated effect size: in this case, $f = 0.25$. As noted in Figure 13-4, G*Power provides the conventional standards for a small, medium, and large effect using a standardized effect size measure called Cohen's f,[13] which is used for situations when more than two means are being compared. Given these parameters, the results show that a total sample size of 207 (or 69 per treatment group) is needed. Assuming a small effect size ($f = 0.1$), a total sample size of 1,269 (or 423 per treatment group) would now be required—a substantial increase.

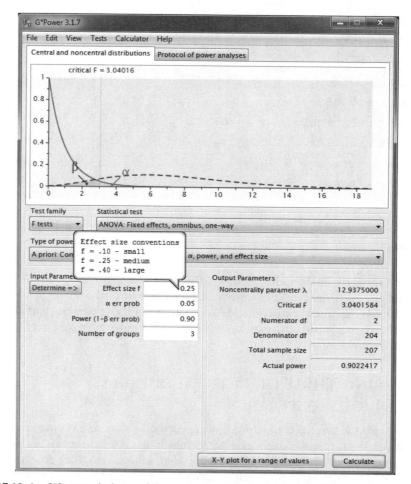

FIGURE 13-4   G*Power calculation of the required sample size for one-way ANOVA.
Courtesy of G*Power.

OTHER CONSIDERATIONS AND ISSUES

Earlier, six pieces of necessary information were considered when performing a sample size calculation based on a power analysis. There are a multitude of additional considerations when calculating sample size. For example, other information may be necessary depending on the study design: (1) the use of paired observations (e.g., a pretest-posttest design with no control group; crossover design) usually requires some information about the correlation between the measurements, and (2) the use of interim analysis of accumulating data in a clinical trial requires a statement in the protocol of the number and timing of planned interim analysis monitoring and the interim monitoring method, as all three can affect the initial sample size estimate.[7,23] Furthermore, investigators may elect to enroll a larger number of subjects than suggested by the sample size calculation to account for potential loss to follow-up as was done by Murdoch et al.[6] in the case presented earlier.

Another consideration is whether there are multiple endpoints or whether subgroup analyses and statistical tests of interaction will be performed. Power analyses are usually performed based on a *single* primary endpoint for the comparison of the main treatment groups of interest. Depending on the situation, the use of multiple endpoints may necessitate the use of a different type of test[24] or the possibility of using an adjusted α level in the sample size calculation to account for the performance of multiple tests.[7] With respect to subgroup analyses and tests of interactions (an interaction between a subgroup variable and a treatment variable implies a treatment effect that varies across subgroups), given that clinical trials are typically powered to detect an overall treatment effect, tests of interaction and for the detection of a treatment effect in subgroups are generally underpowered.[25] If possible, important subgroup analyses and tests of interaction should be defined in the pre-study protocol. Occasionally, studies will be powered to specifically examine interaction effects; see the case above from Bentley and Thacker[3] for an example. Below are a few additional considerations.

CASE-CONTROL AND COHORT STUDIES

The case studies and examples used in this chapter have been based on RCTs, where the treatment groups being compared are created by randomly allocating subjects to receive one or the other treatments under study. The principles and practices of power analysis are readily extended to case-control and cohort studies. For cohort studies, the magnitude of effect the study should be able to detect is usually conceptualized as a relative risk, and for case-control studies, an odds ratio. However, this information is insufficient on its own, because to calculate a sample size for given levels of α and target power, a reference proportion is also necessary. Therefore, the incidence of the outcome in the unexposed group and the prevalence of exposure in the control group (i.e., not cases; those without the outcome of interest) are necessary for performing a power analysis for cohort and case-control studies, respectively.[26] These pre-study estimates serve to inform the variance parameter estimate.

One other consideration for power analyses for these observational studies is the use of groups of unequal size. In a clinical trial, this means having unequal numbers of subjects receiving treatment and control; in a cohort study, it means having a different number of individuals in the exposed and unexposed groups; and in a case-control study, it usually means having more controls than cases. Treatment groups of equal size (i.e., equal treatment allocation) are desirable and generally used in clinical trials, because such an approach maximizes power for a given sample size (although there may be ethical and practical reasons for preferring unequal treatment allocation). The use of unequal group sizes is somewhat more common in case-control and cohort studies, but rarely is there rationale for using ratios larger than 4:1.[26]

DETERMINING VARIANCE

To calculate sample size, investigators need to specify one or more variance estimates. These are sometimes referred to as nuisance parameters, because these parameters are unrelated to the hypotheses and the effect of interest. For continuous outcomes, this may refer to the standard deviation (σ) or variance (σ^2), while for dichotomous outcomes, it is related to the proportion of those with the event in the reference or control group. Along with specifying the minimum difference or effect size to be detected (magnitude of effect), the specification of variances can present investigators with significant challenges. Many recommend the use of a pilot study to obtain variance estimates to use in sample size calculation for the primary study.[17,27] A related alternative is to use an internal pilot design, which allows the required sample size to be re-estimated *during* the conduct of a study using a new estimate of the nuisance parameter from the data already collected.[28] Estimates from prior research and related studies also can be used, but careful consideration needs to be given to ensure that the variance from prior research is the right variance for the planned study; it may be helpful to consult a statistician when trying to determine whether historical data provide a usable variance estimate.[17] Theoretical knowledge and informed judgment are also useful when eliciting a variance. For example, a researcher may first arrive at a range of possible values using a best guess of the maximum and minimum possible values of the outcome variable. To arrive at a rough (and conservative) estimate of the standard deviation, some suggest to divide this range by 3 or 5.[27,29]

SAMPLE SIZE ESTIMATION FOR MORE COMPLEX ANALYSES

The cases and examples provided in this chapter have consisted of the use of power analysis to determine a sample size to detect meaningful *differences between groups*. Power analysis is not restricted to this case; indeed, it can be used to estimate required sample sizes for many different statistical methods, including situations when all dependent and independent variables are continuous or there is a mixture of discrete and continuous independent variables, as is common when conducting multivariable analysis. Thus, power analysis can be used when the hypotheses under consideration are stated like those in Chapter 11, "Simple and Multiple Linear Regression" (i.e., a particular population regression coefficient is equal to zero; all the population regression coefficients are jointly equal to zero; a specified subset of the population regression coefficients are jointly equal to zero). For more information, see Myers, Well, and Lorch.[30]

There are also rules of thumb for various types of regression, which are quite useful when trying to determine sample size requirements when adjusting for many covariates. For example, for linear regression, one rule of thumb is that there should be approximately 15 (some recommend larger values) observations (or subjects) for each predictor variable. There are similar rules of thumb for logistic regression and Cox regression.[31]

Sample size estimation can be performed for any technique, including the ones discussed in this chapter, using *a priori* Monte Carlo simulation methods.[32] This fairly complicated approach is most valuable for very complex analyses. This is the sample size estimation approach used by Kripalani and colleagues[8] in the study mentioned earlier, who examined the effect of a pharmacist intervention on the number of clinically important medication errors per patient (a count variable) using a statistical method called negative binomial regression.

RETROSPECTIVE POWER ANALYSIS

A major assumption up to this point has been that these activities were performed pre-study (*a priori*), or before any subjects were recruited and any data collected. Some recommend the use of power analysis *after* a study has been conducted, in essence calculating power on the basis of the effect size observed in the sample and the final sample size achieved in the study. This approach is called **retrospective power analysis** (retrospective power is also referred to as post hoc power or observed power) and is readily calculated by frequently used statistical software. Despite these recommendations, this attempt at sample size justification through power analysis should be avoided because in the best case scenario it fails to provide any new information, and in the worst case scenario it can be very misleading.

As Hoenig and Heisey nicely describe, observed power does not add any information beyond the results of the statistical test because it is "determined completely by the *p*-value."[33] As the *p*-value of the test decreases, observed power increases and vice versa. Thus, a finding of statistical significance (i.e., a low *p*-value) generally will result in higher observed power, while non-significance generally leads to lower observed power.[18]

Some advocate the calculation of observed power even *with* statistical significance, especially in cases of small sample sizes, to justify one's findings. Such an analysis will not provide the sought-after justification—if the finding is statistically significant, the results of a power analysis will not change that; it is statistically significant.[34] Some also advocate the use of post hoc power following a non-significant finding, oftentimes to justify the non-significant findings (i.e., the reason for the non-significant was because of low power, not the absence of a meaningful effect).[18] Perhaps a worse practice is to combine post hoc power calculations, a non-significant statistical test, and a small observed effect size to provide evidence of strong support for the null hypothesis (i.e., there is no treatment benefit or there is no difference between two treatments). But keep in mind that failing to reject a null hypothesis does not prove that the null is true, no matter what the post hoc power calculation shows. If there is a need to demonstrate that there is no difference of clinical importance between two interventions, then one should use a test for equivalence.[17,33]

SAMPLE SIZE PLANNING USING PRECISION ANALYSIS

In the discussion up until this point, the assumption was that a sample size was being calculated for a hypothesis-testing study. It is also possible to calculate sample sizes when the primary objective is estimation rather than hypothesis testing. In such cases, the researcher is focused on determining a sample size necessary to achieve confidence intervals of a sufficiently narrow width at some fixed confidence level (i.e., 1 − some fixed probability of a type I error). This general approach to sample size determination is referred to as **precision analysis**.[7] As an example, assume that one is interested in calculating the required sample size to arrive at a 95% confidence interval on a mean that extends 0.1σ above and below the point estimate. Suppose the researcher is measuring systolic blood pressure (SBP) in a sample of patients with hypertension, and prior knowledge suggests that the standard deviation for SBP is 20 mmHg. Thus, she wants to find the number of subjects needed such that a 95% confidence interval would be calculated as the sample mean SBP produced in her study ± 2 (i.e., 0.1 × 20). One commonly used equation for this problem is the following:[7]

$$n = \frac{z_{\alpha/2}^2 \sigma^2}{E^2} \tag{5}$$

where z is the two-tailed critical value (i.e., percentile of the standard normal distribution), σ is the standard deviation, and E represents the acceptable amount of error (0.1σ in the present example). Thus, in this example, approximately 385 subjects would be needed:

$$n = \frac{1.96^2 20^2}{(0.1 \times 20)^2} = 384.2 \approx 385 \tag{6}$$

This is easily extended to the situation of binary data (i.e., for a proportion). For example, suppose a researcher is interested in arriving at an estimate of the percentage of students who report current (past 30-day) smoking on a survey. With an error level of + or −4% and a best guess of the population proportion based on prior studies of 0.30, approximately 505 subjects would be needed assuming a 95% confidence interval:

$$n = \frac{z_{\alpha/2}^2 \left[P(1-P)\right]}{E^2} = \frac{1.96^2 \left[0.30(1-0.30)\right]}{(0.04)^2} = 504.2 \approx 505 \tag{7}$$

This approach can also be used for sample size determination when comparing two treatments,[35] for regression coefficients,[36] and many other applications.[32] In these settings, this approach to sample size calculation is referred to as sample size planning for accuracy or accuracy in parameter estimation (AIPE).[32] Given the AIPE framework, it is important to recognize that the two approaches to choosing a sample size discussed in this chapter (i.e., power analysis and precision analysis) can actually be used in a complementary manner in many situations.[36]

SUMMARY AND CONCLUSIONS

Sample size calculation plays a critical role in the planning stage of a study. Such procedures help to ensure that studies have sufficient statistical power to detect effects considered to be of meaningful interest, thereby appropriately using scarce resources. In addition, the process encourages researchers to think critically about many important matters when preparing a research protocol, helping to make sure that the study meets its scientific goals and produces results that have both value and validity. The primary approach used in this chapter involves power analysis, but the use of precision analysis is also demonstrated. Although the computation of a sample size using power analysis requires knowledge of just a small number of basic parameters, it is important that investigators recognize that choosing an effect size of interest and a standard deviation (or variance) in a power analysis requires careful consideration and application of scientific principles. Specification of these parameters is an important task in sample size planning. Depending on the situation and the experience of the research team, consultation with content experts and statisticians may be essential in addition to the conduct of a pilot study. Beyond the basic parameters necessary for performing a pre-study power analysis for sample size estimation, a number of other considerations may influence the calculations and the final sample size estimate. Careful attention to these matters, including the prescription to avoid retrospective power calculations, is important to the conduct of good research, but also in the appropriate interpretation of other studies.

REVIEW QUESTIONS

1. In general, the required sample size for a study increases with (circle one):
   … [increasing/decreasing] variance.
   … [increasing/decreasing] probability of a type I error.
   … [increasing/decreasing] desired target level of power.
   … [increasing/decreasing] size of the effect of interest.

2. Define and differentiate among type I error, type II error, α, β, and power.

3. An investigational drug is being compared with a placebo for the treatment of depression. The study was originally designed to detect a minimum 15% difference in response rates between the groups. Before the start of the study, the investigators are thinking about redefining the magnitude of the effect used in the pre-study power analysis. After substantial debate and consideration, they decide they want to be able to detect a 10% difference in response, as 10% is still clinically meaningful. Holding everything else the same, what effect will this change have on the required sample size? Why?

4. Why should retrospective power analysis be avoided?

5. What are the limitations associated with standardized effect sizes when conducting a pre-study power analysis? When might their use be appropriate?

6. What is the difference between sample size planning using precision analysis and sample size planning using power analysis?

7. Describe the most difficult tasks when performing sample size planning.

8. Revisit the worked example comparing two groups on a dichotomous response variable. Using G*Power and assuming that the researcher proposes to use Fisher's exact test, estimate the sample size necessary to detect a **10% decrease** in the incidence of the primary endpoint (death from cardiac causes or nonfatal myocardial infarction during the perioperative period) associated with beta-blockade using bisoprolol with **90% power**. Assume that standard perioperative care leads to an event rate of 30% and that the researcher wants to conduct a two-sided hypothesis test (test for equality) at the 5% significance level.

9. Using the same assumptions as in question 8, conduct the sample size calculations with the knowledge that the researcher proposes to use a chi-square test of homogeneity. To do this in G*Power, use Test family = "z tests" and Statistical test = "Proportions: Difference between two independent proportions." This works because a two-tailed z-test for the difference between two proportions is mathematically equivalent to the chi-square test of homogeneity.

ONLINE RESOURCES

G*Power 3 website: http://www.gpower.hhu.de

Power Project at the University of Connecticut, Neag School of Education (Ann Aileen O'Connell): http://power.education.uconn.edu/default.htm (An additional resource at this website is a page with links to a number of websites dealing with power analysis, sample size estimation, and other issues in statistics.)

Russell Lenth's power and sample size website: http://homepage.stat.uiowa.edu/~rlenth/Power/index.html

REFERENCES

1. Emanuel E, Wendler D, Grady C. What makes clinical research ethical? *JAMA*. 2000;283(20):2701–2711.

2. Bacchetti P, Wolf L, Segal M, McCulloch C. Ethics and sample size. *American J Epidemiol*. 2005;161(2):105–110.

3. Bentley J, Thacker P. The influence of risk and monetary payment on the research participation decision making process. *J Med Ethics*. 2004;30(3):293–298.

4. Poldermans D, Boersma E, van Urk H, et al. The effect of bisoprolol on perioperative mortality and myocardial infarction in high-risk patients undergoing vascular surgery. Dutch Echocardiographic

Cardiac Risk Evaluation Applying Stress Echocardiography Study Group. *N Engl J Med*. 1999;341 (24):1789–1794.

5. James N, Hussain S, Huddart R, et al. Radiotherapy with or without chemotherapy in muscle-invasive bladder cancer. *N Engl J Med*. 2012;366(16):1477–1488.

6. Murdoch D, Slow S, Scragg R, et al. Effect of vitamin D3 supplementation on upper respiratory tract infections in healthy adults: the VIDARIS randomized controlled trial. *JAMA*. 2012;308(13): 1333–1339.

7. Chow S, Shao J, Wang H. *Sample Size Calculations in Clinical Research*. 2nd ed. Boca Raton, FL: Chapman & Hall/CRC; 2008.

8. Kripalani S, Roumie C, Schnipper J, et al. Effect of a pharmacist intervention on clinically important medication errors after hospital discharge: a randomized trial. *Ann Intern Med*. 2012;157(1):1–10.

9. Bland JM, Altman DG. One and two sided tests of significance. *BMJ*. 1994;309:248.

10. Moyé LA, Tita ATN. Hypothesis testing complexity in the name of ethics: Response to commentary. *J Clin Epidemiol*. 2002;55:209.

11. Kaji A, Lewis R. Are we looking for superiority, equivalence, or noninferiority? Asking the right question and answering it correctly. *Ann Emer Med*. 2010;55(5):408–411.

12. Dasgupta A, Lawson K, Wilson J. Evaluating equivalence and noninferiority trials. *Am J Health-System Pharm*. 2010;67(16):1337–1343.

13. Cohen J. *Statistical Power Analysis for the Behavioral Sciences*. Hillsdale, NJ: Lawrence Erlbaum Associates; 1988.

14. Laird N. Further comparative analyses of pretest-posttest research designs. *Am Stat*. 1983;37:329–330.

15. Norman G. Issues in the use of change scores in randomized trials. *J Clin Epidemiol*. 1989;42(11): 1097–1105.

16. Maxwell SE, Delaney HD. *Designing Experiments and Analyzing Data: A Model Comparison Perspective*. 2nd ed. Mahwah, NJ: Lawrence Erlbaum Associates; 2004.

17. Lenth RV. Some practical guidelines for effective sample size determination. *Am Stat*. 2001;55:187–193.

18. Baguley T. Understanding statistical power in the context of applied research. *Applied Ergonomics*. 2004;35(2):73–80.

19. Eng J. Sample size estimation: how many individuals should be studied? *Radiology*. 2003;227(2): 309–313.

20. Faul F, Erdfelder E, Lang A, Buchner A. G*Power 3: a flexible statistical power analysis program for the social, behavioral, and biomedical sciences. *Behavior Research Methods*. 2007;39(2):175–191.

21. Faul F, Erdfelder E, Buchner A, Lang A. Statistical power analyses using G*Power 3.1: tests for correlation and regression analyses. *Behavior Research Methods*. 2009;41(4):1149–1160.

22. Tunes da Silva G, Logan B, Klein J. Methods for equivalence and noninferiority testing. *Biol Blood Marrow Transplant*. 2009;15(1 Suppl):120–127.

23. Jennison C, Turnbull BW. *Group Sequential Methods: Applications to Clinical Trials*. Boca Raton, FL: Chapman & Hall/CRC; 2000.

24. Dmitrienko A, Molenberghs G, Chuang-Stein C, Offen W. *Analysis of Clinical Trials Using SAS: A Practical Guide*. Cary, NC: SAS Institute; 2005.

25. Assmann S, Pocock S, Enos L, Kasten L. Subgroup analysis and other (mis)uses of baseline data in clinical trials. *Lancet*. 2000;355(9209):1064–1069.

26. Strom BL. Sample size considerations for pharmacoepidemiology studies. In: Strom BL, ed. *Pharmacoepidemiology*. 4th ed. Hoboken, NJ: John Wiley & Sons; 2005:29–36.

27. Kleinbaum DG, Kupper LL, Nizam A, Muller KE. *Applied Regression Analysis and Other Multivariable Techniques*. 4th ed. Belmont, CA: Duxbury Press; 2008.

28. Proschan M. Sample size re-estimation in clinical trials. *Biometrical Journal*. 2009;51(2):348–357.

29. Khamis HJ. Statistics and the issue of animal numbers in research. *Contemporary Topics in Laboratory Animal Science*. 1997;36(2):54–59.

30. Myers JL, Well AD, Lorch RF. *Research Design and Statistical Analysis*. 3rd ed. New York: Routledge; 2010.

31. Vittinghoff E, McCulloch C. Relaxing the rule of ten events per variable in logistic and Cox regression. *Am J Epidemiol*. 2007;165(6):710–718.

32. Maxwell SE, Kelley K, Rausch JR. Sample size planning for statistical power and accuracy in parameter estimation. *Ann Rev Psychol*. 2008;59:537–563.

33. Hoenig JM, Heisey DM. The abuse of power: The pervasive fallacy of power calculations for data analysis. *Am Stat*. 2001;55:19–24.

34. Norman G. Likert scales, levels of measurement and the "laws" of statistics. *Adv Health Sci Educ Theory Pract*. 2010;15(5):625–632.

35. Kelley K, Rausch J. Sample size planning for the standardized mean difference: accuracy in parameter estimation via narrow confidence intervals. *Psychol Methods*. 2006;11(4):363–385.

36. Kelley K, Maxwell SE. Sample size for multiple regression: obtaining regression coefficients that are accurate, not simply significant. *Psychol Methods*. 2003;8:305–321.

SYSTEMATIC REVIEW AND META-ANALYSIS

RICHARD A. HANSEN, RPH, PHD

CHAPTER OBJECTIVES

▸ Define systematic review and meta-analysis
▸ Describe the process of systematic review
▸ Understand the analytical framework for conducting a meta-analysis
▸ Interpret results of a meta-analysis
▸ Understand heterogeneity and bias in meta-analysis
▸ Understand the role of systematic review in research and practice

KEY TERMINOLOGY

Forest plots
Funnel plots
GRADE

Heterogeneity
Meta–analysis
PICOTS

PRISMA
Publication bias
Systematic review

INTRODUCTION

On May 21, 2007, the *New England Journal of Medicine* (*NEJM*) published a systematic review and meta-analysis on the risk of myocardial infarction and death from cardiovascular causes with rosiglitazone, a medication used to treat patients with type II diabetes mellitus.[1] The review found rosiglitazone to be associated with an increased risk of myocardial infarction, and a borderline increase in risk of death from cardiovascular causes. On the same day, the U.S. Food and Drug Administration (FDA) issued a safety alert on rosiglitazone, and this was upgraded to a black boxed warning for heart-related risks later in 2007. This resulted in further clinical research and replication of findings from meta-analysis. In September 2010, the FDA took further action and significantly restricted access to rosiglitazone to only patients with type II diabetes who cannot control their diabetes on other medications. The drug was withdrawn entirely from the market in places such as European countries and New Zealand. The systematic review and meta-analysis published in *NEJM* led to the decline of rosiglitazone, a drug that captured $3.3 billion in U.S. sales in 2006.[2] While controversial, the case of rosiglitazone is one example of how systematic review and meta-analysis can be helpful in understanding the risks and benefits of medications when evidence provided by existing studies is inconclusive or conflicting.

Systematic review is a structured process for identifying and summarizing existing studies that address a specific question. Systematic reviews help patients, healthcare providers, and policy makers understand evidence and formulate best practices.[3] This is especially important given the volume of literature and common challenges that exist in interpreting inconsistent results. Systematic review is especially useful when multiple strong studies are available, but the answers provided by these studies are not in perfect agreement. Systematic review is not useful when there is so much agreement among available studies that the question is already answered, or when too few studies exist so that the question can be answered by review and critique of individual studies. A systematic review should always include a synthesis of included studies, but this synthesis can be qualitative or quantitative. Quantitative syntheses are typically in the form of meta-analysis. When meta-analysis is used, the aim is to produce a single estimate of treatment effect across included studies. In some cases, advanced quantitative methods, such as adjusted indirect comparisons, may be appropriate.

This chapter is divided into two sections. The first section describes the elements of the systematic review process. The second section describes meta-analysis as a method to quantitatively synthesize evidence from studies identified in a systematic review.

SYSTEMATIC REVIEW

A systematic review differs from a traditional narrative review in that it has focused questions, a methods section with clearly defined inclusion and exclusion criteria, and a predefined literature search strategy. A systematic review should use a rigorous approach to identifying and selecting studies in a transparent, reproducible way. The process of conducting a systematic review can be summarized by eight steps (**Figure 14-1**). The first step, and arguably the most important step, is defining focused key questions. In defining key questions, all subsequent aspects of the systematic review will be framed.

Key questions should be important, specific, and reflect uncertainty. Given a general question or area of clinical study, key questions should reflect the type of population, the

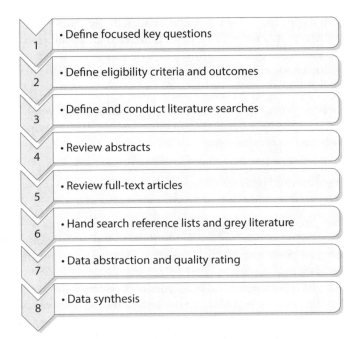

1. • Define focused key questions
2. • Define eligibility criteria and outcomes
3. • Define and conduct literature searches
4. • Review abstracts
5. • Review full-text articles
6. • Hand search reference lists and grey literature
7. • Data abstraction and quality rating
8. • Data synthesis

FIGURE 14-1   Steps in the systematic review process.

type of exposure or intervention, the comparator, and the outcomes to be addressed.[4] For example, an appropriate key question for a systematic review might read:

> *What is the risk of outcome X among adult, community-dwelling patients with condition Y who received intervention A compared with intervention B for at least 3 months?*

This question clearly states that the exposure is intervention A and its being compared with intervention B, and only adult patients with condition Y living in the community that were exposed to these interventions for at least 3 months will be assessed. The A, B, X, and Y in a question like this could be substituted with any number of different possible clinical scenarios.

Research questions, or key questions, should be framed in a way that reflects the intervention and comparison, the population of interest, the outcomes, and the types of data that will be extracted. A useful framework for thinking about this is **PICOTS**, which stands for **P**opulation, **I**ntervention, **C**omparator, **O**utcome, **T**iming, and **S**etting.[5]

> *Population:* includes both the nature of the condition being studied and the underlying characteristics of the population such as age, sex, race, previous treatments, early vs. advanced disease, and other risk factors, such as other common conditions or current medications.

> *Intervention:* refers to the drug, medical procedure, or other healthcare intervention that is being assessed. Considerations about the intervention include dose, duration, frequency, and intensity.

> *Comparator:* outlines whether the intervention is being compared with placebo, compared with usual care with another treatment, or added to an existing treatment. Considerations about the comparator also include dose, duration, frequency, and intensity.

Outcome: is the endpoint measurement, which ideally should reflect a true health outcome that a patient can touch or feel, rather than an intermediate, surrogate endpoint. Considerations in defining outcomes include validation of the measure, sensitivity to change, relevance to the disease, and how the outcome data is collected.

Timing: reflects when the outcome will be measured, and how long measurement will continue. Outcome measurement must consider how responsive the population may be to intervention over time.

Setting: reflects aspects of how health care is being delivered in the population, including access and delivery models, such as urban academic medical centers as opposed to rural primary care.

Once appropriate key questions are framed, the second step is to expand on the inclusion and exclusion criteria and explicitly define eligible outcome measures. An example of how eligibility criteria and outcome measurement might be defined is shown in **Table 14–1**.

Literature search criteria are defined in advance of conducting the search, with the goal of capturing all of the evidence pertaining to the key questions. Searches should be explicit in terms of time frame, language, study type, intervention, condition(s), and characteristics of the population, such as age. Searches should be replicated across multiple databases whenever possible, including databases like Medline, PubMed, Embase, International Pharmaceutical Abstracts (IPA), Cumulative Index to Nursing and Allied Health Literature (CINAHL), and the Cochrane Library. Depending on the nature of the systematic review topic, condition-specific databases also should be used, such as PsychLit for psychiatric research. Results of literature searches typically are imported into reference software such as EndNote, or citations may be managed using specific systematic review software.

After a list of titles and abstracts is identified by the structured literature searches, there are two levels of review. For efficiency, the first level is to review just titles and abstracts. Rigorously conducted reviews typically have each title and abstract reviewed by two independent reviewers, and any study identified as possibly relevant by at least one of these reviewers then moves on for full text review. An alternative approach to this process is to have a single person review all titles and abstracts and have a second reviewer only review those that are recommended for exclusion. This approach minimizes review burden since the second person only has to review the list of possible exclusions and

TABLE 14-1 Example of Eligibility Criteria and Outcome Measures	
Study Eligibility Criteria	**Outcomes of Interest and Specific Measures**
Study Design	All-cause mortality
Head-to-head, double-blind RCTs	Hospital admission
Placebo-controlled, double-blind RCTs	General health status, as measured by:
High-quality systematic reviews	Medical Outcomes Study Short Form 36 (SF36)
Minimum Study Duration	Health-related quality of life, as measured by:
12 weeks	EuroQol-5D (EQ-5D)
Sample Size	Quality of Well-Being (QWB)
At least 40 per group for RCTs	Health Utilities Index (HUI)

RCT = Randomized controlled trial

verify coding for why the study was excluded. All of the studies not excluded after dual review then move on for full text review.

After title and abstract review, full text articles should be obtained for all studies. These full text articles should then be dually reviewed in a manner similar to the abstract review, excluding those that do not meet the defined eligibility criteria and retaining those studies that do meet eligibility criteria. For systematic reviews that have multiple key questions, the full text review process is an appropriate point to identify key question relevance for each study. Studies that have duplicate or overlapping publication (e.g., multiple publications derived from the same study) should be grouped so as not to double count results derived from the same study more than once during data synthesis.

As a quality check of the literature search process, hand-searching the reference lists of included full-text articles is recommended. This process may identify relevant studies that were not identified or indexed in the literature search. Searching the grey literature may also be appropriate. Grey literature includes written materials or reports that are not found in published journals. Examples of grey literature may include technical reports from government agencies, working papers or white papers, conference proceedings, or doctoral theses. Trial registries also may be included as a source of unpublished data. Exclusion of grey literature has been found to lead to exaggerated estimates of intervention benefits,[6,7] although there is a balance in deciding whether or not studies should be included even when they do not report sufficient data to fully assess quality. In some cases, having additional sources of evidence may introduce bias by including evidence of lower methodological quality.[8]

Once all relevant, eligible studies are identified, data are abstracted in a structured evidence table. Abstracting data into an evidence table helps to consistently evaluate and compare studies. An example of an evidence table template that could be used for data abstraction is shown in **Table 14-2**. While the elements abstracted into evidence tables will differ by review topic, typical abstractions will include the following: authors, year of publication, country, funder, study design, eligibility criteria, population characteristics (e.g., age, sex, race/ethnicity, comorbid conditions), whether other treatments were allowed, intervention(s), outcome measures including timing of assessment, and results. Other elements of data abstraction will differ depending on the types of study designs included. For randomized controlled trials, for instance, elements of data abstraction

TABLE 14-2 Example Evidence Table Template					
Author, Year, Country, Funding, Quality Rating	**Study Design, Setting, Eligibility Criteria**	**Participant or Population Characteristics**	**Intervention Details**	**Method and Timing of Outcome Assessment**	**Main Results**
Author, Year (with citation):	Study Design:	Age: n(%) Sex: n(%) Race: n(%) by category	Drugs or intervention description:	Primary Outcome Measures:	Outcome 1:
Country:	Setting:	Disease severity:	Dose:	Timing of Outcome Assessment:	Outcome 2:
Funding:	Eligibility Criteria: *Inclusion:* *Exclusion:*	Concomitant medications allowed:	Duration:		
Quality Rating:					

would also include assessment of the number of patients screened, eligible, and enrolled, as well as withdrawals, withdrawals by reason, and loss to follow-up.

An important part of the systematic review process is assessing quality of component studies. This helps to make sure that studies that meet eligibility criteria but have significant risk of bias and confounding can be excluded from the data synthesis. These poor quality studies may be excluded, but detailed reasons for the quality assessment should be provided. A number of different approaches exist for assessing risk of bias and rating study quality. For example, the U.S. Preventive Services Task Force recommends a relatively subjective rating of good, fair, or poor, taking into consideration elements of internal validity.[9] The Cochrane collaboration focuses on risk of bias as opposed to using a quality rating. They define important elements of consideration as selection bias, performance bias, attrition bias, detection bias, and reporting bias.[9] Many other possible approaches exist, with other common quality rating scales including the Chalmers and Jadad scales.[10]

After abstracting relevant information from the studies and assessing quality (or risk of bias), data can be synthesized and presented. Systematic review presentation should use a diagram to illustrate the flow of information through the different phases of the systematic review. This study flow diagram is sometimes referred to as the Preferred Reporting Items for Systematic Reviews and Meta-Analyses (**PRISMA**) diagram (**Figure 14-2**).[11]

The PRISMA diagram details how studies were identified, the results of abstract screening, the results of full text eligibility assessment including a breakdown of reasons for exclusion, and details of included studies.[11] PRISMA is an evolution of previously used criteria known as QUORUM. The study flow diagram may differentiate included studies by key question, or by studies included in qualitative synthesis as opposed to those included in quantitative synthesis.

The systematic review process helps to identify and evaluate studies that answer a specific key question. In terms of how this is applied to clinical practice, an ongoing challenge is how to assess and communicate the overall strength of a body of evidence in answering a question. Policy makers, clinicians, and patients all have a need for

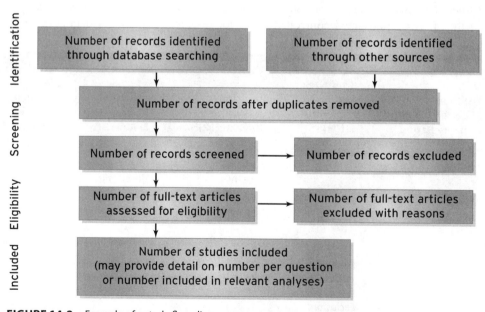

FIGURE 14-2   Example of a study flow diagram.

Source: Reproduced from Moher et al. The PRISMA Statement for Reporting Systematic Reviews and Meta-Analyses of Studies That Evaluate Health Care Interventions: Explanation and Elaboration. PLoS Med. 2009; 6(7): e1000100. doi:10.1371/journal.pmed.1000100

information to help make the best decisions among competing interventions. Conveying the strength of evidence when summarizing reviews can be helpful. One framework for doing this is proposed by the Grading of Recommendations Assessment, Development, and Evaluation (**GRADE**) working group.[12] The GRADE approach recommends evaluating the strength of evidence for each major outcome and for each comparison made. The strength of evidence is evaluated for the body of evidence (rather than component studies) in terms of risk of bias, consistency, directness, and precision. The risk of bias for an evidence base is derived from bias assessment in individual studies. Consistency reflects similarity in the effect sizes across studies. Directness refers to whether the studies assess a single, direct link between the intervention and the outcome. Precision deals with the level of certainty of the effect estimate for a particular outcome. The overall strength of the evidence is then characterized as insufficient, low, moderate, or high. Additional criteria for assessment may include dose-response associations, plausible confounding, strength of association, and publication bias. An example presentation summarizing a GRADE assessment for 11 hypothetical studies of 3 outcome assessments is shown in **Table 14-3**.

META-ANALYSIS

Meta-analysis is the quantitative synthesis of data derived from individual studies that address a key question. Meta-analysis is appropriate when there are multiple studies (usually ≥ 3) identified through a systematic review process. Studies should be of sufficient quality, representing similar populations, interventions, and outcome measures. Meta-analysis is appropriate when results of studies are not so similar that the effect size is already obvious, yet results of studies should not be too dissimilar (i.e., heterogeneity) and indicative of obvious differences in some aspects of the component studies. Data derived from these studies may come in multiple different forms, but commonly data take the form of either a dichotomous or continuous outcome. Dichotomous outcomes may include a variety of different measures such as dead or alive, response or non-response, or meeting goal vs. not meeting goal. Continuous outcomes may include things like mean change in a clinical measure (e.g., blood pressure or total cholesterol) or change in score on a symptom scale. In some cases, measurement across studies might reflect the same construct (e.g., improvement in depression symptoms), but the measurement might be ascertained with different scales that have different properties (e.g., one scale ranges from 0 to 10 while another ranges from 0 to 50). In this case, continuous

TABLE 14-3	Example of GRADE Assessment					
Number of studies; subjects	**Domains pertaining to strength of evidence**					**Strength of evidence**
	Risk of bias; Design/quality	**Consistency**	**Directness**	**Precision**	**Results**	
Outcome 1 3; 210	Medium; RCTs / fair	Consistent	Direct	Precise	Drug A similar to Drug B	Low
Outcome 2 6; 1260	Low; RCTs / 2 good, 4 fair	Consistent	Direct	Precise	Drug A similar to Drug B	High
Outcome 3 2; 1685	High; 1 RCT / fair 1 cohort / fair	Inconsistent	Indirect	Imprecise	Drug A better than Drug B	Insufficient

RCT = Randomized controlled trial

data might be presented as a standardized change using the properties of the scale to adjust the outcome. These data can be reflected using a measure known as Hedge's g.[13]

In the conduct of a meta-analysis, outcome measures must be carefully selected and then data should be abstracted from eligible studies. The following example shows how continuous and dichotomous data could be extracted from studies to allow conduct of a meta-analysis.

CONTINUOUS OUTCOME EXAMPLE

Assume that we have conducted a systematic review and identified five studies that compare treatment A with treatment B in patients with a given disease. In the conduct of these studies, their treatment outcomes were assessed using a symptom scale. Let's assume the scale ranges from 0 to 50 with lower values of the scale reflecting fewer symptoms and higher values of the scale reflecting more symptoms. Using this scale, data can be extracted from the five eligible studies as a continuous outcome (change from baseline to endpoint). Assume that the endpoint is 12 weeks for this example, although not all studies will use the same timing of endpoints, in which case the meta-analysis may need to consider which range of endpoint timing is reasonable to include in the same analysis. For example, is it fair to include data with a 12-week endpoint and compare with data for a 24-week endpoint? These decisions often need to consider the clinical scenario to determine if the symptom score or number of responders is likely to be influenced by the duration of the trial.

For the example of the symptom scale measured as a continuous outcome, an example data extraction is illustrated in **Table 14-4**. Studies 1 through 5 represent a comparison of Drug A with Drug B, with the largest trial including a total of 464 patients (Study 1) and the smallest trial including 189 patients (Study 2). Data from the symptom scale were reported for each study.

For meta-analysis, the mean value of that symptom scale and the standard deviation of the mean were recorded for baseline and endpoint. The mean change in symptom score, if not directly reported in the study, can be calculated by subtracting the mean at endpoint from the mean at baseline. Most studies will directly report a mean change and standard deviation of the mean change, but in cases where these values are not reported, there are approaches to calculating them or, in worst cases, imputing standard deviations based on averages from other studies. The meta-analysis considers the symptom

TABLE 14-4	Example of Continuous Outcome Data for Comparing Mean Symptom Change						
Study	Treatment	Sample Size	Baseline (Mean)	Baseline (SD)	Endpoint (Mean)	Endpoint (SD)	Change (Mean)	Change (SD)
Study 1	Drug A	234	25.2	5.2	11.1	8.4	−14.1	7.5
Study 1	Drug B	230	24.9	5.2	13.1	8.9	−11.8	6.0
Study 2	Drug A	125	25.9	5.9	16.0	7.9	−9.9	10.1
Study 2	Drug B	128	25.8	5.9	18.2	8.1	−7.6	8.7
Study 3	Drug A	128	20.3	3.4	9.9	7.9	−10.5	7.5
Study 3	Drug B	129	20.5	3.4	12.2	8.1	−8.3	6.0
Study 4	Drug A	123	21.4	4.1	10.5	7.9	−10.9	7.5
Study 4	Drug B	122	21.1	3.7	15.1	8.1	−6.1	6.0
Study 5	Drug A	95	19.9	3.6	8.9	7.9	−11.0	4.9
Study 5	Drug B	94	19.9	3.6	11.1	8.1	−8.8	4.8

score change for Drug A from baseline to endpoint, and then compares it with the symptom score change for Drug B from baseline to endpoint. In an unadjusted analysis, for example, we could say that in Study 1 the mean change for Drug A was −14.1, and the mean change for Drug B was −11.8, so the difference in mean change for Drug A vs. Drug B is −14.1 minus −11.8, which is −2.3. The interpretation of this is that Drug A had a 2.3 point greater improvement (since lower scores are better) in symptom score than Drug B. With these numbers, a meta-analysis can be conducted to calculate an overall, pooled weighted mean difference for the comparison of Drug A with Drug B. The meta-analysis calculates all of these differences and then calculates an average estimate across the studies; however, the statistical calculation is not as straightforward as an average. Rather than just an average of the mean differences, the meta-analysis weights each study, usually using the inverse variance as a weight. In other words, each study is weighted in inverse proportion to its variance, which in practical terms usually results in heavier weighting for larger, more precise studies and down-weighting of smaller studies that have lower confidence surrounding the effect estimate. This allows for adjusting for the degree of variance associated with each study.

Table 14–5 shows the statistical output generated from the symptom score example. In this example, however, we note that the largest study was Study 1, and it is assigned a weight of 31.5% in calculating the pooled estimate. The smallest study, Study 5, is assigned a larger weight than expected (25.1%) because it reported a smaller variance than some of the other studies. This may happen contrary to expectations if a smaller study reports an unexpectedly small standard error.

Table 14–5 shows that the pooled estimate of the weighted mean difference across the five studies is −2.672, with a 95% confidence interval of −3.365 to −1.979. Three additional statistics are reported in this analysis. The first is the "Heterogeneity chi-squared," which has a value of 7.23 and a p-value of 0.124. **Heterogeneity** reflects the variation of results of studies included in the meta-analysis. Generally, we want lesser variability in study results and low heterogeneity. If studies represent effect size estimates that are drastically different, then there is a strong plausibility that the studies were conducted in different ways or represent different underlying populations that are influencing results. A chi-squared statistic with a p-value less than 0.05 generally is interpreted as presence of statistically significant heterogeneity. A preferable way to examine heterogeneity is through the I-squared statistic, which is reported as a percentage between 0% and 100%.[14] The higher the I-squared percentage is, the greater the heterogeneity.

TABLE 14-5	Example of Output from a Weighted Mean Difference Meta-Analysis		
Study	**Weighted Mean Difference**	**[95% Conf. Interval]**	**% Weight**
Study 1	−2.300	−3.535 to −1.065	31.50
Study 2	−2.300	−4.625 to 0.025	8.88
Study 3	−2.200	−3.838 to −0.562	17.90
Study 4	−4.800	−6.500 to −3.100	16.61
Study 5	−2.200	−3.583 to −0.817	25.11
I–V pooled WMD	**−2.672**	**−3.365 to −1.979**	**100.00**

Heterogeneity chi-squared = 7.23 (d.f. = 4) p = 0.124
I-squared (variation in WMD attributable to heterogeneity) = 44.7%
Test of WMD = 0: z = 7.56 p < 0.0001
WMD = Weighted mean difference

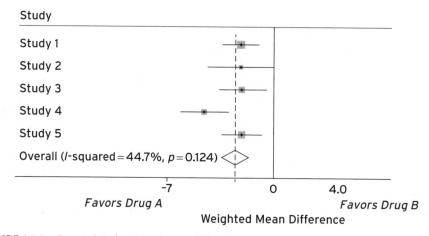

FIGURE 14-3   Forest plot of weighted mean difference meta-analysis.

In this example, the *I*-squared statistic is 44.7%, which suggests a moderate degree of heterogeneity. The results of the forest plot (**Figure 14–3**) may also be used to visually assess heterogeneity. Generally speaking, the less the confidence intervals of individual studies overlap, the higher the heterogeneity.

Forest plots are the primary mechanism for conveying the results of meta-analyses.[15] These figures not only help to illustrate the pooled estimate, but quickly allow assessment of the contribution of each study. For example, in Figure 14-3, we see the point estimate for each study represented by a square (■), with the horizontal lines representing the confidence intervals for that study. The diamond represents the overall pooled estimates, with the size of the diamond (or sometimes confidence interval bars) representing the lower and upper confidence intervals. For this example, Drug A had a statistically significant greater overall reduction (improvement) in symptoms scores than Drug B since the 95% confidence interval of the overall pooled estimate does not cross zero. While statistically significant, clinical significance of this 2.7 point difference on the symptom scale would need to be interpreted.

DICHOTOMOUS OUTCOME EXAMPLE

Using the previous example with a continuous outcome measure, assume that for the purposes of measuring symptom improvement in clinical studies, the scale is often categorized so that scores less than 15 are classified as responders to treatment. Now the data can be treated as dichotomous (i.e., response or non-response). The dichotomized data are shown in **Table 14–6**.

Dichotomous data such as these can be used to calculate an odds ratio (OR) or relative risk (RR). In this example, the odds of response for a given study arm is calculated as the number of patients who responded divided by the number of patients who did not. For Drug A in Study 1, the odds of response is 180/54 = 3.333. For Drug B in Study 1, the odds of response is 134/96 = 1.396. The OR is calculated as odds of response with Drug A over the odds of response with drug B, or 3.333/1.396 = 2.388.

Alternatively, the relative risk can be calculated as the number of patients who respond divided by the total number of patients. For Drug A in Study 1, the risk (of response) is 180/234 = 0.769. For Drug B in Study 1, the risk (of response) is 134/230 = 0.583. The RR (sometimes referred to as risk ratio) is calculated as the risk with Drug A over the risk with Drug B, or 0.769/0.583 = 1.320. The statistical output for an RR meta-analysis of symptom responders is shown in **Table 14–7**. Generally, the results of analyses using the OR as opposed to the RR will be similar when the outcome of interest is uncommon. When the overall event rate is higher (as in the symptom responder example), the OR is inflated when compared with the RR.[16] The example shown here represents a relatively common event (response) and, therefore, the OR is inflated compared with the RR.

The output of the RR meta-analysis appears similar to the output for the weighted mean difference, except this time the study estimates reflect the relative rate of response with Drug A over the relative rate of response with Drug B. The pooled estimate for this example suggests that the relative risk of responding is statistically significantly better with Drug A than Drug B (RR = 1.22; 95% CI 1.13–1.33). Had the RR (and upper bounds of the 95% CI) been less than 1, Drug B would have been favored. The pooled RR is again weighted with the relative contribution of each study, which in essence can be calculated as follows: (RR Study 1 × % Weight Study 1) + (RR Study 2 × % Weight Study 2) + (RR Study 3 × % Weight Study 3) + (RR Study 4 × % Weight Study 4) + (RR Study 5 × % Weight Study 5). The forest plot for this meta-analysis is illustrated

TABLE 14-6 Example of Dichotomous Outcome Data for Comparing Mean Symptom Change

Study	Treatment	Sample Size	Number with Response	Number with No Response	Odds of Response
Study 1	Drug A	234	180	54	3.333
Study 1	Drug B	230	134	96	1.396
Study 2	Drug A	125	90	35	2.571
Study 2	Drug B	128	75	53	1.415
Study 3	Drug A	128	100	28	3.571
Study 3	Drug B	129	100	39	2.564
Study 4	Drug A	123	70	53	1.321
Study 4	Drug B	122	60	62	0.968
Study 5	Drug A	95	80	15	5.333
Study 5	Drug B	94	60	34	1.765

TABLE 14-7 Example of Output from a Relative Risk Meta-Analysis

Study	Relative Risk	[95% Conf. Interval]	% Weight
Study 1	1.320	1.159 to 1.504	28.29
Study 2	1.229	1.024 to 1.474	16.97
Study 3	1.086	0.945 to 1.247	25.86
Study 4	1.157	0.913 to 1.467	10.84
Study 5	1.319	1.107 to 1.572	18.05
D+L pooled RR |	**1.222**	**1.125 to 1.328**	**100.00**

Heterogeneity chi-squared = 5.11 (d.f. = 4) p = 0.276
I-squared (variation in RR attributable to heterogeneity) = 21.7%
Estimate of between-study variance tau-squared = 0.0020
Test of RR = 1: z = 4.73 p < 0.0001
RR = Relative risk

in **Figure 14-4**. Note that the *I*-squared estimate of heterogeneity is only 21.7% in this analysis as compared with the 44.7% observed in the weighted mean difference analysis. This shows that how data are interpreted and categorized can sometimes influence our assessment of things like heterogeneity.

The analyses presented here are simplified for the purposes of demonstrating concepts of meta-analysis. In reality, meta-analyses are more complicated than they have been described here. For example, the calculations for the pooled analysis would be done using the natural log of each estimate since relative measures such as the RR and OR are asymmetric with complex standard error formulas (e.g., negative relationships are indicated by values between 0 and 1, and positive relationships are indicated by values from 1 to infinity). Additional choices that will influence analyses include whether a fixed or random effects model is used. The fixed effects model assumes that variability across studies is due to random variation, while the random effects model assumes that there is a different underlying effect for each study, and the analysis takes this into consideration as an additional source of variation. The output illustrated in Table 14-7 reflects a random effects analysis, with the tau-squared representing the estimate of between-study variance. Underlying aspects of the topic and data may drive choice of a fixed vs. random effects analysis. Otherwise, random effects analyses are generally viewed as the more conservative analysis.

When conducting and interpreting a meta-analysis, there is always the concern for publication or other forms of selection bias.[17,18] **Publication bias** is the most widely acknowledged form of bias in meta-analysis. It results from the likelihood that studies with positive findings are more likely to be published (at least in common, reputable journals), and these published findings are more likely to be identified and included in a systematic review and meta-analysis. Seeking out unpublished data and including trial registries can help overcome this. But, as discussed earlier in this chapter, these sources often do not provide sufficient data to assess internal and external validity of a study (i.e., quality/risk of bias), and including studies of uncertain quality can introduce selection bias.[8]

Several approaches are available to assess risk of publication bias. The most common is a visual assessment of risk of bias using a funnel plot. **Funnel plots** are scatter plots illustrating the relationship between treatment effect estimates from individual studies

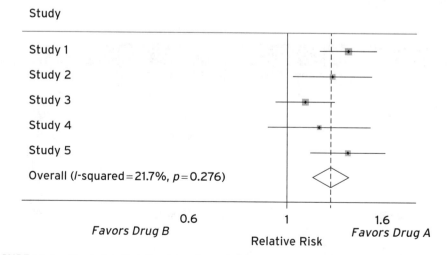

FIGURE 14-4 Forest plot of relative risk meta-analysis.

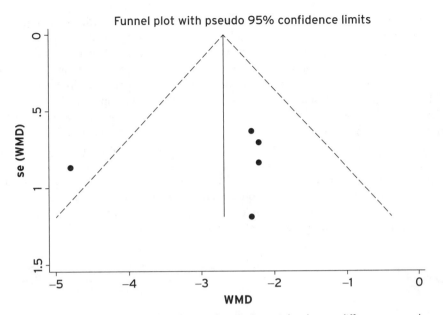

FIGURE 14-5   Funnel plot for test of publication bias in the weighted mean difference example.

and precision (e.g., standard error or variance).[19] For example, **Figure 14-5** shows the funnel plot for the weighted mean difference meta-analysis depicted in Table 14-5 and Figure 14-3.

The plot illustrates the relationship between each study's effect estimate (the weighted mean difference on the *X*-axis) and the standard error of the weighted mean difference (*Y*-axis). The funnel plot adds a pseudo 95% confidence interval (dashed lines). This shows that if all studies fall within this pyramid, then there is little visual risk of publication bias. In this example, because a study falls outside this pyramid, there is visual evidence for the possibility of publication bias. Additional statistics can be used to assess publication bias, such as Egger's test[20] or the Begg and Mazumdar rank correlation test.[21] Both the Egger and Begg tests did not identify statistically significant publication bias in the symptom score example ($P = 0.67$ and $P = 0.22$, respectively).

SUMMARY AND CONCLUSIONS

Systematic review and meta-analysis can be powerful tools for reviewing and synthesizing clinical evidence. These tools are particularly important given the volume of information that needs to be reviewed in making evidence-based decisions. For the primary care clinician, for example, an estimated 7,287 related articles are published each month, and it would take a clinician an estimated 627.5 hours each month to keep up with this information.[22] It is impossible and unrealistic for any clinician to dedicate this time to keeping their practice up-to-date, and this supports the need for ongoing, well-conducted systematic review and meta-analysis in evidence-based medicine.[3] Systematic reviews and meta-analyses also are of growing interest as the number and types of interventions expand. In many cases, competing interventions have not been directly compared, and meta-analytic techniques known as indirect comparisons can help to guide decision making.[23]

Systematic review and meta-analysis have become valuable with increasing interest in comparative effectiveness research. The review of existing studies using systematic review and meta-analysis sometimes is referred to as secondary comparative effectiveness research, which is advantageous because it is more efficient than primary comparative effectiveness research (the conduct of new studies to compare one intervention with another). In the United States, for instance, examples of widespread use of systematic review and meta-analysis include the Drug Effectiveness Review Project (DERP)[24] and the Agency for Healthcare Research and Quality's (AHRQ) Effective Health Care Program. The DERP program uses systematic review and meta-analysis to help guide policy decisions for participating state Medicaid programs. Similarly, the AHRQ program conducts systematic reviews and meta-analyses as a clinical decision–making resource for patients, providers, and policy makers. Many others are using these methods for synthesizing clinical evidence. Understanding how to interpret results of these studies is critical for healthcare professionals and policy makers.

REVIEW QUESTIONS

1. How is a systematic review different from a traditional, narrative review?
2. What is PICOTS, and how is it relevant to systematic review?
3. What is the PRISMA diagram, and how is it used in systematic review?
4. How is GRADE different from quality assessment of individual trials?
5. What is a meta-analysis, and when is a meta-analysis appropriate?
6. Describe measures of heterogeneity that are used in meta-analysis.
7. What is publication bias, and how is it assessed in meta-analysis?

ONLINE RESOURCES

Agency for Healthcare Research and Quality (AHRQ) Effective Health Care Program: http://www.effectivehealthcare.ahrq.gov/index.cfm

Preferred Reporting Items for Systematic Reviews and Meta-Analyses (PRISMA): http://www.prisma-statement.org/

Systematic Reviews: Centre for Reviews and Dissemination Guidance for Undertaking Reviews in Healthcare: http://www.york.ac.uk/inst/crd/pdf/Systematic_Reviews.pdf

REFERENCES

1. Nissen SE, Wolski K. Effect of rosiglitazone on the risk of myocardial infarction and death from cardiovascular causes. *N Engl J Med*. 2007;356(24):2457–2471.
2. Nissen SE. The rise and fall of rosiglitazone. *European Heart Journal*. 2010;31(7):773–776.
3. Mulrow CD. Rationale for systematic reviews. *BMJ*. 1994;309(6954):597–599.
4. Counsell C. Formulating questions and locating primary studies for inclusion in systematic reviews. *Ann Intern Med*. 1997;127(5):380–387.
5. Haynes R. Forming research questions. In: Haynes R, Sacket D, Guyatt G, Tugwell P, eds. *Clinical Epidemiology: How to do Clinical Practice Research*. 3rd ed. Philadelphia, PA: Lippincott Williams & Wilkins; 2006;3–14.
6. McAuley L, Pham B, Tugwell P, Moher D. Does the inclusion of grey literature influence estimates of intervention effectiveness reported in meta-analyses? *Lancet*. 2000;356(9237):1228–1231.
7. Conn VS, Valentine JC, Cooper HM, Rantz MJ. Grey literature in meta-analyses. *Nursing Res*. 2003;52(4):256–261.

8. Egger M, Juni P, Bartlett C, Holenstein F, Sterne J. How important are comprehensive literature searches and the assessment of trial quality in systematic reviews? Empirical study. *Health Technol Assess*. 2003;7(1):1–76.

9. U.S. Preventive Services Task Force. Procedure Manual; AHRQ Publication No. 08-05118-EF. 2008; http://www.uspreventiveservicestaskforce.org/uspstf08/methods/procmanual.htm. Accessed September 15, 2012.

10. Armijo-Olivo S, Stiles CR, Hagen NA, Biondo PD, Cummings GG. Assessment of study quality for systematic reviews: a comparison of the Cochrane Collaboration Risk of Bias Tool and the Effective Public Health Practice Project Quality Assessment Tool: methodological research. *J Eval Clin Prac*. 2012;18(1):12–18.

11. Moher D, Liberati A, Tetzlaff J, Altman DG. Preferred reporting items for systematic reviews and meta-analyses: the PRISMA statement. *J Clin Epidemiol*. 2009;62(10):1006–1012.

12. Owens DK, Lohr KN, Atkins D, et al. AHRQ series paper 5: grading the strength of a body of evidence when comparing medical interventions—agency for healthcare research and quality and the effective health-care program. *J Clin Epidemiol*. 2010;63(5):513–523.

13. Hedges L. Distribution theory for Glass's estimator of effect size and related estimators. *J Educ Stat*. 1981;6(2):107–128.

14. Higgins JP, Thompson SG, Deeks JJ, Altman DG. Measuring inconsistency in meta-analyses. *BMJ*. 2003;327(7414):557–560.

15. Lewis S, Clarke M. Forest plots: trying to see the wood and the trees. *BMJ*. 2001;322(7300):1479–1480.

16. Deeks JJ, Higgins JP, Altman DG. Chapter 9: Analyzing data and undertaking meta-analyses. In: Higgins JP, Green S, eds. *Cochrane Handbook for Systematic Reviews of Interventions. Version 5.0.1.* The Cochrane Collaboration, 2008. Available from www.cochrane-handbook.org.

17. Dickersin K, Min YI, Meinert CL. Factors influencing publication of research results. Follow-up of applications submitted to two institutional review boards. *JAMA*. 1992;267(3):374–378.

18. Egger M, Smith GD. Bias in location and selection of studies. *BMJ*. 1998;316(7124):61–66.

19. Sterne JA, Egger M. Funnel plots for detecting bias in meta-analysis: guidelines on choice of axis. *J Clin Epidemiol*. 2001;54(10):1046–1055.

20. Egger M, Davey Smith G, Schneider M, Minder C. Bias in meta-analysis detected by a simple, graphical test. *BMJ*. 1997;315(7109):629–634.

21. Begg CB, Mazumdar M. Operating characteristics of a rank correlation test for publication bias. *Biometrics*. 1994;50(4):1088–1101.

22. Alper BS, Hand JA, Elliott SG, et al. How much effort is needed to keep up with the literature relevant for primary care? *JMLA*. 2004;92(4):429–437.

23. Glenny AM, Altman DG, Song F, et al. Indirect comparisons of competing interventions. *Health Technol Assess*. 2005;9(26):1–134, iii–iv.

24. Neumann PJ. Emerging lessons from the drug effectiveness review project. *Health Aff (Millwood)*. 2006;25(4):W262–271.

SECTION

3

PRINCIPLES OF DRUG LITERATURE EVALUATION

PRINCIPLES OF EVIDENCE-BASED MEDICINE

JEFFREY T. SHERER, PHARMD, MPH, BCPS

CHAPTER OBJECTIVES

- ▸ Define evidence-based medicine
- ▸ Identify the steps involved in evidence-based medicine
- ▸ Illustrate the purpose of evidence-based medicine
- ▸ Identify the hierarchy of evidence
- ▸ Discuss strengths and limitations of evidence-based medicine

KEY TERMINOLOGY

Clinical expertise
Clinical significance
Evidence
Evidence–based medicine

External validity
Hierarchy of evidence
Internal validity

Patient values and
    preferences
PICO

INTRODUCTION

With increasing disease complexities and treatment options, there is need to incorporate emerging clinical evidence into decision making to provide safe, cost-effective, high-quality patient care. The best approach to dealing with a clinical situation is not always apparent, and it is not possible to know the right thing to do in all situations. Evidence-based medicine (EBM) provides a scientific framework for asking and answering clinical questions to meet the needs of patients in a variety of settings. **Evidence-based medicine** has been initially defined as "a systemic approach to analyze published research as the basis of clinical decision making."[1] This definition emphasized the use of research evidence to patient care. This is a paradigm shift in patient care from experience and expertise emphasis to incorporation of evidence in patient care.

The most recent and widely accepted definition of EBM incorporates evidence along with clinical experience and patient preferences into the decision-making process to increase the likelihood that the patient will receive helpful interventions and decrease the likelihood of them receiving interventions that are likely to be harmful or ineffective. **EBM** is now defined as "the integration of best research evidence with clinical expertise and patient values."[2] While the specific area of practice or discipline is sometimes used in the description such as evidence-based pharmacy or evidence-based nursing, this chapter will use the broad definition of "medicine" to reflect the delivery of health care in general. This chapter will cover the history of EBM and its purpose. The steps involved in EBM are presented along with the various types of evidence that may be incorporated. Finally, the advantages and disadvantages of EBM are discussed.

HISTORY AND EVOLUTION OF EBM

Since antiquity, knowledge and skills regarding the delivery of health care have generally been passed from one generation of practitioners to the next. This clinical experience approach to patient care, which often includes incorporating background information about anatomy, physiology, and pharmacology along with the clinical experience gained from previous encounters with patients, is fraught with peril due to its nonsystematic, potentially biased nature. A second approach dating to around the turn of the 19th century is to base care on experimental physiology.[3] Using animal models, the presumed cause of a disease was elucidated and a treatment that was thought to address that particular cause was delivered (**Figure 15-1**). The main problem with using this approach in isolation is that it put too much emphasis on the question of "why *should* this treatment work?" and not enough on the question of "*does* this treatment work?"

The next approach, and one that can be thought of as the historical underpinning behind modern EBM, is the "numerical method" pioneered by French physician Pierre Charles Alexandre Louis in the mid-1800s.[4] At a Paris hospital, Louis collected data on patient outcomes from procedures such as bloodletting, a popular treatment for a number of varied ailments including pneumonia, yellow fever, and liver problems. He concluded, not surprisingly to our modern sensibilities, that bloodletting was at best of no use and at worst harmful. This systematic, numerically based approach to observing what *did* happen rather than what *should have* happened was an important early step in the

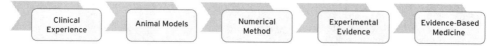

FIGURE 15-1   Evolution of evidence-based medicine.

field of clinical epidemiology, which is essentially the incorporation of numerical data into clinical decision making.

A large step in the evolution of what is now called EBM was provided largely by Archibald Cochrane, who actively promoted use of experimental evidence for patient care. Cochrane was a British physician who served in the Mediterranean Theater during World War II, where he was captured by Axis forces. While in deplorable conditions at a prisoner-of-war camp in Greece, Cochrane, who in his own writings stated that he was skeptical about many interventions used at the time, managed to perform a rudimentary clinical trial to attempt to convince his captors that symptoms fellow prisoners were experiencing were due to a vitamin deficiency.[5] While not the first clinical trial—the general concept goes back to early recorded history—Cochrane's efforts to seek out and organize experimental evidence, especially after the conclusion of the war and his return to practice in the United Kingdom, was an important step in EBM.

The term "evidence-based medicine" is relatively new, having been created at Canada's McMaster University in the late 1980s.[1] The initial term referred to the use of "a systemic approach to analyze published research as the basis of clinical decision making" according to McMaster University Internal Medicine residency coordinator, Gordon Guyatt. The terminology and the practices of critical appraisal and the use of clinical research for patient care expanded quickly, with the first appearance in the published literature in the early 1990s.[6] In 1992, an organization called the Evidence-Based Medicine Working Group published a seminal article in the *Journal of the American Medical Association* titled "Evidence-Based Medicine: A New Approach to Teaching the Practice of Medicine."[7] In 1996, Sackett and colleagues defined EBM as "making the conscientious, explicit, and judicious use of current best evidence in making decisions about the care of individual patients."[8]

EBM TODAY

By the end of the 1990s, EBM was taught and practiced widely. Most medical and other health professions schools teach at least the basics of how to practice in an evidence-based manner. Furthermore, guidance in the principles and practice of EBM is also commonly provided in many postgraduate training programs such as pharmacy and medical residencies. As these trainees have become practitioners, they have often carried forward an enthusiasm for EBM and imparted it to the next generation. The current practice of EBM involves incorporating evidence, along with clinical experience and patient preferences, into patient care, consistent with a widely accepted definition of EBM as "integration of best research evidence with clinical expertise and patient values."[2]

Evidence refers to findings from clinical research, especially from patient-centered research, that are relevant to patient care.[2] It includes findings from systematic reviews, applied research from laboratories, and clinical research from experimental and observational studies. It is essentially new research information, usually presented numerically, that helps inform decision making. New evidence replaces old and sometimes well-accepted evidence to provide safe and effective care based on the evolved scientific evidence.[2] This is a paradigm shift from the use of just traditional knowledge and experience to incorporation of research evidence to patient care. With evolving evidence from applied and clinical research, there is a need for clinicians to be current and critical about research to practice EBM. The gathering and appraising of evidence are major components of EBM.

Clinical expertise involves using clinical skills and previous experience to evaluate evidence and the patient's health status and preferences.[2] It is the insight and intuition acquired by a seasoned clinician through extensive interactions with patients and seeing the outcomes obtained from various interventions. Pharmacists have extensive skill and experience in issues related to pharmacotherapy and clinical services. This expertise can help understand and apply relevant research evidence to patient care. This involves discerning relevant and non-relevant information and understanding patient expectations based on personal observations. Experience can be especially paramount in patient care when there is limited or a lack of scientific evidence. This trial-and-error approach based on just experience can be beneficial sometimes, but its non-systematic nature may lead to bias.

Patient values and preferences refer to "collection of goals, expectations, predispositions, and beliefs that individuals have for certain decisions and their potential outcomes."[2] Patient preferences are relative values on healthcare choices by patients based on beliefs, attitudes, and cultural and spiritual factors. It affects patients' desires to avoid certain health outcomes and willingness to undergo specific treatments. In recent years, "patient-centered care" has become synonymous with delivery of health care that reflects patient values and preferences. The Institute of Medicine (IOM) has defined patient-centered care as "care that is respectful of and responsive to individual patient preferences, needs, and values and [ensures] that patient values guide all clinical decisions."[9] The federal government has specifically created the Patient-Centered Outcomes Research Institute (PCORI) to fund research that incorporates patients' values and their input in healthcare decisions.[10]

All three parts—scientific evidence, clinician expertise, and patient values and preference—are vitally important, and a common misconception about EBM is that the research evidence somehow trumps the other factors. Historically, a model where all three factors were of equal importance has largely been followed. Some have recently advocated from a shift to a different model where patient preferences, available evidence, and the clinical state and circumstances are weighted equally with a fourth factor, clinical expertise, which helps with decision making in all of these areas (**Figure 15–2**).[11]

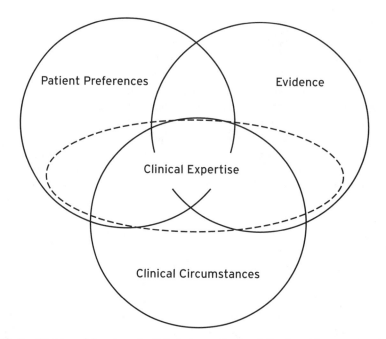

FIGURE 15-2   Newer model on the role of clinical expertise in relation to evidence and patient status and preferences.

Reproduced from Haynes RB, Devereaux PJ, Guyatt GH. Clinical expertise in the era of evidence-based medicine and patient choice. *Evidence Based Medicine*. 2002;7:36-38 with permission from BMJ Publishing Group Ltd.

This model specifically includes clinical state and circumstances separate from expertise to provide objective evaluation of patient health status and clinical setting. The clinical state is the reason for medical intervention and a critical component in clinical decision making. Clinical circumstance refers to the setting, such as primary, secondary, or tertiary care, in which care is provided. Clinical expertise is the application of clinician skills and knowledge with research evidence and patient clinical status and preferences to deliver high-quality patient care. It can be thought of as evaluating evidence, patient clinical status, and patient preferences in order to balance often conflicting or incomplete information to provide the best possible care. For example, providing enough correct and usable information for the patient to be able to make properly informed choices based on their own values would be considered clinical expertise. Whether this approach is an improvement on the previous one remains to be seen, but in any event it does emphasize the critical role that clinical expertise plays in practice even when a strongly evidence-based template is used.

Without clinical experience, it may be difficult to determine whether a given piece of evidence is applicable to a given situation or patient. Without high-quality evidence, clinicians are forced to rely on their own nonsystematic observations and experiences, which may be biased and incorrect. Without input from patients about their beliefs and desires, clinicians run the risk of doing things *to* patients rather than *for* patients. By incorporating all three factors, clinicians can increase the likelihood that the patient will receive safe and effective care that helps in ways that are important to them. The idea of incorporating evidence into decision making has spread widely beyond health care, including education and even sports.[12]

STEPS IN PRACTICING EBM

EBM provides a framework to wade through literature and find high-quality, relevant information that can be applied in practice at the bedside or policy level. It seeks to incorporate research findings along with clinical experience and patient preferences in order to make better healthcare-related decisions. These decisions can cover a number of different areas, such as treatments including drugs, screening, diagnostic tests, and prognosis. In the field of pharmacy, decisions mostly involve pharmacotherapy, but many other applications such as the evidence surrounding expanded pharmacy services also exist. In general, EBM involves four main steps (**Figure 15-3**).

Some include a fifth step, which is assessing how well the individual is performing steps one through four and determining how to improve the process in the future. The following sections describe in detail each of the steps using an example.

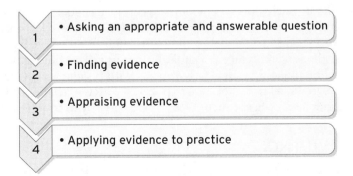

1 • Asking an appropriate and answerable question

2 • Finding evidence

3 • Appraising evidence

4 • Applying evidence to practice

FIGURE 15-3   Steps in EBM.

ASKING AN ANSWERABLE QUESTION

Asking answerable clinical questions is the first and a vitally important step in practicing EBM. Without a properly structured question, the clinician can easily become lost and frustrated.

PICO Model

Most advocates of EBM suggest the use of what is known as the **PICO** method, where P stands for Patient, Population, Program, or Problem, I stands for Intervention, C stands for Comparison, and O stands for Outcome.[13] Without following the PICO model, it is easy to go adrift. For example, say the clinician is seeing a patient in a clinic setting and needs to review the patient's pharmacotherapeutic regimen and make appropriate recommendations. If the patient has a diagnosis of heart failure, then asking "What is the best treatment for heart failure?" will result in a woefully inadequate literature search. However, by following the structure of the PICO model, much better answers can be located.

To ask an answerable clinical question, it is first necessary to define the group the clinician is interested in. If the question is in reference to a specific patient, what important characteristics does the patient have? Is he/she an adult or a child? What disease state(s) do they have? The P in PICO can also refer to other subjects. For example, if the clinician is looking to gather information on the effectiveness of a certain program or policy or is just seeking general information about a population with a certain disease state, then these can be the P in the clinical question. In the above-cited example, the clinician might notice that the patient in the clinic is an elderly patient with a low ejection fraction (i.e., systolic heart failure). Incorporating this information into the question rather than searching for "heart failure" is likely to find more relevant information.

The next aspect to asking a good clinical question is to determine what intervention is of interest. As pharmacists, the intervention of interest is usually pharmacotherapy. However, non-drug treatments, diagnostic or prognostic tests, and other interventions also are relevant. For example, a clinician may be interested in the angiotensin-converting enzyme (ACE) inhibitors, so this would need to be incorporated into the question.

A good question will need something to compare to the intervention of interest. In pharmacy, this is usually the standard (active) treatment or a placebo. Other comparisons, such as simply no treatment, may also be appropriate. In the previous example, the clinician may be interested in how ACE inhibitors compare to other vasodilators such as an alpha-adrenergic blocker.

Finally, it is necessary to specify the outcome the clinician is most interested in. Whenever possible, this outcome should be something that is relevant to patients such as death, hospitalization, major illness, or decreased quality of life. Laboratory tests, vital signs, and the like are rarely the best outcomes to consider. A good rule of thumb is that if it is not something a patient would complain about, it is probably a less-than-ideal outcome. In the previous example, since patients with systolic heart failure have a decreased life expectancy, choosing mortality as a clinically important outcome makes sense.

Thus, the clinical question: In elderly patients with systolic heart failure, do ACE inhibitors reduce mortality in comparison to placebo? This is much more likely to result in a successful search for evidence than "What is the best way to treat heart failure?"

FINDING EVIDENCE

The second step in the EBM process is finding evidence. This usually consists of searching the published literature through a bibliographic database such as PubMed, the

| BOX 15-1 | **Example of an Appropriate and Answerable Question** |

In elderly patients with systolic heart failure, do angiotensin-converting enzyme inhibitors reduce mortality in comparison to placebo?

Cumulative Index to Nursing and Allied Health Literature (CINAHL), and others. Depending on the depth at which the clinician wants to probe and how much time exists to do so, manually skimming through reference lists in identified relevant trials may turn up other pieces of evidence not revealed in the literature search. Millions of peer-reviewed articles are published every year. Nobody, even in a highly specialized area of practice, is able to prospectively keep up with the literature in their field. This often makes it necessary to answer questions on the fly rather than collecting information in advance to use in case it becomes needed ("just in time" versus "just in case" information). As technology continues to develop, access to relevant resources is vital to practice EBM at the bedside. This includes electronic devices that allow clinicians to find evidence and access critical reviews on common topics that have been performed previously by others.

Continuing with the example clinical question, the clinician could then go search the literature using a bibliographic database such as PubMed, incorporating the terms angiotensin-converting enzyme inhibitor, placebo, and heart failure. While an in-depth discussion of searching bibliographic databases is beyond the scope of this chapter, the results of this literature search could be limited to clinical trials and meta-analyses in humans to dramatically decrease the number of citations that would need to be reviewed and assessed.

Many other resources are also available. The Cochrane Database of Systematic Reviews contains hundreds of reviews and meta-analyses covering a large number of clinical questions and is an invaluable resource. Several schools and organizations have catalogs of critically appraised topics that include common questions or situations where the search for and appraisal of primary literature has already been performed. Chapter 16, "Introduction to Drug Literature" provides detailed discussions on sources of drug literature.

| BOX 15-2 | **Example of Sources of Finding Evidence** |

PubMed (http://www.ncbi.nlm.nih.gov/pubmed/)
Cochrane (http://www.cochrane.org/cochrane-reviews)

APPRAISING EVIDENCE

The third step in the process is appraising evidence. It is important to note that this is a *part* of EBM rather than its entirety. Much time is spent in training health professionals to evaluate evidence, and this is inarguably a critically important step, but without understanding and being proficient at the other steps in the process, even the best literature evaluator will not likely be able to incorporate evidence into practice effectively. Although appraising observational studies and randomized controlled studies is discussed in later chapters in this text, a few especially important points are covered here.

One of the main goals in appraising a piece of evidence is assessing its internal validity. **Internal validity** is the degree to which a study establishes a cause-and-effect relationship between the intervention (or exposure, depending on the type of study) and the outcome.[14] It is a function of the design and execution of the study and may be threatened by many factors. For example, the internal validity of a randomized controlled trial could be adversely affected by such things as lack of (or problems with) randomization or variation from the study protocol. If the internal validity of a study is poor, then the results simply cannot be believed. In many cases, the clinician is best served by severely discounting the results of the study or ignoring them altogether. However, every study has flaws that do not necessarily mean that the results should not be believed.

Not all evidence is created equal. Over the years, a system has emerged to rank various types of evidence based on freedom from bias, scientific reliability, and clinical usefulness (**Figure 15-4**). This is termed as the **hierarchy of evidence**. Systematic reviews or meta-analyses of randomized controlled trials are believed to contain the most accurate and believable results. At the other end of the spectrum, case series, case reports, and expert opinions are felt to be the least accurate. This is not to say that these lower forms of evidence are useless. Indeed, in many cases, they may be all that is available or the only ethical study design. Still, given conflicting evidence from different study types, it is generally thought that the study design that is higher on the spectrum is probably the more believable result.

The use of observational study designs (i.e., case-control and cohort studies) in clinical decision making is especially debatable given the widespread acceptance of the randomized controlled trial in evaluating drugs and other therapeutic interventions. Because treatments in an observational study are not randomly assigned, it introduces an increased risk of bias (selection and confounding) and the possibility of systematic differences in outcomes between the groups. In many cases, observational and experimental studies provide similar findings. In others, they do not.[15] Given the frequent lack of "real world" settings for randomized controlled trials and their extreme expense,

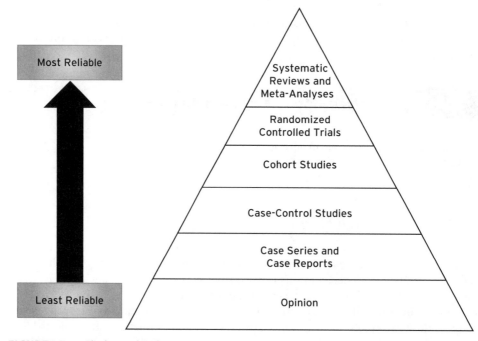

FIGURE 15-4 The hierarchy of evidence.

interest in using observational trials to assess the effectiveness of drug therapy is high. In particular, the recent surge in funding for comparative effectiveness research, which seeks to evaluate therapeutic alternatives in a real-world setting, has great importance for the future of EBM.[16]

BOX 15-3	**Example of Appraising Evidence**

The clinician reviews each relevant piece of information found, particularly considering their internal and external validity. When conflicting information is found, the searcher considers the hierarchy of evidence, giving additional weight to systematic reviews and clinical trials and less weight to opinion and non-randomized studies.

APPLYING EVIDENCE

Applying evidence to the patient or policy at hand is the final step in the process of EBM. In many ways, it is also the most complicated and open to judgment. One factor that must be considered is the external validity of the study. **External validity** refers to the degree to which the results of the study can be extrapolated to other populations.[14] This is critical in determining whether the results of the study can be applied to the individual patient about whom the question was asked in the first place. For example, if the clinician is searching for information about how to treat systolic heart failure in adults, a study evaluating treatments for other types of heart failure (e.g., diastolic) or in other populations (e.g., neonates) is unlikely to provide useful information. While there are few hard-and-fast rules, a good rule of thumb is to look at the inclusion and exclusion criteria for a particular study to determine if the individual patient in question would have qualified to enroll in it. If the answer is no, then great caution should be exercised before believing the study findings are likely to be true for that individual.

Determining whether the findings of a study are clinically significant, statistically significant, neither, or both is also important. **Clinical significance** means that the results of the research are important enough that they should be considered when making decisions about patient care. Findings that are statistically significant (unlikely to be due to chance) may not be clinically important if the magnitude of the difference is small. Given a large enough sample size, tiny differences between two arms in a clinical trial may be statistically different, but the difference may not be large enough for a clinician to prefer that intervention. Furthermore, other factors (adverse effects, cost, convenience, etc.) may make the statistically "better" intervention a less desirable choice.

For example, given a large enough sample size, a clinical trial comparing two drugs to decrease hospitalizations due to heart failure may find that there is a small reduction (0.5% per year) in one group versus the other, and that this difference is highly unlikely due to chance ($P = 0.001$). However, most clinicians would not deem this difference in the risk of hospitalization in a year to be of great clinical importance, so factors such as which drug is less expensive, easier to take, or better tolerated would likely be more important.

Small p-values themselves cannot allow the clinician to determine whether a difference between groups is large enough to be of clinical importance. Very small p-values say only that the difference observed is highly unlikely to be due to chance, not that the difference is clinically important. Conversely, occasionally authors or others claim that study findings are clinically important even though the conclusions do not achieve statistical significance. This has to be avoided. The lack of statistical significance means the role of chance cannot be ruled out, so it is premature to claim that the findings should be applied to patients. Most often this result happens when a study is underpowered, and the most appropriate course of action at that point is to do an additional study with a larger sample size so that small but clinically important differences are more likely to be detected if they truly exist.

Finally, patients' goals, desires, and values must be incorporated into the process. This requires dialogue with patients to understand their beliefs, values, experiences, and expectations regarding the treatment and outcomes. Health beliefs are often driven by social, cultural, and ethical norms. Incorporating these into the decision-making process requires active sharing and involvement in healthcare choices. For example, some patients may have a strong preference for an intervention that they feel is more "natural" than an alternative. This does not mean that the patient should automatically receive this intervention, but it should be part of the dialogue along with other important factors such as the amount and quality of evidence supporting that intervention and the clinician's experiences.

The terminology *shared decision making* has recently come into use when discussing the incorporation of patient preferences into evidence-based decision making.[17] It includes three major components.[18] The first is that a dialogue should exist between the patient and healthcare professional. The second is that this dialogue should include discussions about various options and likely outcomes. Finally, the patient and the healthcare professional should come to a consensus about what action is most appropriate at that point in time. Shared decision making and, more broadly, the overall incorporation of patient preferences into the EBM paradigm reflect one of the foremost principles of medical ethics: that patient autonomy must be respected.

The fifth step would involve an assessment of how well the approach worked for answering this particular question. This would most likely consist of the clinicians reflecting on what parts of the process worked well and what was difficult. It may also involve other individuals auditing and providing feedback about how well the clinician is adhering to recommended practices.

BOX 15-4	Example of Applying Evidence

The clinician evaluates how closely the patient about whom the question was asked resembles the average patient in the study and whether the patient would have been eligible for enrollment. The clinician also considers other clinical options available to treat heart failure, the patient's preferences, other drugs or diseases that may affect outcomes, and the clinical experience to determine whether the patient is likely to benefit from this intervention.

ADVANTAGES OF EBM

There are many advantages of EBM. The first and possibly largest advantage is that it attempts to find and incorporate interventions that work, not that *should* or *seem to* work. For example, interventions such as antiarrhythmic therapy for patients who are post–myocardial infarction and having premature ventricular contractions or patients with osteoporosis who take sodium fluoride to increase bone density *should* experience reduced mortality and fractures, respectively. However, when these interventions were studied, more deaths and more fractures were observed.[19,20] By increasing the likelihood that patients will receive helpful interventions and not receive harmful interventions, patient well-being will be improved.

A clinician who is proficient in the principles of EBM can also use the concepts to become better at keeping up with new information as it is published. Someone who is well versed in study designs, how to appraise a study, and how to apply the results of a study to practice should be more efficient in choosing articles to read than an individual who is less skilled in these areas.

Additionally, the implementation of a more evidence-based approach can help foster communication. A clinician who is adept at the evidence-based approach will have the terminology to explain and understand difficult concepts in the previously mentioned areas (i.e., study design, validity, and application). Furthermore, a good background in evidence-based practice can help the clinician see flaws in others' (and their own) thinking and better interact with sales representatives.

LIMITATIONS OF EBM

EBM has limitations that need to be recognized and appreciated. It primarily focuses on *whether* an intervention works, not how it *might* work. This has fewer implications for clinical practice than it does for basic science, since improving patient outcomes is a worthy goal regardless of whether it is well understood *why* certain interventions work. In basic science, where understanding the pathophysiologic and pharmacologic underpinnings are vital, the process and approach are less useful.

Another limitation of EBM is that it requires knowledge, skills, and support mechanisms to practice it effectively. Just like other factors needed for effective clinical practice including knowledge of anatomy, pathophysiology, pharmacology, pharmacotherapeutics, and skills in communicating and assessing patients, the ability to practice EBM is something that is not innate. The philosophy, steps, and processes must be imparted by someone who is familiar with them. Additionally, access to systems with which to search for and evaluate evidence, preferably at the point of care, are also necessary. The EBM process can be often labor intensive and time consuming. With busy clinical practices, it may not translate to practice due to practical considerations. As the benefits of EBM are becoming more widely known and its precepts continue to be incorporated into healthcare education, these limitations should continue to diminish.

Some individuals perceive EBM as "cookbook medicine" and a threat to their clinical autonomy. This is unfortunate. Enough gray areas exist in medicine that there will always be a need for practitioners who practice the art. EBM can help identify areas where there is clearly a best thing to do, freeing up clinicians to tackle the more difficult or less clear areas.[21] It has been suggested that guidelines especially are similar to cookbooks, but that a good practitioner—like a good chef—will use that as the basis for providing good care or a good meal rather than starting from scratch and improvising a recipe every time.

Finally, many important questions do not have sufficient evidence to adequately inform clinical decision making. For example, heart failure with preserved left ventricular function is common, and yet little information to guide treatment exists.[22] While this can be frustrating, it is still necessary to provide the best care possible for patients, even when evidence is lacking. Furthermore, by explicitly acknowledging gaps in the evidence, it is possible to identify priorities in future research in order to close these gaps.

Despite its limitations, the reality is that there are no better alternatives than EBM. Many proposed alternatives recommend approaches such as combining things like clinical judgment and pathophysiologic rationale with empirical evidence,[23] but even the most diehard proponents of EBM do not believe that empirical evidence is the only important factor. If it was, a more appropriate name would be "medicine by evidence alone" rather than "evidence-based medicine," which is intended to incorporate clinical experience, patient values, and other factors. Even with its flaws, and analogous to Winston Churchill's famous quip about democracy, EBM is the worst approach that has ever been tried, except for all the others. Some of the main advantages and disadvantages of EBM are listed in **Table 15-1**.

TABLE 15-1 Advantages and Disadvantages of EBM

Advantages of EBM	Disadvantages of EBM
Attempts to increase the likelihood of receiving interventions that are efficacious	Does not address why an intervention does or does not work
Attempts to decrease the likelihood of receiving interventions that are inefficacious or harmful	Requires specialized knowledge and skills to practice effectively
Allows clinicians to better keep up with new literature and developments	May be perceived as "cookbook medicine"
Increases critical thinking skills	Many questions lack available evidence

ROLE OF THE PHARMACIST IN EBM

Pharmacists can and should play a highly active and important role in practicing EBM as well as encouraging and teaching other healthcare providers to do so. This is especially true since pharmaceuticals are such an important therapeutic resource in modern medicine. Because of their unique background and training, pharmacists who are skilled at EBM can be highly valued members of the healthcare team. Physicians and nurses generally value pharmacist recommendations, and it is easier to convince other providers when the recommendations are based on principles of EBM.

Additionally, pharmacists should be proficient at EBM because of the evolving nature of health care, especially pharmacotherapy. The introduction of new drugs and the development of new indications for older drugs mean that much of what clinicians learn in their training quickly becomes outdated. Being skilled in the concepts of EBM makes it far easier to keep up with the changing landscape and makes it more likely that the patients for whom the pharmacist is responsible receive the best care possible.

Pharmacists can play a vital role in evidence-based prescribing to improve the quality of pharmaceutical care. The challenges that have been identified in evidence-based prescribing are mainly related to evidence including availability, timely access, and translation.[24] Pharmacists can be valuable resources in ensuring the availability of evidence relevant to patient care, especially in complex pharmacotherapy cases. Often, considerations such as available time in patient care and expertise in interpretation and applications of evidence can hinder EBM in clinical practice. Pharmacists can assist decision makers in taking care of access and translational aspects of pharmacotherapy evidence. In this information age, pharmacists are in a strong position to take the lead for ensuring evidence-based pharmacotherapy because of their knowledge, skills, and experience.

SUMMARY AND CONCLUSIONS

EBM is paradigm shift in delivering patient care from clinician-based care to evidence-based care that incorporates scientific evidence with clinical expertise and patient preferences. All three are vitally important in providing high-quality patient care. The major advantage of this approach to practice is that it increases the likelihood that patients will receive interventions that are effective and will not receive interventions that are ineffective or even harmful. EBM is a four-step process that involves asking answerable questions, finding evidence, appraising evidence, and applying that evidence to practice. While EBM does have some limitations, these are often overstated and the impact of these limitations can often be minimized by a skilled practitioner. Pharmacists can be highly valued members of the healthcare team because their background and training can help them to easily integrate research evidence with clinical expertise and patient values, especially for pharmacotherapy.

REVIEW QUESTIONS

1. What factors other than the results of research studies must be incorporated into evidence-based medicine?
2. What advantages does evidence-based medicine have over other approaches?
3. Why has evidence-based medicine increased in importance and popularity over the past few decades?
4. Describe the hierarchy of evidence and how this hierarchy was established.
5. What is the difference between statistical significance and clinical significance?
6. What is the Cochrane Database of Systematic Reviews, and how can it help clinicians deliver evidence-based care?
7. What are some limitations to evidence-based medicine, and how can these limitations be minimized?

ONLINE RESOURCES

The Cochrane Collaboration: http://www.cochrane.org
Evidence-Based Medicine Toolkit: http://www.ebm.med.ualberta.ca/Ebm.html
McMaster University Evidence-Based Practice Resources: http://hsl.mcmaster.ca/resources/topic/eb/
Oxford University Evidence-Based Medicine Tools: http://www.cebm.net/index.aspx?o=1023
Progress in Evidence-Based Medicine: http://jama.jamanetwork.com/article.aspx?articleid=182722

REFERENCES

1. Claridge JA, Fabian TC. History and development of evidence-based medicine. *World J Surg.* 1995;29(5):547–553.
2. Sackett DL, Strauss SE, Richardson WS, et al. *Evidence-Based Medicine: How to Practice and Teach EBM.* London: Churchill-Livingstone; 2000.
3. Shoja MM, Tubbs RS, Loukas M, Shokouhi G, Ardalan MR. Marie-François Xavier Bichat (1771–1802) and his contributions to the foundations of pathological anatomy and modern medicine. *Ann Anat.* 2008;190:413–420.
4. Best M, Neuhauser D. Pierre Charles Alexandre Louis: master of the spirit of mathematical clinical science. *Qual Saf Health Care.* 2005;14:462–464.
5. Cochrane AL. Sickness in Salonica: my first, worst, and most successful clinical trial. *BMJ.* 1984;289:1726–1727.
6. Guyatt GH. Evidence-based medicine. *ACP Journal Club.* 1991;114:A-16.

7. Evidence-Based Medicine Working Group. Evidence-based medicine: a new approach to teaching the practice of medicine. *JAMA*. 1992;268:2420–2425.

8. Sackett DL, Rosenberg WM, Gray JA, Haynes RB, Richardson WS. Evidence-based medicine: what it is and it isn't. *BMJ*. 1996;312:71–72.

9. Patient-Centered Outcomes Research Institute. Patient-Centered Outcomes Research. Available at: http://www.pcori.org/research-we-support/pcor/. Accessed April 15, 2013.

10. Patient-Centered Outcomes Research Institute. National Priorities for Research and Research Agenda. Available at: http://www.pcori.org/assets/PCORI-National-Priorities-and-Research-Agenda-2012-05-21-FINAL.pdf. Accessed April 15, 2013.

11. Haynes RB, Devereaux PJ, Guyatt GH. Clinical expertise in the era of evidence-based medicine and patient choice. *Evidence Based Medicine*. 2002;7:36–38.

12. Beane B, Gingrich N, Kerry J. How to take American health care from worst to first. *New York Times*. October 24, 2008:A31.

13. Schardt C, Adams MB, Owens T, Keitz S, Fontelo P. Utilization of the PICO framework to improve searching PubMed for clinical questions. *BMC Med Inform Decis Mak*. 2007;7:16.

14. Slack MK, Drauglis JR. Establishing the internal and external validity of experimental studies. *Am J Health-Syst Pharm*. 2001;58:2173–2184.

15. Ray JG. Evidence in upheaval: incorporating observational data into clinical practice. *Arch Intern Med*. 2002;162:249–254.

16. Schumock GT, Pickard AS. Comparative effectiveness research: relevance and applications to pharmacy. *Am J Health-Syst Pharm*. 2009;66:1278–1286.

17. Barratt A. Evidence based medicine and shared decision making: the challenge of getting both evidence and preferences into health care. *Patient Education Counseling*. 2008;73:407–412.

18. Charles C, Gafni A, Whelan T. Decision-making in the physician-patient encounter: revisiting the shared treatment decision-making model. *Social Sci Med*. 1999;49:651–661.

19. The Cardiac Arrhythmia Suppression Trial (CAST) Investigators. Preliminary report: effect of encainide and flecainide on mortality in a randomized trial of arrhythmia suppression after myocardial infarction. *New Engl J Med*. 1989;321:406–412.

20. Riggs BL, Hodgson SF, O'Fallon WM, et al. Effect of fluoride treatment on the fracture rate in postmenopausal women with osteoporosis. *N Engl J Med* 1990;322:802–809.

21. Reinerstein JL. Zen and the art of physician autonomy maintenance. *Ann Intern Med*. 2003;138:992–995.

22. Hunt SA, Abraham WT, Chin MH, et al. 2009 focused update incorporated into the ACC/AHA 2005 Guidelines for the Diagnosis and Management of Heart Failure in Adults: a report of the American College of Cardiology Foundation/American Heart Association Task Force on Practice Guidelines. *Circulation*. 2009;119:e391–479.

23. Tonelli MR. Integrating evidence into clinical practice: an alternative to evidence-based approaches. *J Eval Clin Pract*. 2006;12:248–256.

24. Mamdani M, Ching A, Golden B, Melo M, Menzefricke U. Challenges to evidence-based prescribing in clinical practice. *Ann Pharmacother*. 2008;42(5):704–707.

INTRODUCTION TO DRUG LITERATURE

McKenzie C. Ferguson, PharmD, BCPS

Erin M. Timpe Behnen, PharmD, BCPS

CHAPTER OBJECTIVES

- ▸ Describe the systematic approach to searching for drug information
- ▸ Explain the differences between primary, secondary, and tertiary literature
- ▸ Discuss strengths and weaknesses of primary, secondary, and tertiary literature
- ▸ Describe common and reputable sources of medical literature
- ▸ Identify and appraise clinical practice guidelines
- ▸ Utilize common bibliographic databases to locate evidence
- ▸ Discuss ways to identify the quality of information found on the Internet

KEY TERMINOLOGY

Boolean operators
Clinical practice guidelines
Compendium
Cost-benefit analyses
Cost-effective analyses
Cost-minimization analyses
Cost-utility analyses

Exploding
Focused search
Meta-analysis
Non-systematic review
Peer review process
Pharmacoeconomic
    studies

Pharmacoepidemiology
Prescribing information
Primary literature
Secondary literature
Systematic review
Tertiary literature
Truncation

INTRODUCTION

New drug information is published every day, and this enormous amount of accumulated information creates a need for efficiency when searching for information. The provision of drug information is a fundamental responsibility of every practicing pharmacist, and the knowledge and skills to access it effectively and efficiently are essential. The need for efficiency when searching for drug literature is imperative. An organized, logical, and focused approach to the request will enable the clinicians to spend less time searching and more time evaluating the quality of information. This is what ultimately leads to improvements in patient care and patient-oriented outcomes.[1] This involves providing comprehensive, accurate information in a timely manner so as to provide high-quality patient care.

Evidence-based medicine is the foundation for providing high-quality medical and pharmaceutical care. Finding appropriate evidence is a critical step in implementing evidence-based practices. This chapter will outline the systematic approach to searching for drug literature, further discuss the importance of efficiency in searching, and explain how to identify high-quality evidence. The different types of drug literature will be reviewed, including examples of each and methods for evaluation of the material and advantages and disadvantages of each type. How to properly select a resource for a specific clinical question will also be addressed. Lastly, a discussion of using the Internet for drug information is included.

SYSTEMATIC APPROACH TO DRUG INFORMATION REQUESTS

A systematic approach is needed to efficiently search drug information for drug information requests (see **Figure 16-1**).[2–4] This approach includes obtaining appropriate background information about the requestor and the request, determining and categorizing the question, developing a search strategy, evaluating the information found, formulating a response, and providing appropriate follow-up and documentation.

Once a drug information request is received, it is important to first obtain the demographics of the requestor, such as contact information and practice setting, so an appropriate response can be generated and documented. Next, it is essential for pharmacists to inquire as to whether the request is for a specific patient and, if so, to obtain all necessary patient-specific information. For example, an initial question about the indications for use of paroxetine may be assumed to be for an adult, when in fact it could be intended for use in adolescents or even during pregnancy. Before an accurate search can begin, enough background information must be acquired to adequately define and refine the initial request. This includes obtaining appropriate background information specific to the type of question. For example, a question about medication use during pregnancy needs to consider the timing of drug administration (e.g., trimester, anticipated duration of use) and complicating factors.

After obtaining background information, the request should be categorized to help develop a search appropriately focused to specialty resources. Classifying a drug information request is the process of choosing which themes a drug information request conveys (e.g., pediatric, pregnancy/lactation, drug interaction, dosing). **Table 16-1** includes a list of example classifications. This process will provide a prompt for specific background questions that should be asked, dictate which resources are the best place to begin searching, and provide a method for tracking types of requests.[2–4]

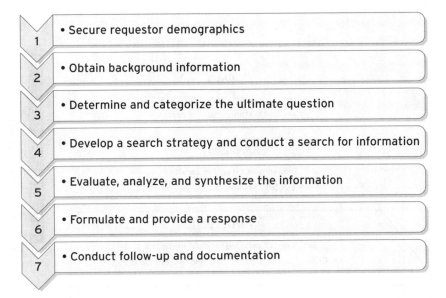

1 • Secure requestor demographics

2 • Obtain background information

3 • Determine and categorize the ultimate question

4 • Develop a search strategy and conduct a search for information

5 • Evaluate, analyze, and synthesize the information

6 • Formulate and provide a response

7 • Conduct follow-up and documentation

FIGURE 16-1   Systematic approach to responding to a drug information request.

Data from Watanabe AS, McCart G, Shimomura S, Kayser S. Systematic approach to drug information requests. *Am J Hosp Pharm.* 1975;32(12):1282–1285.; Fischer JM. Modification of the systematic approach to answering drug information requests. *Am J Hosp Pharm.* 1980;37(4):470,472,476.; Nathan JP, Gim S. Responding to drug information requests. *Am J Health Syst Pharm.* April 15, 2009;66(8):706–711.

TABLE 16-1 Examples of Ways to Classify Drug Information Requests		
Adverse Drug Reaction	Drug Use Policy	Poison/Toxicology
Allergy	Economics/Cost	Policy/Procedure
Alternative Medicine	Immunization	Pregnancy/Lactation
Compounding/Manufacturing	Investigational Drug	Product Availability
Contraindications/Warnings	IV Therapy	Product Identification
Dose	Legal/Regulatory	References/Monographs
Drug Interaction	Pediatrics	Route of Administration
Drug Shortages	Pharmacokinetics	Stability/Compatibility
Drug Therapy/Therapeutics	Pharmacology	Tablet/Capsule Identification

Once the drug information request is clearly defined, tertiary, secondary, and primary sources (described in **Figure 16–2**) are reviewed. The approach begins with a search of the broadest and most easily accessible information first, such as a compendium or a textbook (i.e., tertiary). Depending on the classification of the request, specialty resources might be consulted. If the response can be fully addressed using general information resources, then the search ends successfully. If not, the initial search of information is supplemented with strategic searches in indexing/abstract services, such as MEDLINE (i.e., secondary), to obtain additional information. Original research evaluation from a journal article (i.e., primary literature), the direct source of original information, is sometimes required to add sufficient detail to a response.[2,5] This overall approach to a drug information search focuses on specific resources and ultimately saves time.

Once all relevant information has been gathered, evaluation and synthesis of a response can take place. The response should be directly tailored to the requestor in his preferred format. All responses should be formally documented. Also, follow-up with the requestor is critical to maintaining credibility and documenting outcomes.[1,5]

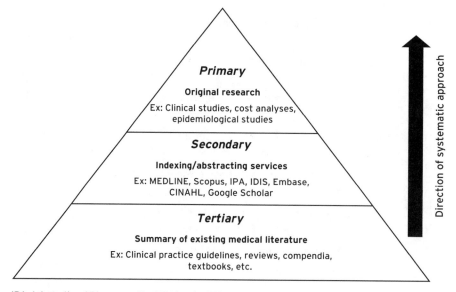

IPA—International Pharmaceutical Abstracts; IDIS—Iowa Drug Information Service; CINAHL—
Cumulative Index to Nursing and Allied Health Literature

FIGURE 16-2 Systematic approach to searching for drug information.

QUALITY OF MEDICAL LITERATURE

Because medical literature is published in abundance, it is important to know how to distinguish low- from high-quality information. Though much of this comes with experience and familiarity with certain areas of specialty, there are ways to independently assess for high-quality literature by evaluating authors, timing of the publication, and peer review process. Up-to-date, peer-reviewed, and currently referenced information written by authors with expertise are basic indicators of quality.

Authors should be evaluated for expertise in the area of publication. If a publication is authored by a non-expert, then the reliability of the information should be scrutinized for accuracy. In situations where a non-clinician authors the resource, real-world application and feasibility should be further assessed. Author credentials that reflect a team-based approach to care (e.g., physicians, nurses, pharmacists, allied/public health professionals) may also be appropriate, depending on the subject.

The timeliness of publication needs to account for a couple factors. One of these is how the information is published. Comprehensive textbooks are generally not updated more frequently than every 3 to 4 years, whereas online information can be updated daily. Also, in situations where information in the specialty area changes frequently, the frequency of publication will likely be more often. Some texts might publish monthly or quarterly supplements as a way to update a previously published resource.

The **peer review process** involves one or more independent reviewers to assess the written content before publication. This process strengthens the quality of literature. It is usually conducted by a volunteer expert in the same field and focuses on content and quality. Clear advantages of peer review are that it ensures the work is of a certain standard, allows for experts to make sure that all relevant information is discussed, and is thus typically more trustworthy than non-peer-reviewed publications.[6,7] The disadvantages are that it slows the publication process and overall dissemination of important information, and the process relies on experts to provide a high-quality critique.[6]

TYPES OF LITERATURE

TERTIARY LITERATURE

The first step in the systematic approach to searching is in tertiary resources. Examples of tertiary literature include clinical practice guidelines, review articles, compendia, and textbooks or other general reference materials (**Table 16–2**).[5] In **tertiary literature**, the condensed information from primary sources is organized in a format that facilitates efficiency. Because tertiary resources are a synthesis of existing medical literature, their relevance and significance are based on their ability to evaluate established knowledge. Evaluation of tertiary resources is important, as not all resources are created equally. For the individual practitioner, the choice of which resources to consult and purchase will depend greatly on the area of clinical practice and budget. Frequency of publication, depth and scope of information, and ease of use are a few key considerations.[5]

Clinical Practice Guidelines

Evidence-based medicine working groups are often key driving forces in the movement of information from the literature into actual clinical practice.[8] One such use of evidence-based medicine is in the creation of clinical practice guidelines. The Institute

TABLE 16-2 Examples of Tertiary Literature		
Tertiary Resource	**Common Examples/Sources**	**Website/URL (if applicable)**
Clinical Practice Guidelines	National Guideline Clearinghouse	www.guidelines.gov
	National Institute for Health and Care Excellence (NICE)	http://www.nice.org.uk/
	MEDLINE search (e.g., PubMed)	http://www.ncbi.nlm.nih.gov/pubmed
	Organizational websites (e.g., Infectious Disease Society of America)	http://www.idsociety.org/Index.aspx
Review Articles	MEDLINE search (e.g., PubMed)	http://www.ncbi.nlm.nih.gov/pubmed
	Cochrane Database of Systematic Reviews	
Compendia	American Hospital Formulary Service Clinical Pharmacology Drug Facts & Comparisons Drug Information Handbook Lexicomp Micromedex	
Textbooks	*Pharmacotherapy: A Pathophysiologic Approach* *Goodman and Gilman's The Pharmacological Basis of Therapeutics*	
Prescribing Information (i.e., package inserts)	DailyMed	http://dailymed.nlm.nih.gov/dailymed/about.cfm
	Manufacturer's websites Package labeling	

of Medicine defines **clinical practice guidelines** as "systematically developed statements to assist practitioner and patient decisions about appropriate health care for specific clinical circumstances."[9] Guidelines can highlight key clinical considerations for choosing effective strategies, reduce unnecessary healthcare costs, and avoid error. The best quality guidelines continually review the medical literature and summarize the best current evidence. This increases the validity of the guidelines.[9] Guidelines focus on a specific clinical problem, articulate relevant issues when treating the patient with that problem, assemble the medical literature, assign values to the evidence, and generate clinical recommendations. High-quality guidelines use expert panels in the development process. Often, these multidisciplinary panels involve physicians, nurses, and pharmacists among others dedicated to the improvement of public health. Panel members are authoritative experts within the area of practice without bias to recommend one treatment over another. Furthermore, panel members with expertise in quality measurement and reporting, healthcare policy and administration, and health informatics may be included. Scheduled guideline review should be a continuous process whereby information is updated as needed based on the latest, highest-quality evidence.[9]

Countries such as the United States and the United Kingdom have public-access websites entirely dedicated to the dissemination of guidelines.[10] In the United States, the National Guideline Clearinghouse (NGC) is an initiative of the Agency for Healthcare Research and Quality (AHRQ) with the mission to provide healthcare professionals accessible mechanisms for obtaining objective evidence and clinical practice guidelines.[11] In the United Kingdom a similar agency exists—the National Institute for Health and Clinical Excellence. Guidelines can also be located within organizational websites (e.g., National Heart, Lung, and Blood Institute, Infectious Disease Society of America, American Diabetes Association), but they can sometimes be difficult to locate. Lastly, another way to search is with indexing/abstracting databases, where filters can often be set to find guidelines.

The quality of clinical practice guidelines can be highly variable. For this reason, it is important that healthcare professionals understand how to assess the quality of this resource. The process of guideline development is a key determinant of overall quality. Validity, reliability/reproducibility, clinical applicability, and flexibility are some indicators of quality. Guidelines that use a defined methodology are preferred, with background into the scope of the clinical problem, specific methods used to synthesize the evidence, discussion of the evidence, rationale for the strength of recommendation, and a link to high-quality, current references. Clinical studies are the foundation for the best evidence-based guidelines and are thus more objective than opinion or consensus guidelines. In addition, guidelines that are peer-reviewed and that present recommendations and evidence relevant to patient care are considered to be both relevant and valid.[9,12,13]

Well-defined grading systems for assigning levels of evidence are important to help the healthcare professional independently evaluate the strength of the recommendation. The Grades of Recommendation, Assessment, Development and Evaluation (GRADE) approach to quality of evidence incorporates the hierarchy of clinical evidence along with the chance for different types of bias to lower or raise the quality of evidence. The strength of recommendations grading system differentiates strong versus weak recommendations based on high, moderate to low, and low quality of evidence.[14]

Systematic Reviews

A systematic review, a focused review of existing literature, can be considered either primary or tertiary literature. The assembly of already-established knowledge qualifies it as a tertiary resource, whereas the scientific investigation and statistical evaluation of multiple studies (i.e., meta-analysis) lends itself to being defined as a primary source. As defined previously, **systematic review** is a structured process for identifying and summarizing existing studies that address a specific question. It involves selection of studies based on defined inclusion and exclusion criteria and a pre-defined literature search strategy. **Meta-analysis** is a quantitative synthesis of data derived from individual studies (usually ≥ 3) identified through a systematic review process. The Cochrane Collaboration is an international network of qualified experts that prepare evidence-based Cochrane Reviews, searchable in the Cochrane Database of Systematic Reviews, which is part of the Cochrane Library of resources.[15] Cochrane Reviews are considered very reputable sources due to strict guidelines for ensuring that only the highest quality of evidence is reviewed. These reviews can be presented in protocol format (methods for a planned review) or as a systematic review (e.g., meta-analysis).

Non-Systematic Review Articles

A common tool for researching background information on a topic is a general review article. A **non-systematic review** is a tertiary resource that reviews a specific topic but differs from a systematic review in that the methodology is not based on structured, predefined literature search strategy. The topic may be a review of a particular disease state and associated treatment options. The advantage with these review articles is that if they are current to the area of practice, they can update the reader with a review of the current medical literature and new treatment strategies, some of which may not yet be incorporated in clinical practice guidelines.

Compendia

A **compendium** is a summary of information on a particular subject such as drug information; many drug compendia exist, including Micromedex, Facts and Comparisons, Lexicomp, and Clinical Pharmacology. Most are available online and in print. Additionally, compendia are available for use on portable devices for point-of-care access. Drug information compendia tend to be organized in monograph format, with consistent, specific section headings for each drug. This is usually the first place to look for drug information, as these publications attempt to emulate the key characteristics that make them desirable resources, including accessibility, ease of use, and frequent updates.

Textbooks

Textbooks are another tertiary resource constructed on factual knowledge from the medical literature. They are designed to provide comprehensive and structured information to students and practitioners for teaching and learning purposes. Textbooks are widely used to obtain valuable basic medical information regarding diagnoses and treatment. Pharmacotherapeutic textbooks place additional emphasis on pharmacological treatment of disease. Specialty textbook resources can be valuable sources of information relevant to a particular area of practice such as Mandell's *Principles and Practice of Infectious Diseases* or *Nelson Textbook of Pediatrics*.

Prescribing Information from Manufacturers

Pharmaceutical industry materials are also a source for drug information. **Prescribing information** is a compilation of Food and Drug Administration (FDA)–approved information as submitted by the manufacturer as part of the New Drug Application (NDA) and contains information regarding the efficacy and safety of the drug on the basis of evidence from clinical studies. Prescribing information is synonymous with "package insert" or "prescription drug labeling" and exists to aid healthcare providers in proper prescribing. The FDA regulates the format of this information so that it is consistent for all new drug approvals. According to the FDA, all prescribing information must be informative and accurate, not promotional, false, or misleading, and must not imply claims for which evidence is lacking. The latest revisions to the format include an upfront *Highlights* and *Contents* section (i.e., table of contents) for easier navigation. The FDA also has a database, DailyMed, for indexing the most current prescribing information; however, it does not currently contain labeling information for all FDA-approved prescription drugs.[16]

Important limitations exist with prescribing information. First, it may not represent all of the available medical evidence associated with the drug, which may include clinical studies with non-industry sponsors or support. Also, more studies (published or unpublished) may have been conducted since the last labeling approval. Second, prescribing information is unable to detail non-FDA-approved information such as additional indications for use. Assuming that reasonable and supportive evidence is available in the medical literature, "off-label" use may be appropriate.

Another method of retrieving drug information from pharmaceutical industry is through direct communication with the manufacturer, often through a medical information department or specialist. Medical information specialists are staffed by healthcare professionals such as pharmacists and nurses, and they are sometimes able to access more drug information than what is included in prescribing information. Information regarding off-label uses, differing dosage regimens, extended stability, use in alternative populations (e.g., pediatrics, elderly), different routes of administration, and adverse reactions can be obtained from a medical information department. The information provided by these departments is often regulated by the FDA.

ADVANTAGES AND DISADVANTAGES OF TERTIARY LITERATURE

Ease of use and convenience are the key reasons tertiary resources are the first step to searching for information. Also, most tertiary sources are authored by experts, and information can be found using these resources without pursuing a secondary search. However, because tertiary literature is a condensed version of information from primary sources, it may be incomplete. Specific information might require additional searching. Also, given that drug information is published at a rapid pace depending on the frequency of publication, the information may become outdated quickly, especially for textbooks. Bias and misinterpretation of research are also concerns with tertiary literature, which enforces the need for critical evaluation by clinicians.

BOX 16-1	**Example Case 1 (Tertiary)**

A medical camp is being planned by your pharmacy organization to provide dental and pharmacy services to patients. You need to investigate what options exist for the most economical antibiotic for prophylaxis of a tooth extraction in a patient with a true penicillin allergy.

Search Strategy

The systematic approach uses tertiary resources first in your search for drug information. Before looking in compendia, you must first investigate what antibiotic options exist for treating a tooth extraction in patients with a penicillin allergy. This focuses your search to clinical practice guidelines. Once you determine your options, you can then look in applicable compendia or other resources for pricing information.

SECONDARY LITERATURE

Secondary literature sources act as an intermediary between primary and tertiary literature, and directly link the researcher to both original research articles and reviews. The most common format of secondary literature is an indexing/abstracting service, which is often referred to as a secondary database and is usually accessed electronically.[5] Examples of secondary databases with a focus on pharmacy and biomedical literature are MEDLINE/PubMed, International Pharmaceutical Abstracts (IPA), Iowa Drug Information Service (IDIS), SCOPUS, Embase, Cumulative Index to Nursing and Allied Health Literature (CINAHL), and Google Scholar, among many others (**Table 16-3**).[3,17–20]

When a request cannot be fully answered using tertiary resources, secondary literature is the next step in the searching process. When a search is conducted, results are presented as a list of bibliographic citations (i.e., indexing) with or without abstracts. All secondary databases are unique in format, search methods, and content. Some databases index/abstract articles from medical literature, whereas others also include professional meeting abstracts.

It is important to choose an appropriate secondary database to search. Because the databases differ in time frame, literature coverage, source country, and area of specialty, it is essential that the researcher search the most relevant database for the request. For example, Embase provides coverage of European, non-English, and pharmacology and toxicology journals in addition to MEDLINE coverage. Often, a complete search may require searching in multiple databases. Many databases index historical literature. The importance of knowing the earliest indexing year will aid in evaluating the information in such a context. Equally important is how frequently the secondary literature is updated. Given the pace of medical literature publication, it is imperative that newly published literature is indexed in a timely manner. Secondary databases vary greatly

TABLE 16-3 Examples of Secondary Databases for Drug Information [3,17–20]		
Secondary Resource	**Content**	**Coverage**
MEDLINE	Free online citation database of biomedical and life science journals by National Library of Medicine; 100% MEDLINE coverage; PubMed includes 100% MEDLINE plus in-process, ahead-of-print citations, and others	1946–present
SCOPUS	Subscription database; 100% MEDLINE coverage plus literature from the life sciences, physical sciences, social sciences, and humanities	Pre-1996 (some coverage back to 1823)
Embase	Subscription database; 100% MEDLINE coverage plus more coverage of European, non-English, and pharmacology and toxicology journals	1947–present
International Pharmaceutical Abstracts (IPA)	Subscription database; it includes abstracts about drug use and development from health journals	1970–present
Google Scholar	Free; links to scholarly publications but not specific to any discipline (links to articles, theses, books, abstracts, professional societies, universities, and other websites)	Unknown

in their literature coverage. Some databases specialize in certain areas of practice. For example, Reactions Weekly is a secondary database solely focused on literature related to adverse drug reactions. Information is derived from journals, case reports, scientific meetings, media releases, and regulatory agencies. Other databases such as MEDLINE/PubMed, SCOPUS, and Embase search a broad scope of biomedical literature.

Search methodology also differs in secondary databases. This can be important because several databases cover similar content, so ease of accessibility and searching becomes an important factor in choosing which database to use. The majority of secondary literature is available online so accessibility, currency of published information, and ease of use have improved dramatically.

General Guidance for Efficient Secondary Searching

The most effective way to ensure a comprehensive search is performed is through a well-organized search strategy (**Table 16-4**). This comes with appropriate training, experience, and understanding of biomedical literature. It is important to recognize that a search may need to be revised several times to ensure satisfaction with the results found. As a result, keeping an organized record of completed searches is critical to prevent duplication and maintain efficiency.[7]

There are two main ways to search for secondary literature. One is through a controlled vocabulary thesaurus, and the other is to search by keywords. Many databases index literature according to controlled vocabularies. This system ensures that each piece of medical literature is indexed to a set of specific terms so that when a search is completed, no relevant citations are omitted. As an example, MEDLINE indexes according to Medical Subject Headings (MeSH). Emtree is another controlled vocabulary that operates as a life science thesaurus. The advantages to searching within controlled vocabularies are that relevant literature is unlikely to be missed, and irrelevant literature is avoided. Secondary databases differ widely in the ways a search is performed using the controlled vocabulary. For example, in PubMed/MEDLINE, the search within the MeSH database must be selected; in Ovid MEDLINE, it is automatically linked to MeSH terms.

Searching through controlled vocabularies is often preferred; however, there are situations when searching by keywords is appropriate. A keyword search will find any literature that uses that search term in the appropriate field such as Title or Abstract. Limitations to searching in this manner are that the search results may not be relevant to your intended search and other pertinent literature could be missed. For example, a keyword search using the term "non–insulin-dependent diabetes" will miss relevant articles that index according to the term "type 2 diabetes." However, some situations

TABLE 16-4   General Guidance to Efficient Secondary Searching[7]
Keep an organized record of completed searches.
Use a controlled vocabulary thesaurus when available (e.g., MeSH terms in PubMed).
Avoid use of keywords except in some situations (e.g., it is the only option for searching, newly published literature, clinical trial acronym, etc.).
Combine search terms with appropriate Boolean operators (i.e., AND, OR, NOT).
Use truncation as necessary to search for part of a word (e.g., inhal$)
Use limits and/or topic subheadings as needed to focus a search.
Search "related articles" when applicable.

do warrant searching by keywords. Some databases do not index according to controlled vocabularies, so searching by keywords is the only option. Also, newly published articles may not yet be indexed according to these vocabularies. Some terms have no appropriate term in the controlled vocabulary. For example, clinical trial acronyms (e.g. PLATO study, ACCORD trial) are often only found via keyword search in appropriate fields. When a keyword search is necessary, it is important that terms are spelled correctly and generic drug names are used. It is also important to recognize that several searches may need to be completed to consider all synonyms and alternative terms.

Combining search terms by using Boolean operators is another useful way to search. **Boolean operators** are search words that are used to connect keywords based on mathematical logic. The most common are AND, OR, NOT. Each operator uniquely adjusts the search of multiple terms. The AND operator is used to combine two terms together to focus literature on results containing both terms. This can be useful if too many citations result from searching with a single term. The OR operator is helpful if you are getting too few results with a single term, as it will look for results using either term. Lastly, combining terms with NOT will help reduce results with unwanted characteristics.[7]

Truncation is another method that searches for part of a word to search for secondary literature. For example, a keyword search for "randomiz★" will search for all literature that contains the root "randomiz" so results including randomize, random-ized, randomization, and randomizing will be found. Databases may use different symbols to designate truncation. Truncation must be used cautiously so that the root word does not serve as a prefix for several unrelated words (e.g., "pharm★": pharmacy, pharmaceutics, pharmacology, pharmacoeconomic).[7]

Limits and filters offer an additional way to search for literature. Many databases offer the ability to limit or filter a search to a specific type of article (e.g., clinical trial, practice guideline), a specific time frame, or language, among many others. Limits offer the advantage of focusing the search. However, they should also be used only as the search dictates so that relevant literature is not omitted. For example, unless there is a need for recent literature, it wouldn't be good to limit the search to only articles from the last 5 years. Likewise, many databases contain English abstracts with useful information, so limiting to only English articles could remove some relevant foreign results.

There are several alternative ways to search for medical literature aside from those already described. Search terms often have several subheadings linked to the main term. For example, the MeSH term for enoxaparin has subheadings for administration/dosage, adverse effects, chemistry, economics, and toxicity, among others. Broadly focused medical databases usually have the option of exploding or focusing a search. By **exploding** a term, all of the subheadings are included in search results, whereas a **focused search** on one or more subheadings results in literature focused to that subheading. Some databases have features to search "related articles." This can be helpful if you have only a few relevant results and want similar articles. Also, searching reference lists within the articles themselves can help find relevant literature. This is formally known as the "network method" and is especially useful if not much literature is found through the secondary search process.[7]

Advantages and Disadvantages of Secondary Literature

Secondary searching enables the practitioner to retrieve comprehensive published medical literature specific to a topic. Advantages are that many different sources for finding secondary literature are available. Most of the secondary sources are available via

BOX 16-2	**Example Case 2 (Secondary)**

You are working in a community pharmacy and a physician has contacted you. The physician would like to know if any medications should be adjusted post-surgery in a patient who has recently had gastric bypass surgery.

Search Strategy

A search of compendia would be warranted with this question to find pharmacokinetic information related to the specific medications. In addition, a Cochrane Review might be available relevant to the request. In this case, however, you would also want to search in secondary literature. The most appropriate secondary resources would ideally be broad in biomedical and science contexts, as you suspect this question will have a lot to do with pharmacokinetic parameters. For this reason, you search MEDLINE, SCOPUS, or Embase to find information related to this question. A good review article or some primary literature would be very helpful to address this request.

the Internet, thus allowing them to be continually updated. These are easy to use and timely. Depending on the scope of the request and the needs of the researcher, different resources may be preferred for a search as well as searching multiple databases. However, these differences can also be advantageous. Each has unique features that can greatly enhance search strategies, and thus becoming familiar with these processes is important. Additionally, some secondary biomedical databases require costly subscriptions, with the exception of PubMed, which is freely available.

PRIMARY LITERATURE

Primary literature is the foundation on which all other literature sources are built. **Primary literature** is original research that can be published or unpublished work. Using primary literature is often the final step in the search for drug information because it is the most specific type of literature.[21]

Clinical Studies

Clinical research, according to the National Institutes of Health (NIH), includes patient-oriented research, epidemiological and behavior studies, and health services research.[21] Clinical studies are those conducted in humans to evaluate a number of different outcomes including the etiology or mechanisms of disease, diagnosis, prevention, interventions for disease management, or safety. Clinical research findings are based on a clinical trial, cohort study, or case-control study, among many other study designs.

Pharmacoeconomic Studies

Clinical studies that describe and analyze the costs and consequences of drug therapy are considered **pharmacoeconomic studies**. However, a true pharmacoeconomic study is not only a cost analysis (i.e., costs of drug therapy), but also an evaluation of drug costs in addition to the impact on health outcomes. Several types of pharmacoeconomic studies exist: cost-effective analysis (CEA), cost-minimization analysis (CMA), cost-utility analysis (CUA), and cost-benefit analysis (CBA).[22,23]

    Cost-effective analyses measure cost per unit health outcome in natural units (e.g., years of life saved, symptom-free days, etc.). This type of analysis makes it useful for clinicians to measure the cost impact when health outcomes are improved.[22,23] Differences in costs among comparable drug therapies are evaluated with **cost-minimization analyses**. The disadvantage with this type of study is that it cannot compare differences among drug therapies that have different outcomes.

Cost-utility analyses (CUA) attempt to assign "utility" weights to quality outcomes so that the impact can be measured in relation to cost (e.g., quality-adjusted life years). A CUA is able to compare outcomes related to morbidity, which can be useful when evaluating outcomes where mortality is not always the primary health outcome of concern (e.g., cancer chemotherapy).[22,23] In **cost-benefit analyses**, a monetary value is placed on both the costs of therapy and the beneficial health outcomes. The advantage is that it allows for direct comparisons between the costs of treatment and the costs saved with improved outcomes. In this way, different outcomes can be compared because they are ultimately all evaluated in terms of cost. The disadvantage, however, is that placing a monetary value on health outcomes can be a challenge (e.g., quality of life).[22,23]

Pharmacoepidemiologic Studies

Pharmacoepidemiology is the application of principles of epidemiology to evaluate pharmaceutical products and services. In other words, it is the study of the potential impact of drug therapy or clinical services in large numbers of patients. These types of studies use observational designs like cohort and case-control designs to evaluate the safety and effectiveness of outcomes of drug therapy or clinical services in large patient populations.[24,25]

Other Sources of Primary Literature

Professional meeting abstracts and proceedings, theses, and patents are also considered primary sources of information. Meeting abstracts and proceedings may be published in some secondary databases and may be available online via the professional organization. Similarly, specific databases exist to search for theses and dissertations, which are often a required component of graduate school studies for a master's degree and a doctoral degree, respectively. A patent is another source of original information that is a property right granted by the U.S. government to exclude others from making, using, or selling an invention for a finite amount of time.[26]

EVALUATION OF PRIMARY LITERATURE

Expertise is needed to properly evaluate primary literature. An evaluation of the full piece of literature with a critique of strengths and limitations is needed before assuming that the information can influence patient care management. This requires evaluation of types of research, methodologies, bias, ethical principles, data analysis, and statistics. Biomedical literature evaluation is a lifelong skill that challenges clinicians to critique and understand the evidence before implementation.

ADVANTAGES AND DISADVANTAGES OF PRIMARY LITERATURE

Advantages of using primary literature include the ability to obtain complete, detailed, and the most relevant information about a topic that allows the researcher to independently evaluate the information. Also, new biomedical literature is published every day,

BOX 16-3	Example Case 3 (Primary)

As a hospital pharmacist working in the Emergency Department, you get a request to investigate whether nebulized naloxone is a viable and effective treatment option for overdose in a pediatric patient in transit to the hospital.

Search Strategy

For this question, you spot-check compendia for any off-label information, but nothing relevant is found. You then suspect you are going to need to look in a secondary database for primary literature. In this case, you search MEDLINE and CINAHL for literature related to this request. You end up finding only one case report detailing its use and limitations, as most of the literature on this topic is related to intranasal administration vs. nebulization.

making it the most current source for information. Disadvantages are that it requires the researcher to conduct a comprehensive search to obtain truly relevant research findings that are translatable to patient care. Furthermore, it takes a significant amount of time and expertise to conduct a full evaluation of primary literature.

INFORMATION CYCLE

Publication of medical literature is a lengthy process. Primary literature can take several months to a year to complete the publication process, including the time from initial review, peer review, editing, and proofreading. Once through the process, a journal article is published. The time at which an article becomes indexed into a secondary literature source can vary; however, most secondary databases are updated frequently (e.g., daily or weekly). This enables the clinicians to quickly locate newly published articles in a timely manner or even ahead of print. The time for an article to be referenced in tertiary literature can be longer due to the length of an additional publication process. This is especially true for print tertiary sources, including textbooks, as they are often updated as a new edition every 3 to 4 years. However, many electronic tertiary drug information databases are updated on a regular basis. This information cycle keeps practitioners abreast of the latest medical advancements and clinical studies.

DRUG LITERATURE ON THE INTERNET

With increasing information on the Internet, the way practitioners search for medical information has dramatically changed. The quality of information found via the Internet is highly variable. Finding credible information on the Internet can be accomplished using the same indicators previously described. Quality can also be partially assessed by the domain of the website.[27] Other factors for evaluating information on the Internet include author disclosures; lack of advertisements; presence of code of conduct and/or quality seals; reputable, current sources of the information; and the last date of revision.[28,29]

The ease of accessing information on the Internet is largely why most practitioners use it as a core resource. Clinical practice guidelines, prescribing information, and information from government agencies (e.g., the Centers for Disease Control [CDC] and the Food and Drug Administration [FDA]) are all easily accessible. Electronic tertiary and secondary databases are accessed via the Internet, many of which require a subscription, and journal portals provide open access or subscribed access to articles. Given the breadth of information that can be found on the Internet, however, it is imperative that practitioners know how to evaluate the material found.

SEARCH ENGINES

Though Internet search engines are often just starting points for a search, the number and quality of results can greatly impact the overall information found. For example, Wikipedia is a less credible source of medical and drug information on the Internet due to the lack of expertise, limited or no peer review, and its ability to be updated.[30] Google Scholar and PubMed are two secondary search engines freely available, in addition to government-sponsored websites such as those from the National Library of Medicine (NLM) and the Agency for Healthcare Research and Quality (AHRQ).

EVALUATION

Unfortunately, no standard criteria exist for establishing the quality of health information from the Internet. Websites are not mandated to certain quality standards, nor do they have to undergo peer review. In general, website suffixes ending in .gov (i.e., government sponsored) and .edu (i.e., educational institutions) are scored higher in terms of quality versus .org (i.e., noncommercial organizations) and .com (i.e., commercial organizations) sites.[27,30] Professional organization websites are common reasons for healthcare professionals to use the Internet to obtain clinical practice guidelines and best practice recommendations.

Many Internet quality/rating instruments have been developed; however, many of them do not list criteria for quality evaluation and others eventually cease to operate.[29] Health on the Net Foundation (HON) is a not-for-profit, non-governmental agency that aims to ensure reliable and credible medical information is published on the Internet. The HON Code, which is affixed to all certified websites, is available for free and holds websites to basic ethical standards for presentation of information and ensuring that sources are cited.[31] Though this certification does not rate information quality, nor does it ensure that information is 100% accurate, it is one way to begin to evaluate quality.

Quality assessment involves evaluation of the source of information, formal certifications, and also an independent review by the clinical practitioner with respect to publication authors, timing of publication, and peer review. This is due to the subjectivity of how quality can be defined.[32] Often, authorship of content is not reported on a website, but some reputed websites like WebMD provide detailed author information. Currency of information should also be evaluated, as many websites do not list a clearly visible "date updated." Accuracy of content should be able to be confirmed by references. Peer review is often limited or absent for most websites. Credibility of authorship, privacy policy, disclosure, and bias (funding source, conflicts of interest, advertisements, etc.) are also indicators of information quality.[30]

SUMMARY AND CONCLUSIONS

Medical literature is the foundation for the practice of evidence-based medicine. Pharmacists are routinely asked to provide comprehensive drug information in a timely manner to other healthcare providers. As such, it is important for pharmacists to use a systematic approach when responding to requests to address the appropriate question, and maintain efficiency and documentation. An organized approach to searching for information via the use of tertiary, secondary, and primary literature is essential. Efficient searches in bibliographic databases aim to locate the best evidence in a timely manner. Knowing how to properly evaluate the quality of these resources and information from the Internet, including clinical practice guidelines, is an important skill for all pharmacists and other clinicians.

REVIEW QUESTIONS

1. What are the steps of the systematic approach to a drug information request?
2. What is the approach to searching for drug information?
3. List examples of tertiary resources.
4. When assessing the quality of Internet resources, what needs to be considered?
5. What are ways to search for clinical practice guidelines?
6. What are ways to effectively and efficiently search for secondary literature?

ONLINE RESOURCES

Agency for Healthcare Research and Quality: http://www.ahrq.gov/
DailyMed: http://dailymed.nlm.nih.gov/dailymed/about.cfm
Drugs@FDA: http://www.accessdata.fda.gov/scripts/cder/drugsatfda/index.cfm
PubMed Tutorials: http://www.nlm.nih.gov/bsd/disted/pubmed.html

REFERENCES

1. American Society of Health-System Pharmacists. ASHP guidelines on the provision of medication information by pharmacists. *Am J Health-Syst Pharm.* 1996;53:1843–1845.
2. Watanabe AS, McCart G, Shimomura S, Kayser S. Systematic approach to drug information requests. *Am J Hosp Pharm.* 1975;32(12):1282–1285.
3. Fischer JM. Modification of the systematic approach to answering drug information requests. *Am J Hosp Pharm.* 1980;37(4):470,472,476.
4. Nathan JP, Gim S. Responding to drug information requests. *Am J Health Syst Pharm.* April 15, 2009;66(8):706–711.
5. Watanabe AS, Conner CS. *Principles of Drug Information Services: A Syllabus of Systematic Concepts.* Hamilton, IL: Hamilton Press; 1978.
6. Ascione FJ. *Principles of Scientific Literature Evaluation Critiquing Clinical Drug Trials.* Washington, DC: American Pharmaceutical Association; 2001.
7. Timmins F, McCabe C. How to conduct an effective literature search. *Nursing Standard.* 2005;20(11):41–47.
8. Evidence-Based Medicine Working Group. Evidence-based medicine. A new approach to teaching the practice of medicine. *JAMA.* 1992;268(17):2420–2425.
9. Field MJ, Lohr KN, eds. *Clinical Practice Guidelines: Directions for a New Program.* Washington, DC: National Academies Press; 1990.
10. National Institute for Health and Care Evidence. Available at: http://www.nice.org.uk/. Accessed August 25, 2012.
11. Agency for Healthcare Research and Quality, National Guideline Clearinghouse. Available at: http://www.guidelines.gov/. Accessed August 25, 2012.

12. Hayward RS, Wilson MC, Tunis SR, Bass EB, Guyatt G. Users' guides to the medical literature. VIII. How to use clinical practice guidelines. A. Are the recommendations valid? The Evidence-Based Medicine Working Group. *JAMA*. 1995;274(7):570–574.

13. Wilson MC, Hayward RS, Tunis SR, Bass EB, Guyatt G. Users' guides to the Medical Literature. VIII. How to use clinical practice guidelines. B. What are the recommendations and will they help you in caring for your patients? The Evidence-Based Medicine Working Group. *JAMA*. 1995;274(20):1630–1632.

14. Guyatt GH, Oxman AD, Vist GE, et al, GRADE Working Group. GRADE: an emerging consensus on rating quality of evidence and strength of recommendations. *BMJ*. 2008;336(7650):924–926.

15. The Cochrane Collaboration. Available at: http://www.cochrane.org/about-us. Accessed October 13, 2012.

16. An Introduction to the Improved FDA Prescription Drug Labeling. Available at: http://www.fda.gov/downloads/Training/ForHealthProfessionals/UCM090796.pdf. Accessed August 18, 2012.

17. U.S. National Library of Medicine. Available from: http://www.nlm.nih.gov/pubs/factsheets/medline.html. Accessed October 13, 2012.

18. SCOPUS. Available at: http://www.info.sciverse.com/UserFiles/sciverse_scopus_content_coverage_0.pdf. Accessed October 13, 2012.

19. Embase: Biomedical Database. Available at: http://www.embase.com/info/what-is-embase/coverage. Accessed October 13, 2012.

20. International Pharmaceutical Abstracts. Available at: http://www.ovid.com/webapp/wcs/stores/servlet/product__13051_-1_13151_Prod-109_____PDP. Accessed October 13, 2012.

21. National Institutes of Health. Available at: http://grants.nih.gov/grants/policy/hs/glossary.htm. Accessed September 15, 2012.

22. Rascati KL. *Essentials of Pharmacoeconomics*. Baltimore, MD: Lippincott Williams & Wilkins; 2009.

23. Grauer D, Lee J, Odom T, Osterhaus J, Sanchez L, Touchette D, eds. *Pharmacoeconomics and Outcomes*. 2nd ed. Kansas City, MO: American College of Clinical Pharmacy; 2003.

24. Fletcher RH, Fletcher SW, Wagner EH. *Clinical Epidemiology: The Essentials*. 3rd ed. Philadelphia, PA: Lippincott Williams & Wilkins; 1996.

25. DiPietro NA. Methods in epidemiology: observational study designs. *Pharmacotherapy*. 2010;30(10):973–984.

26. The United States Patent and Trademark Office. Available at: http://www.uspto.gov/inventors/patents.jsp. Accessed September 15, 2012.

27. Ansani NT, Vogt M, Henderson BA, et al. Quality of arthritis information on the Internet. *Am J Health Syst Pharm*. 2005;62(11):1184–1189.

28. Kunst H, Groot D, Latthe PM, Latthe M, Khan KS. Accuracy of information on apparently credible websites: survey of five common health topics. *BMJ*. 2002;324(7337):581–582.

29. Gagliardi A, Jadad AR. Examination of instruments used to rate quality of health information on the Internet: chronicle of a voyage with an unclear destination. *BMJ*. 2002;324:569–573.

30. Brunetti L, Hermes-DeSantis E. The Internet as a drug information resource. *US Pharmacist*. 2010;35(1):Epub.

31. Health on the Net Foundation. Available at: http://www.hon.ch/home1.html. Accessed September 30, 2012.

32. Wilson P. How to find the good and avoid the bad or ugly: a short guide to tools for rating quality of health information on the Internet. *BMJ*. 2002;324:598–600.

EVALUATING CLINICAL LITERATURE: AN OVERVIEW

Jill T. Johnson, PharmD, BCPS

CHAPTER OBJECTIVES

▸ Describe a stepwise approach to appraising published literature
▸ Understand the clinical relevance of study objectives
▸ Evaluate appropriateness of design and methods for study objectives
▸ Evaluate methods of analysis and interpretation of results
▸ Differentiate between clinical and statistical significance in the medical literature

KEY TERMINOLOGY

a priori	Composite endpoints	Surrogate endpoints
Clinical endpoints	Number needed to harm	
Clinical significance	Number needed to treat	

INTRODUCTION

Critical appraisal of medical literature by clinicians as a tool to improve patient care has evolved since the late 1970s.[1] It introduced a change in the practice paradigm based on knowledge and evolving medical literature rather than on traditional medical authority or anecdotal cases. Although early adoption of evidence-based medicine (EBM) was not readily accepted for various reasons, it has now become a mainstay of the way many clinicians practice. Sometimes, the term "evidence-based" is used incorrectly by authors of research funded by for-profit agencies, such as pharmaceutical manufacturers. Such research is often interpreted in favor of the industry product when compared to research funded by not-for-profit organizations.[2,3] Therefore, the ability to critically evaluate medical literature empowers clinicians with enlightened skepticism and the ability to identify biases and errors, including inappropriate control interventions, surrogate outcomes, publication bias, and other types of biases, misleading conclusions, and other false interpretations.

A clinician's ability to deliver the best possible patient care by applying evidence and providing treatment based on sound scientific principles reflects the importance of critical appraisal skills in clinical practice. This chapter will provide an overview of how to critically evaluate medical literature. Beginning with evaluating the clinical research question, the chapter will provide a stepwise approach in appraising research articles. This will include evaluating study design, methods, and statistical analysis. The chapter will particularly emphasize the interpretation of results in the context of patient care. It will also provide specific considerations in evaluating therapy and harm, and it will conclude with general considerations for clinicians for other biases in publications and their implications.

GENERAL FORMAT OF AN ARTICLE

Although there are several variations in presenting research evidence, most articles published in the medical literature today have four sections to help guide the reader: introduction, methods, results, and discussion (IMRaD). In addition to the above sections, a research paper usually includes an abstract and references.[4]

ABSTRACT

The abstract is the first part of the publication, although it is typically the last part written by the authors. Abstracts summarize, in a limited number of words, the aims of the research, the methods used to conduct the study, the results, and study conclusions. From the abstract, the reader can discern the study design and methodology including study population, intervention or exposures, and the outcomes for the primary and secondary endpoints. Based on the key study results, a sentence or two finalizes an abstract and summarizes the conclusions. The abstract should not be relied on to make a clinical decision because it does not provide sufficient detail to ascertain whether the findings are relevant to a population or person. Rather, an abstract should be used to decide whether the article is relevant for decision making, and if so, then the entire article should be evaluated to determine whether the results should be applied.

INTRODUCTION

The introduction includes pertinent background information to justify why the research was done and describes what is already known about the topic to date. Moreover, this section allows the author to point out gaps in the current knowledge or flaws in prior work in the field. The most important parts of the introduction are the rationale for the current experiment/observation and clearly defined research objectives that allow the clinician to properly critique the study design.

Methods

The methods section describes the researcher's process for how the experiment or observational study was conducted. It typically includes detailed information on study sample, study setting, interventions or exposures, randomization (if any), outcome assessments, study instruments, evaluations used, sample size, primary data collection or secondary data source, and statistical analysis. Details in the methods section should be adequate for the research to be reproduced.

The study population, described in the methods section, includes inclusion and exclusion criteria for research subjects. Variables often include age, diagnosis, gender, clinical and physical status, and ethnic background. The specific details regarding experimental or observational study design are included to inform readers about randomization (if any), control group, and timeline of study design. It also discloses whether the research was performed at a single site or at multiple centers. If the design is retrospective, details of the data source are included. For a prospective study, details of data collection are provided.

For prospective studies, the methods section describes what drug treatment was given, how it was administered (e.g., route, dose, frequency), and the process and frequency of monitoring. For observational research, the details of drug exposure definition and measurement details are provided. Outcome measurements should be described in detail including reliability and validity of measurement for the primary or secondary endpoints. For the primary endpoint, the study should be powered with enough research subjects and provide sufficient follow-up to find a difference, if there is a difference. Secondary endpoints are stated *a priori* (before the study begins) so that they can be measured systematically. The final part of the methods section contains the statistical analysis information. The methods of analyses, including statistical tests used to analyze the data, are specified. The researcher specifies the alpha level to find a statistical difference and often includes the sample size and power assumptions for the study.

Results

The results section reports the research findings including descriptive details of study sample, key findings of primary analyses, and any secondary or sub-group analyses findings. This section typically presents the facts and data without interpretation. The statistical significance is reported along with the results in the form of text, tables, and figures. For clinical trials, the results section usually consists of three sections: the patient baseline characteristics; the results of how effective the drug was; and, lastly, how safe it was, relative to the control group. For observational research, the results section includes a description of study sample, adjusted and unadjusted findings, and any subgroup or sensitivity analyses.

Discussion

The discussion section allows the researcher to interpret the research findings; however, the author should avoid reciting the results section. The core discussion should focus on the findings of the primary objective. The discussion section includes a general explanation of the research findings and allows comparison of findings with previous research or other relevant research. Possible explanations for consistencies or inconsistencies from previous research should be provided. The study implications for practice and/or policy could enhance the discussion by providing valuable information for translating research into practice. The study limitations and directions for future research should be included.

REFERENCES

The references are listed at the end of a research article. They typically are listed in the order in which they occur. Scientific journal articles follow the American Medical Association (AMA) format. This allows the reader to pull the original publication, if needed.

CRITICALLY APPRAISING A RESEARCH ARTICLE

A systematic approach is needed to critically review research articles. It provides a balanced method to evaluate all aspects of research to ensure validity and reliability of research findings. Although there are several aspects to evaluate, most of the evaluation is focused on certain critical components.[5] This systematic evaluation described below provides a general framework to critically appraise any research article using the list of nine questions, irrespective of study design (**Table 17–1**).

TABLE 17-1 Nine Questions for Critical Appraisal of a Research Article

1. Is this a clinically relevant research study?
   a. Does this research add to the medical literature?
   b. Is the research objective relevant to practice?

2. Is the study design appropriate to address the research question?
   a. Does it use appropriate experimental or observational design?
   b. Is the design an improvement over previous designs?

3. Are the recruitment and selection of the study sample explained clearly?
   a. How was the study sample recruited and selected?
   b. Is the study sample relevant to the research objective?

4. Are the study methods appropriately explained?
   a. Are the methods of randomization or observation methods explained?
   b. Are there any methods used to reduce bias?

5. Are the endpoints relevant for patient care?
   a. Are clinical outcomes relevant?
   b. Did they explain how and when the outcomes were measured?

6. Are the statistical analyses appropriate for the study?
   a. Are the statistical analyses appropriate for the design?
   b. Is the sample size adequate for the research question?

7. What are the key research findings?
   a. Is the key research finding statistically significant?
   b. How large is the effect?
   c. Are findings consistent with clinical rationale and previous literature?

8. Are there any study limitations?   a. Were there limitations in sample, design, and analyses that limit the research findings?

9. How can the research findings be used in practice?
   a. Can the findings be generalized to other populations?
   b. Should the findings be incorporated into practice?

1. IS THIS A CLINICALLY RELEVANT RESEARCH STUDY?

Even if the article represents a well-done research project, if it is not relevant, it is not useful for clinical practice. If the research would not change what the clinician would otherwise have chosen to do, then the relevance of the research could be questioned. If the research implies that a new treatment should be used in the clinical scenario and that treatment is not already being used, then relevance is established. Clinical relevance refers to the applicability and usefulness of research to clinical practice.

a. Does this research add to the medical literature?

Even if the article is not representative of research that makes a substantive new contribution to the larger body of evidence, the work may still enhance the ability to generalize to a new population or at least increase the confidence in the validity of previous research.[6] For example, in the late 1990s, carvedilol was the topic of the U.S. Carvedilol Trial.[7] Carvedilol was introduced for use in patients with chronic systolic heart failure and ejection fractions of $\leq$ 35%, a population in whom clinicians previously believed that beta-blockers were contraindicated due to negative inotropic effects, but showed an unexpected survival benefit in just 6 months. Subsequently, other beta-blocker trials were published that contributed to the literature, some showing benefit [8-10] and one not showing benefit.[11] This additional evidence was still relevant to patient care because it helped establish that general beta-blockade may not provide survival benefit and that specific beta-blockers should be used if that particular endpoint is to be achieved.

b. Is the research objective relevant to practice?

The research objective must be relevant to practice in the way that results could be applied and the outcome would be meaningful to a patient. For example, lowering LDL in and of itself does not necessarily lower cardiac events. Hence, any drug touting an LDL-lowering ability may not be relevant to practice. Consider estrogen replacement therapy (ERT) in postmenopausal women discussed previously. ERT lowers LDL but does not translate in practice to lower cardiac events as once presumed.[12,13] Therefore, the research objective is relevant to practice when the objective is to measure something meaningful to real practice and real patients. A research objective seeking to answer the question about the impact of a treatment on a clinically relevant outcome must measure the outcome rather than an endpoint that may not answer the question; otherwise, there is a risk of it not being relevant.

2. IS THE STUDY DESIGN APPROPRIATE TO ADDRESS THE RESEARCH QUESTION?

There are several research designs that are appropriate for a research question. The research should select the best research design that addresses the research question. Often the current state of knowledge determines the appropriateness of study design. Early studies tend to use explorative designs, whereas later studies use analytical design to test a hypothesis.

a. Does it use appropriate experimental or observational design?

The type of question a researcher seeks to answer determines the best study design to yield the answer to the research question (**Table 17–2**).[14] Therapy and diagnosis questions are best answered by randomized controlled trails (RCTs), as they minimize bias

TABLE 17-2	Type of Evidence to Best Answer a Research Question[14]
Type of Research Question	**Best Type of Study to Answer the Research Question**
Diagnosis	Prospective, blind comparison to the gold standard
Therapy	Meta-analysis of randomized controlled trials (RCTs), systematic reviews of included RCTs, or RCT
Prognosis	Cohort study > case-control > case series
Harm	RCT > cohort > case-control > case series
Prevention	RCT > cohort > case-control > case series

and leave only the intervention as the sole difference. Harm is measured best by RCTs; but observational designs like cohort or case–control are valuable alternatives when there are ethical or practical concerns for evaluating medication safety. Likewise, prognosis questions are measured by an observational design. Prevention questions, such as efficacy of intermittent pneumatic compression on preventing venous thrombosis, are best answered by RCTs. However, devices such as these are difficult, if not impossible, to use to blind the research participants. Therefore, observational design provides an answer that may be more biased than an RCT, but still allows for an association of benefit (or detriment) to be established.

b. Is the design an improvement over previous designs?

If a previous trial design was observational, the new data from an RCT are likely more believable and perhaps closer to the truth than the older data. Remember, EBM uses the current best evidence. For example, in the 1990s, it was thought that estrogen replacement therapy (ERT) was a good idea for postmenopausal women to decrease cardiovascular disease. Thousands of women were prescribed estrogen for a decade or more based on observational and epidemiologic data that showed that LDL was reduced when they were prescribed ERT. Consequently, in 1996, ERT was included in the American College of Cardiology guidelines for this purpose. Studies used to support the guideline said that "observational studies indicate that estrogen therapy does reduce mortality in women with moderate and severe coronary disease."[15] Subsequently, in 1998, Hulley et al. published a landmark RCT in the *Journal of the American Medical Association* that randomized a secondary prophylaxis population of postmenopausal women to estrogen plus progestin (in those with a uterus) or placebo.[12] Unlike the observational studies, this study actually measured coronary heart disease events and myocardial infarction. During year 1, the event rate was higher for the ERT group. However, over the subsequent 4 years, the rate leveled off. The end result was that no benefit for ERT was observed.[12,13] Using the ERT example, observational designs showed a reduced risk of coronary disease.[16] Once well-designed RCTs were completed, the better-quality evidence trumped the old evidence, and it was concluded that ERT has no benefit on cardiovascular disease.[12,13]

3. Are the Recruitment and Selection of the Study Sample Explained Clearly?

The recruitment and selection of the study subjects should be explained in detail for both experimental and observational research. Inclusion and exclusion criteria specify which population was studied and which attributes they could or could not have to be eligible for entry into the study. Study results can be applied to individuals who are similar to those study subjects representing the results of the trial. This requires examining the inclusion criteria and evaluation of baseline characteristics of the study population. The method used for recruitment of patients should be clearly specified, including details of promotional strategies and incentives provided. The sources and locations of the study sample should also be provided.

a. How was the study sample recruited and selected?

The manner in which the study sample was recruited and selected is determined largely by the inclusion and exclusion criteria. Further information may include whether subjects came from an outpatient clinic or were discharged from a hospital. In an RCT, recruitment methods should include details about promotional material used to identify patients and allocation concealment. Failing to conceal the random allocation process may introduce selection bias and potentially result in a non-randomized trial. A trial has adequate concealed allocation or blinding if all investigators are unaware of future treatment allocations and have no control over randomization.[17] If the trial does not state that some form of concealed allocation was used, it is a more conservative assumption to conclude that allocation concealment was *not* used. Descriptive information regarding the individual sites of a multiple center study can be included. For observational research, the applications of selection (inclusion and exclusion) criteria in prospective and retrospective research should be provided. The details of data source and collection can help to define the source population. The issue of random selection of subjects in observation research becomes relevant only for generalization purposes.

b. Is the study sample relevant to the research objective?

It is important to ask this relevance question because it pertains to applicability of the results. If a research question pertains to an elderly population, the study must enroll geriatric patients. Pediatric enrollees or younger adults may not be likely to experience the same results. For example, the MEDENOX trial compared the use of enoxaparin 20 mg and 40 mg to placebo in medically ill patients to determine if either was effective for reducing venous thrombosis (VTE).[18] Enoxaparin 40mg was effective for reducing VTE in the population. However, the mean age of the population was 72 years of age with risk factors predisposing them to VTE. If a research objective does not relate to the study sample, this diminishes the validity and applicability of the study findings.

4. Are the Study Methods Appropriately Explained?

The research methods should provide details of study design and methodology including randomization/observation methods and any methods used to minimize the bias. The specifics of study design are often described using a figure with detailing regarding the timing of intervention/exposure and outcomes. Methodological details include the data collection and measurement process, and definitions of primary objective-efficacy and safety outcome measures.

a. Are the methods of randomization or observation methods explained?

The randomization process should be described in detail and may include specifics such as the drug–placebo ratio and variables for which, if any, stratification was performed. Randomization helps to ensure that similar groups are being compared without either/

any group having a prognostic advantage at baseline. Baseline differences in the study groups may compromise the validity of study results. The clinician must decide whether the magnitude of difference, if there is any, would likely change the results to the degree that a different decision regarding therapy may be made.

The flaw with not randomizing treatment assignments is the potential for other factors to suppress any sign of treatment effect. Many factors determine the clinical outcome of an individual (e.g., severity of illness, other known and unknown prognostic factors). For example, in a case in which the researchers expect that smoking history could affect the trial results and they would like to ensure that smoking history is not a confounding variable, randomization can be stratified to ensure equal numbers of smokers in each of the groups being compared. For observational research, the specifics of design (cohort or case-control) and methodology including data sources and collection, operational definition of exposure, outcome, and key predictors should be provided. Techniques such as matching for sample selection and prospective data collection for measurement of confounders can help to strengthen the study design.

b. Are there any methods used to reduce bias?

In clinical research, common biases include investigator bias, selection bias, performance bias, attrition bias, and detection bias. Randomization minimizes most of these biases. Other techniques such as blinding and statistical approaches can also help to minimize biases. If applied systematically, preconceived opinions of the treatment, whether favorable or not, could undermine randomization and skew the results. Although the terms "double blinding" or "single blinding" are often used, it is usually more helpful for the reader if the author explains exactly who was unaware of the treatment assignment. However, blinding does not provide bias reduction in a trial aimed at showing non-inferiority. The issues of confounding and selection bias are significant in observational research. Any confounder that could bias the study results should be measured and statistically adjusted. The statistical approaches like multivariable analyses, matching, sensitivity analyses, and other advanced techniques should be explained in observational research.

5. ARE THE ENDPOINTS RELEVANT FOR PATIENT CARE?

The selection of relevant endpoints is critical, as it has important implications for patient care. The endpoints should be valid and reliably measured to ensure the relevance of study findings. Clinical endpoints are more relevant than surrogate endpoints. For example, a trial showing that a drug prolongs the time it takes for the doubling of serum creatinine in a population with diabetes implies that the drug lessens detrimental kidney effects. However, measuring the rate of patients being placed on dialysis or needing renal transplant actually measures the rate of detrimental kidney effects without having to infer from surrogate endpoint data. Retrospective observational studies may have issues in including reliable and valid endpoints. These should be carefully evaluated before the study implementation.

a. Are clinical outcomes relevant?

Clinical endpoints

Clinical endpoints are outcomes that represent disease or symptoms. **Clinical endpoints** are direct measures of how a patient feels, functions, or survives. They are expected to predict the effect of therapy. Examples may include death, disease (myocardial infarction, stroke), or symptoms (pain, bleeding). They typically are understood by a layperson without interpretation by a medical professional. By contrast, surrogate endpoints may correlate with clinical endpoints; however, there is no guarantee that they will. In clinical research, finding out the effect on the clinical endpoint is the goal. The question of relevance is related to the extent of improvement and determining whether the amount of improvement warrants use of the new therapy.

Surrogate endpoints

Surrogate endpoints are used as an outcome measure in a clinical trial when the clinical endpoint of interest is too difficult or too expensive to measure routinely and when it is thought that the surrogate marker correlates well enough to justify its use as a substitute. **Surrogate endpoints** are indirect measures of clinically meaningful endpoints. Often lab measurements such as cholesterol levels or CD4 count are used as surrogates for clinically meaningful endpoints. For surrogate endpoints to be considered valid, there should be substantial evidence of causal relationship between change in the surrogate and change in the clinically important outcome. The problem with some surrogate endpoints is that to prove the surrogate endpoint is adequate, one has to conduct research using an actual clinical endpoint or provide evidence from previous research.[19]

Composite endpoints

Composite endpoints are outcomes that capture the number of patients experiencing one or more of several outcomes. Many trials use composite endpoints, and the outcome is considered to have been achieved when any one of the components included in the composite has been reached. Three assumptions are important to remember for a composite endpoint to be meaningful. First, the individual components must be clinically meaningful and of similar importance to the patient. A composite endpoint that contains non-fatal myocardial infarction, non-fatal stroke, and sudden cardiac death with resuscitation includes similarly meaningful events. By contrast, a composite endpoint that contains myocardial infarction, ischemic stroke, and rehospitalization due to heart failure does not include similarly important outcomes. In many cases, the weakest component skews the results to create an apparent difference between treatment groups when a difference may not exist between the more similar outcomes. When large variations exist between components, the composite endpoint should not be used. Second, the effect on each component should be biologically plausible. Last, the components should go in the same direction. When the composite endpoint is affected positively overall but the individual components give mixed results, the clinician is left confused about whether to use that agent. For example, in the LIFE trial comparing losartan and atenolol in hypertension, the primary composite endpoint of cardiovascular (CV) mortality, stroke, and myocardial infarction resulted in a hazard ratio of 0.87 (95% CI 0.77–0.98) with losartan vs. atenolol.[20] However, when the components were considered individually, no statistical significance in CV mortality was seen, a statistically significant advantage was seen with stroke, and a non-significant *increase* was seen with MI.

b. Did they explain how and when the outcomes were measured?

The validity and reliability of outcome measurement should be explained in detail. The operational definitions of all relevant endpoints should be provided. The authors should also explain the schedule of outcome measurements for both experimental and observational research. Often an accompanying figure illustrates the schedule of events; however, in the absence of such illustration, adequate description in the text should allow the reader to sketch a map representing a schedule of how each research subject was followed. Closer follow-up that one group receives compared to the other group can weaken the inferences drawn from the results. For example, if a new anticoagulant that does not require international normalized ratio (INR) monitoring was compared to warfarin, which requires every 4 weeks monitoring, the closer follow-up of the warfarin patients could introduce bias either for or against the results that warfarin produces. The closer follow-up might allow for detection of bleeding episodes that might go undetected in the less closely monitored group. Ascertainment bias, which this represents, introduces a systematic distortion in measuring how frequently an event occurs due to the manner the data are collected.

6. ARE THE STATISTICAL ANALYSES APPROPRIATE FOR THE STUDY?

Statistical analyses are used to assess and account for chance and random errors. This includes descriptive analyses of baseline characteristics of study groups and comparisons of study endpoints using various statistical techniques. The sample size should be sufficient to detect clinical, meaningful differences between the study groups.

a. Are the statistical analyses appropriate for the design?

The choice of a statistical test is determined by several factors including the research question type of dependent variable, number of study groups, sample size, and other statistical rationales (**Table 17–3**). The justification of statistical tests should be explained by the authors along with the statistical assumptions. The level of significance is often set at 5%, and a *p*-value of less than 5% is considered statistically significant. Although RCTs often require simple statistical approaches, analysis for observational research requires multivariable analyses or other advanced statistical methods to assess and control for possible confounders and effect modifiers.

TABLE 17-3 Common Statistical Tests in Clinical Research			
Purpose	**Nominal Outcome**	**Ordinal Outcome**	**Interval/Ratio Outcome**
To compare repeated measures in a single group	McNemar test	Wilcoxon signed ranks test	Paired *t*-test
To compare two groups	Chi-square	Mann–Whitney *U* test	Two-sample *t*-test
To compare three or more groups	Chi-square	Kruskal–Wallis ANOVA	Analysis of variance (ANOVA)
To assess correlation between variables		Spearman correlation	Pearson correlation
To examine predictors or assess relationships	Logistic or Cox regression	Linear/logistic regression	Linear regression

b. Is the sample size adequate for the research question?

Sample size depends on four variables: type I and type II error rates, data variability, σ^2, and treatment effect size, d. In many clinical trials, treatment effect size is the clinically important difference expected to be produced between two groups.[21] Failure to show a difference between groups may be related to sample size or one or more assumptions used to estimate sample size. Other possible explanations for failing to show a difference could be the desire to show too big a difference between groups or trying to show the difference with too much certainty. By contrast, if a pre-specified outcome showed a statistically significant effect, it should be concluded that the finding is valid, even if the sample size was incompletely recruited. These considerations are relevant for both experimental and observational research.

7. What Are the Key Research Findings?

The key findings should focus on the primary objective. Both statistical and clinical significance of the findings should be evaluated to determine the relevance of the findings. A researcher may show statistical significance but fail to show a clinician that a meaningful difference can be achieved. It may be valuable for a clinician to have an idea of what minimally important difference would be needed to persuade him or her to use a drug in a patient prior to analyzing the results of the trial. Just because a trial has a "statistically significant" finding does not equate to a "substantial" benefit. Again, these considerations are relevant for both experimental and observational research.

a. Is the key research finding statistically significant?

Statistical significance is typically indicated by a p-value—the probability of finding the results of the study, assuming the null hypothesis is true. A p-value of ≤ 0.05 in a study is an indication of statistical significance—evidence against the null (e.g., the null hypothesis is that outcomes are equal in treatment and control groups). It either meets statistical significance or it doesn't. A p-value of > 0.05 means that there is not sufficient evidence to reject the null hypothesis or to conclude that the two treatments are different on the outcome. When there is sufficient evidence (usually $p \leq 0.05$), the findings are considered statistically significant. Once statistical significance is established, clinical significance should be examined. "Statistically significant" does not imply that the results are necessarily more important. "Statistically significant" should never be automatically interchanged with "substantial."

b. How large is the effect?

In many studies, the difference in clinical endpoints between groups is a key factor in determining the strength of the finding. **Clinical significance** refers to change in efficacy or safety that is clinically meaningful in practice. The major factors in determining what is "meaningful" are extent of change and type of clinical endpoint. What seems like a small 2% difference in mortality between groups may still affect a large number of individuals depending on how common the diagnosis is. However, 2% difference in blood pressure may not be clinically significant, even if it is statistically significant. Treatment effect is reported in several different ways. The absolute risk reduction (ARR) or absolute risk increase (ARI), depending on the direction, is one way. In a clinical trial measuring the benefit or detriment one treatment arm has over another, the ARR or ARI can be calculated. It is the difference between the rate of events for one arm of a trial and the rate of events for the other arm. Subsequently, the reciprocal of the ARR or the ARI is the **number needed to treat** (NNT) or the **number needed to harm**

BOX 17-1	**Clinical Scenario[24]**

The Randomized Aldactone Evaluation Study (RALES) enrolled 1,663 patients with NYHA Class III/IV patients and assigned 841 to placebo and 822 to spironolactone. All-cause death occurred in 386 (45.9%) placebo patients and 284 (34.5%) spironolactone patients. The ARR was 11.4%, or 0.114. The NNT was 1/0.114, or nine patients. For every nine patients like those enrolled in the RALES trial taking spironolactone instead of placebo, one all-cause death will be prevented.[24] The interpretation of whether spironolactone should be used in this setting requires some clinical judgment. It would be nice if, for every one patient treated, one patient would benefit. For various reasons, all drugs do not work in everyone. Overall, an NNT of nine is a worthwhile drug therapy, but other issues must be considered.

The NNH is calculated the same way. In the same RALES trial, 9% of men developed gynecomastia in the spironolactone group while only 1% of the placebo arm reported it. This results in an NNH of 13 for the adverse event gynecomastia. Therefore, when weighing whether to use the drug in a similar population, the input of the patient must be considered. In cases in which patient input is not applicable, the NNT and NNH form the risk-benefit decision for the prescriber. If roughly every 9th person will avoid death while every 13th person will suffer from gynecomastia, and there is no way to discern who they will be, a patient should be given the option whether or not to use the drug.

(NNH), respectively. The NNT is the number of patients needed to be treated with a therapy to prevent an event from occurring. The NNH refers to number of patients who would need to be treated to cause harm or an adverse event.

c. Are findings consistent with clinical rationale and previous literature?

The consistency of study findings strengthens the research evidence. This requires evaluation of previous research and pharmacological rationale to explain the study findings. Although this is important in experimental research, it is critical in observational research. Years ago, a trial comparing losartan to captopril in heart failure patients concluded that there was a statistically significant improvement in all-cause mortality with losartan over captopril.[22] The biologic plausibility was missing, as was support from previous literature. Subsequently, a similar yet larger trial with longer follow-up compared the drugs to each other again in a similar population.[23] The results from this stronger, higher-quality evidence did not support the findings of the first trial. When an inconsistent finding of this type occurs, a clinician should question whether a difference truly exists and should follow the current best evidence. Observational research often requires multiple studies across diverse study populations for the findings to be considered as credible evidence because of inherent biases.

8. Are There Any Study Limitations?

Research is always constrained for practical and scientific reasons. These include study sample, study design and methodology, and analyses. The research findings should always be evaluated in the context of study limitations. Some limitations are small and may not limit the study findings; other limitations may be large and may warrant some constraints regarding applicability of study findings.

a. Were there limitations in sample, design, and analyses that limit the research findings?

Study limitations are any research constraints that diminish the validity and/or restrict the generalizability of the results. Limitations can include flaws in study design including the failure to recruit enough study subjects such that power is reduced. Any factor that reduces the internal validity (methodological flaws) or the external validity (generalizability) is considered a limitation of the study. The extent of these limitations should be evaluated and should be factored in applying the research findings to practice and policy. Often observational research has more study limitations than experimental research due to inherent biases in study design. Consequently, observational research is lower than experimental designs in the hierarchy of evidence.

9. How Can the Research Findings Be Used in Practice?

Often, research findings can be used in similar types of patients in whom the research was conducted. It may not be reasonable to expect the same results from a clinical trial using an adult, non-elderly sample would translate to an elderly population. In some cases, similar results may occur; however, to assess the effects in the elderly population, the trial should be performed in that population. In addition, the utility of the research in patient care is based on the considerations of internal validity and strength of study findings.

a. Can the findings be generalized to other populations?

Extrapolating research findings to populations in whom the treatment has not been tested is questionable. In some cases, it may be reasonable to extrapolate research findings, but the reality exists that the results may not be reproducible in a different population or one with different variables. For example, the use of beta-blockers in heart failure is limited to carvedilol, metoprolol succinate, and bisoprolol largely because another beta-blocker, bucindolol, was tried and failed to show the benefit. This prevented extrapolation to other beta-blockers for this use. By contrast, angiotensin-converting enzyme inhibitor (ACE) use in heart failure does not seem to suffer the same restrictions, possibly because each agent that has been tried thus far has provided a sufficient effect to reasonably allow clinicians to extrapolate the results to other ACE inhibitors in the absence of trials in each and every ACE inhibitor. The true effect will remain unknown for individual drugs until the treatment is tested in the actual population.

b. Should the findings be incorporated into practice?

Several considerations should be made before incorporating research findings into practice. First, the study design and methods from which the results came should be critically appraised. The internal validity considerations are paramount in translating evidence into patient care. The strength of the findings based on NNT and NNH can help to implement EBM. If the new findings are beneficial over the standard of practice and there is less harm, implementation of the findings should be put into practice. If the new findings are beneficial over the standard but there is more harm, an individual judgment must be made to determine if the detriment in the form of adverse effects is worth it to achieve the benefit the new finding offers.

GENERAL CONSIDERATIONS

In addition to scientific and methodological considerations, clinicians should keep in mind that other general factors can undermine the research findings. Addressing the following additional questions can help to provide a well-rounded evaluation of the research under consideration.

1. Is This a Peer-Reviewed Paper?

Non-peer-reviewed publications occur in newspapers, magazines, or journals and are written by any self-proclaimed expert without review by experts in the field. Peer-reviewed journals publish articles that have been reviewed and edited by experts and professionals in the field who are familiar with the topic and can provide meaningful, rigorous, scientific critiques of the article prior to publication.

2. Who Funded the Research?

Those who fund the research often have input into the research. Whether the funding agency maintains the decision to publish, controls ownership of the data, or pays the researcher in some way could influence the analysis of the data. Research supported by industry is interpreted by their authors differently than that is supported by not-for-profit agencies. Financial competing interests have been shown to influence the authors' conclusions. Some factors that lead to misconstrued interpretation of the data are inappropriate control interventions such as imbalanced dose comparisons, the use of surrogate endpoints, publication bias, and incomplete or misleading descriptions of the research findings.

One study that analyzed 12 clinical trials to assess the association between competing interests and authors' conclusions found that those with competing financial interests more commonly favored the experimental intervention. The same association was not found for those with competing personal, academic, or political interests.[3,25] Another study that assessed 370 randomized drug trials found that trials funded by for-profit organizations had a more than five-fold increased odds of recommending the experimental drug as the drug of choice compared with trials funded by nonprofit organizations.[2]

Publication bias is the publishing of trial results of positive trials while not publishing trial results that show no difference or negative results. It leads to a body of literature with skewed findings. Industry-funded research has a vested interest in showing positive results and not in showing no difference or negative results in clinical trials. The peer-review process has shown a less than stellar ability to mitigate the problem. One study testing the peer-review process found that a fabricated manuscript with a positive finding was more likely to be recommended for publication than an otherwise identical manuscript that showed no difference.[26]

In 1997, Congress passed the Food and Drug Administration Modernization Act, which created a public resource that required federally or privately funded clinical trials conducted under investigational new drug applications (INDs) to be registered. In 2000, the National Institutes of Health National Library of Medicine released the website ClinicalTrials.gov.[27] Many major medical journals will not publish unless the trial is registered with ClinicalTrials.gov before the entry of the first study subject. The public is able to see the progress of such trials and expects results to be published regardless of the direction of the findings.

3. Are There Any Conflicts of Interests?

Conflicts of interest (COIs) can occur in many ways. Research can be conflicted based on its funding as well as relationships between the investigators and the sponsor. Funding of research can produce a COI by inserting financial incentive to influence results by paying the researchers directly, providing free supplies or drugs, or supporting their research programs in academia. The potential for a financial COI exists when there is a financial incentive (real or perceived) that could potentially influence the research results. Examples of such potential COIs include sponsor inducements to the investigators (speaking opportunities, enrolling incentives, etc.) that are outside the support provided for the conduct of the study. Financial COIs may arise if the investigators or their immediate families have a relationship with the sponsor or potentially stand to gain from the results of the trial. Supervisory COIs can occur when a supervisor has an ulterior motive, financial or otherwise, for the employee's research to produce biased results. Sometimes these COIs may be managed by inserting a safe haven for the employee researcher, thereby minimizing influence by the supervisor. A COI, in and of itself, does not invalidate the research findings. At a minimum, the potentially conflicted party should disclose the conflict so the reader can put the results into context.

SUMMARY AND CONCLUSIONS

Articles published in the medical literature are written in similar formats, usually using IMRaD structure, regardless of study design, which helps the reader to develop an information expectation even before critically appraising the publication. The type of research question determines the best study design to answer a research question. Systematically appraising the medical literature, regardless of the study design, helps a clinician address issues that may otherwise be overlooked. Using these nine critical appraisal questions provided may help the clinician to read with a critical eye and develop skills to discern high-quality evidence from low-quality evidence. Deciding to incorporate research findings into practice is critical, and several important considerations should be made before subjecting an individual to a new treatment, diagnostic test, or prognostic category. Lastly, becoming aware of bias that can enter into research is the first step in mitigating the bias. Once a clinician knows what to look for, a decision can be made about whether or not to apply the evidence to practice.

REVIEW QUESTIONS

1. Discuss the key components of IMRaD format.
2. Explain key considerations for evaluating appropriateness of design and methods for study objectives.
3. Differentiate the use of surrogate endpoints from the use of clinical endpoints.
4. What are three assumptions for composite endpoints to be useful to the reader to be able to apply trial results?
5. What are some key considerations for applying research findings into practice?
6. Discuss some general factors that can undermine the research findings.

ONLINE RESOURCES

Introduction to Health Technology Assessment: http://www.nlm.nih.gov/nichsr/hta101/ta101_c1.html
Study design and choosing a statistical test, BMJ online: http://www.bmj.com/about-bmj/resources-readers/publications/statistics-square-one/13-study-design-and-choosing-statisti

REFERENCES

1. Guyatt G, Rennie D. *Users' Guides to the Medical Literature*. Chicago: AMA Press; 2004:xvi.

2. Als-Nielsen B, Chen W, Gluud C, Kjaergard LL. Association of funding and conclusions in randomized drug trials: a reflection of treatment effect or adverse events? *JAMA*. 2003;290:921–928.

3. Kjaergard LL, Als-Nielsen B. Association between competing interests and authors' conclusions: epidemiological study of randomised clinical trials published in the *BMJ*. *BMJ*. 2002;325:249.

4. Pakes GE. Writing manuscripts describing clinical trials: a guide for pharmacotherapeutic researchers. *Ann Pharmacother*. 2001;35:770–779.

5. Guyatt G, Sackett DL, Cook DJ. Users' guides to the medical literature: how to use an article about therapy or prevention; are the results of the study valid? *JAMA*. 1993;270(21):2598–2601.

6. Young JM, Solomon MJ. How to critically appraise an article. *Nature Clinical Practice*. 2009;6(2):82–91.

7. Packer M, Bristow MR, Cohn JN, et al. The effect of carvedilol on morbidity and mortality in patients with chronic heart failure. *N Engl J Med*. 1996;334:1349–1355.

8. Packer M, Coats AJS, Fowler MB, et al. Effect of carvedilol on survival in severe chronic heart failure. *N Engl J Med*. 2001;344:1651–1658.

9. MERIT-HF Study Group. Effect of metoprolol CR/LX in chronic heart failure: metoprolol CR/XL randomized intervention trial in congestive heart failure. *Lancet*. 1999;353:2001–2007.

10. CIBIS-II Investigators and Committees. The cardiac insufficiency bisoprolol study II (CIBIS-II) a randomized trial. *Lancet*. 1999;353:9–13.

11. The BEST Investigators. A trial of the beta-blocker bucindolol in patients with advanced chronic heart failure. *N Engl J Med*. 2001;344:1659–1667.

12. Hulley S, Grady D, Bush T, et al. Randomized trial of estrogen plus progestin for secondary prevention of coronary heart disease in postmenopausal women. *JAMA*. 1998;280:605–613

13. Grady D, Herrington D, Bitttner V, et al. Cardiovascular disease outcomes during 6.8 years of hormone therapy; Heart and Estrogen/Progestin Replacement Study follow-up (HERS II). *JAMA*. 2002;288:49–57.

14. Types of questions and types of studies. Available at: http://www.hsl.unc.edu/Services/Tutorials/EBM/Supplements/QuestionSupplement.htm. Accessed October 16, 2012.

15. Ryan TJ, Anderson JL, Antman EM, et al. ACC/AHA Guidelines for the management of patients with acute myocardial infarction: executive summary. *Circulation*. 1996;94:2341–2350.

16. Grady D, Rubin SM, Petitti DB, et al. Hormone therapy to prevent disease and prolong life in post-menopausal women. *Ann Intern Med*. 1992;117:1016–1037.

17. Forder PM, Gebski VJ, Keech AC. Allocation concealment and blinding: when ignorance is bliss. *MJA*. 2005;182(2):87–89.

18. Samama MM, Cohen AT, Darmon JY, et al. A comparison of enoxaparin with placebo for the prevention of venous thromboembolism in acutely ill medical patients. *N Engl J Med*. 1999;341:793–800.

19. Senn S, Barnett V. *Statistical Issues in Drug Development*. 2nd ed. Chichester: John Wiley & Sons; 2007.

20. Dahlof B, Devereux RB, Kjeldsen SE, et al. Cardiovascular morbidity and mortality in the losartan intervention for endpoint reduction in hypertension study (LIFE): a randomized trial against atenolol. *Lancet*. 2002;359:995–1003.

21. Study design and choosing a statistical test. BMJ online. Available at: http://www.bmj.com/about-bmj/resources-readers/publications/statistics-square-one/13-study-design-and-choosing-statisti. Accessed January 4, 2012.

22. Pitt B, Segal R, Martinez FA, et al. The ELITE Study Investigators. Randomised trial of losartan versus captopril in patients over 65 with heart failure (evaluation of losartan in the elderly study, ELITE). *Lancet*.1997;349:747–752.

23. Pitt B, Poole-Wilson PH, Segal R, et al. Elite II Investigators. Effect of losartan compared with captopril on mortality in patients with symptomatic heart failure: randomized trial—the losartan heart failure survival study ELITE II. *Lancet*. 2000;3555:1582–1587.

24. Pitt B, Zannad F, Remme WJ, et al. The effect of spironolactone on morbidity and mortality in patients with severe heart failure. *N Engl J Med*. 1999;341:709–717.

25. Evidence-Based Medicine Working Group. Progress in evidence-based medicine. *JAMA*. 2008;300(15):1814–1816.

26. Emerson GB, Warme WJ, Wolf FM, Heckman JD, Brand RA, Leopold SS. Testing for the presence of positive-outcome bias in peer review. *Arch Intern Med*. 2010;170(21):1934–1939.

27. History, policies, and law. ClinicalTrials.gov website. Available at: http://www.clinicaltrials.gov/ct2/about-site/history#CongressPassesLawFDAMA. Accessed October 16, 2012.

EVALUATING RANDOMIZED CONTROLLED TRIALS

ERIN M. TIMPE BEHNEN, PHARMD, BCPS

MCKENZIE C. FERGUSON, PHARMD, BCPS

CHAPTER OBJECTIVES

▸ Identify and describe the use of formal criteria to assess quality of randomized trials

▸ Assess validity issues in randomized trials

▸ Apply general criteria to evaluate methodological rigor in randomized trials

▸ Evaluate common biases in randomized trials

▸ Interpret and apply key findings in clinical practice

KEY TERMINOLOGY

Chalmers scale
Construct validity
Composite endpoint

Consolidated Standards
  of Reporting Trials
  (CONSORT)

Jadad scale

INTRODUCTION

Randomized controlled trials can provide the strongest evidence when they are well designed and conducted. Unfortunately, poor study design and methodology may produce misleading results and clinical evidence that may ultimately impact treatment decisions reaching patients.[1] Several studies have evaluated the conduct and reporting of randomized controlled trials and have found that more than half of those analyzed had missing or incomplete key information regarding methods used for allocation of patients, blinding, reporting a defined primary endpoint, and calculation of a sample size.[2-6] This highlights the importance of critical evaluation of clinical trials by clinicians.

Treatment considerations are often based on the evidence derived from randomized controlled trials. Although these trials are designed to provide the strongest evidence for patient care, any flaw in study design and implementation can undermine the results and ultimately affect the evidence base. Clinicians should be able to identify the flaws in study design and implementation and further evaluate the impact of the flaws on the results. Patient care treatment decisions require a thorough understanding of the evidence in the context of current practice, study design and implementation, and patient specific considerations. Chapter 4 provided details regarding the conduct of randomized trials. This chapter will identify guidelines for standard reporting of randomized controlled trials and will describe scales and checklists available for assessing randomized trials. Factors to consider when evaluating internal and external validity and other issues for critically evaluating randomized controlled trials will be outlined and applications to an example article will be included. Finally, considerations for application of randomized controlled trial findings to patient care will be described and applied.

CRITERIA FOR EVALUATING AND REPORTING CLINICAL TRIALS

STANDARDIZED REPORTING REQUIREMENTS

Previously, biomedical journals recommended various formatting and content requirements in their guidelines for author submissions. However, in 1979, a group of medical journal editors, now known as the International Committee of Medical Journal Editors (ICMJE), published the Uniform Requirements for Manuscripts Submitted to Biomedical Journals to improve consistency of reporting.[7] This document provided standard requirements for manuscript preparation in an effort to improve accuracy and clarity of reports in the medical literature. These include standard requirements for manuscript preparation and submission, and statements on overlapping publications and obligation to publish negative studies. Standards related to ethical issues with publishing (e.g. criteria for authorship) were added later. In addition to assisting authors and editors, this standardization of formatting allowed for readers to have specific expectations of the articles they were reading. The Uniform Requirements have been adopted by hundreds of medical journals.[7]

The latest reporting requirement of randomized trials is the **Consolidated Standards of Reporting Trials (CONSORT)** Statement, a minimum set of standards that are evidence-based for preparing reports of randomized controlled trials. The initial CONSORT statement in 1996 was the result of a meeting of medical editors, clinical researchers, epidemiologists, and methodologists from across the nation who developed an evidence-based checklist of items. If these items were not included in randomized trials, then it could result in biased findings. The checklist includes 25 items of standard requirements that appear in **Table 18–1**.[8] Revised CONSORT Statements were published in 2001 and 2010 and extensions for additional designs (e.g., non–inferiority and equivalence trials, cluster trials, and pragmatic trials) and interventions (e.g., herbal medicine interventions, non–pharmacological treatment interventions, and acupuncture interventions) are also available.[8–10] The CONSORT Statement was endorsed by the ICMJE and has been endorsed by more than half of the core medical journals found in the *Abridged Index Medicus* on PubMed.[9]

TABLE 18-1   Consort 2010 Checklist of Information to Include when Reporting a Randomised Trial*

Section/Topic	Item No	Checklist item	Reported on page No
Title and abstract			
	1a	Identification as a randomised trial in the title	____
	1b	Structured summary of trial design, methods, results, and conclusions (for specific guidance see CONSORT for abstracts)	____
Introduction			
Background and objectives	2a	Scientific background and explanation of rationale	____
	2b	Specific objectives or hypotheses	____
Methods			
Trial design	3a	Description of trial design (such as parallel, factorial) including allocation ratio	____
	3b	Important changes to methods after trial commencement (such as eligibility criteria), with reasons	____
Participants	4a	Eligibility criteria for participants	____
	4b	Settings and locations where the data were collected	____
Interventions	5	The interventions for each group with sufficient details to allow replication, including how and when they were actually administered	____
Outcomes	6a	Completely defined pre-specified primary and secondary outcome measures, including how and when they were assessed	____
	6b	Any changes to trial outcomes after the trial commenced, with reasons	____
Sample size	7a	How sample size was determined	____
	7b	When applicable, explanation of any interim analyses and stopping guidelines	____
Randomisation:			
Sequence generation	8a	Method used to generate the random allocation sequence	____
	8b	Type of randomisation; details of any restriction (such as blocking and block size)	____
Allocation concealment mechanism	9	Mechanism used to implement the random allocation sequence (such as sequentially numbered containers), describing any steps taken to conceal the sequence until interventions were assigned	____
Implementation	10	Who generated the random allocation sequence, who enrolled participants, and who assigned participants to interventions	

Section/Topic	Item No	Checklist item	Reported on page No
Blinding	11a	If done, who was blinded after assignment to interventions (for example, participants, care providers, those assessing outcomes) and how	——
	11b	If relevant, description of the similarity of interventions	——
Statistical methods	12a	Statistical methods used to compare groups for primary and secondary outcomes	——
	12b	Methods for additional analyses, such as subgroup analyses and adjusted analyses	——
Results			
Participant flow (a diagram is strongly recommended)	13a	For each group, the numbers of participants who were randomly assigned, received intended treatment, and were analysed for the primary outcome	——
	13b	For each group, losses and exclusions after randomisation, together with reasons	——
Recruitment	14a	Dates defining the periods of recruitment and follow-up	——
	14b	Why the trial ended or was stopped	——
Baseline data	15	A table showing baseline demographic and clinical characteristics for each group	——
Numbers analysed	16	For each group, number of participants (denominator) included in each analysis and whether the analysis was by original assigned groups	——
Outcomes and estimation	17a	For each primary and secondary outcome, results for each group, and the estimated effect size and its precision (such as 95% confidence interval)	——
	17b	For binary outcomes, presentation of both absolute and relative effect sizes is recommended	——
Ancillary analyses	18	Results of any other analyses performed, including subgroup analyses and adjusted analyses, distinguishing pre-specified from exploratory	——
Harms	19	All important harms or unintended effects in each group (for specific guidance see CONSORT for harms)	——
Discussion			
Limitations	20	Trial limitations, addressing sources of potential bias, imprecision, and, if relevant, multiplicity of analyses	——
Generalisability	21	Generalisability (external validity, applicability) of the trial findings	——
Interpretation	22	Interpretation consistent with results, balancing benefits and harms, and considering other relevant evidence	——
Other information			
Registration	23	Registration number and name of trial registry	——
Protocol	24	Where the full trial protocol can be accessed, if available	——
Funding	25	Sources of funding and other support (such as supply of drugs), role of funders	——

*We strongly recommend reading this statement in conjunction with the CONSORT 2010 Explanation and Elaboration for important clarifications on all the items. If relevant, we also recommend reading CONSORT extensions for cluster randomised trials, non-inferiority and equivalence trials, non-pharmacological treatments, herbal interventions, and pragmatic trials. Additional extensions are forthcoming: for those and for up to date references relevant to this checklist, see www.consort-statement.org.

Reproduced from the CONSORT Group. CONSORT 2010 Statement. Available at http://www.consort-statement.org/consort-statement/

The standardized reporting mechanisms help readers to critically evaluate clinical trials. With standardization, readers may expect that specific information, including clear descriptions of methodology, should appear and where to find that information within the article. Although the standardized reporting tools may help in easily identifying biases and flaws, they cannot conclude implications for patient care. Clinicians must weigh all of the items and put the information in context to determine implications on patient care. To thoroughly evaluate randomized controlled trials, clinicians must assess study validity (both internal and external) to determine applicability of the study results to current clinical practice.

QUALITY ASSESSMENT SCALES FOR RANDOMIZED TRIALS

Although the standardized reporting requirements were developed to improve reporting in the medical literature, more rigorous expectations for publishing and evaluating randomized trials were sought. By 1995, a total of 25 scales, with a range of 3 to 34 items, and 9 checklists, with a range of 4 to 57 items, were reported in the literature to evaluate the quality of randomized controlled trials. The scales included scored components that assessed varying degrees of trial characteristics and provided an overall score, whereas the checklists assessed the presence or absence of certain qualities of randomized trials. All of the scales and checklists varied widely from each other, with some designed to evaluate any trial and others developed for specific areas (e.g. arthritis and pain). Additionally, testing of the scales for validity and reliability varied.[11] Some of the scales have been used more frequently than others.

The most frequently used scale with the most rigorous development is the Jadad scale.[12] The **Jadad scale** was originally developed to assess pain research and includes only three items related to descriptions of sequence generation, blinding methodology, and withdrawals and dropouts. The reliability of this scale has been tested in various settings. The second most cited and adapted scale is the Chalmers scale.[13] This 32-item scale was originally designed to assess studies using aspirin in patients with cardiovascular disease. The **Chalmers scale** assesses descriptions of methodology, statistical analysis, and presentation of results. The most commonly used scales for evaluating randomized controlled trials are briefly described in **Table 18-2**.

While all of the criteria to evaluate quality of clinical trials vary in length, all include items addressing blinding, sequence generation, and dropouts or withdrawals.[12–19] The tools vary in the assessment of validity and reliability issues, with the scale by Jadad et al. having been studied the most. These tools assess methodology of randomized controlled trials to evaluate the quality of reporting; this helps in determining the likelihood that the results are valid. Although checklists and scales are useful and often used to evaluate quality, they cannot identify all potential study design and implementation flaws. Also, checklists and scales cannot incorporate the weight of flaws in the final assessment of study findings.

VALIDITY

Study validity refers to the quality of research evidence regarding the effect of treatment on patient outcomes.[20] Both internal (causality) and external (generalization) validity must be evaluated and weighed to determine the validity of results in a randomized controlled trial.

The article "Dabigatran versus Warfarin in the Treatment of Acute Venous Thromboembolism" published in *New England Journal of Medicine* is used to identify and apply concepts of internal and external validity in randomized controlled trials. Briefly, this randomized, double-blind, non-inferiority trial compared effectiveness and safety

TABLE 18-2	Common Tools for Evaluating Clinical Trials[12-19]	
Name	Number of Scale Items	Description of Items
Jadad Scale[12]	3	Sequence generation, blinding methodology, and withdrawals and dropouts.
Chalmers Scale[13]	32	Methodology, statistical analysis, and presentation of results.
Delphi List[14]	9	Treatment allocation, baseline characteristics, eligibility criteria, blinding, defining the primary outcome, and using intention-to-treat analysis.
van Tulder List[15]	11	Randomization, allocation, blinding, withdrawals, and use of an intention-to-treat population.
Cochrane Risk of Bias Tool[16]	7	Random sequence generation, allocation, blinding, and selective reporting.
Centre for Evidence-Based Medicine Critical Appraisal of Randomized Controlled Trials[17]	5	Randomization, allocation, intention-to-treat, measure of objectives, and treatment effect sizes.
National Institute for Health and Clinical Excellence (NICE) and Scottish Intercollegiate Guidelines Network (SIGN) Methodology Checklists for Randomized Controlled Trials[18,19]	NICE–23 SIGN–29	Allocation practices, blinding, attrition bias, performance bias, and detection bias.

of dabigatran and warfarin in the treatment of patients with pulmonary embolism (PE) or deep vein thrombosis (DVT).[21]

Internal Validity

Randomized controlled trials are used to investigate causality of an intervention on an outcome. In a study that is internally valid, randomization, measurement, and assessment of the variables are conducted appropriately to arrive at accurate results. There are many factors that can lead to decreased internal validity. As discussed in Chapter 4, these factors include: history, maturation, testing, instrumentation, statistical regression, selection, attrition, and diffusion or imitation of treatments.[22] Randomization and standardization in methodology assist with decreasing threats to internal validity. Baseline characteristics, often described in tables, and potential effects of dropouts should be reviewed to ensure similarities between the treatment groups. Most of the factors influencing internal validity would be minimized in the dabigatran study due to the randomization of treatments. Maturation, selection, and regression could occur, but these would be similar in the two groups due to randomization. The characteristics of the study groups were similar to each other due to randomization. All patients in the study were treated similarly in requirements for international normalized ratio (INR) monitoring, symptom evaluations, and follow-up visit schedules. Testing and instrumentation may not be an issue as both treatment groups went through the same process of assessments. Most patients in this study adhered to the study regimen (98%).

History could have been a factor if there was a significant change in the clinical practice guidelines for treatment of venous thromboembolism, but this did not occur. In regards to attrition, only small numbers of patients dropped out of the study in both arms, which would not likely result in a change in overall group characteristics.[21] A clinician must evaluate each of the threats to internal validity and determine if any may have influenced the results and by how much.

EXTERNAL VALIDITY

Randomized controlled trials incorporate a relatively small group of participants who are meant to represent a much larger group of everyone to whom the intervention may be applied. External validity of a study allows for the application of the causal relationship results evaluated in the study to be generalized to the larger population irrespective of different types of person, place, and time. Various factors may decrease the external validity or the ability to generalize the study results to others. These factors may include interaction of selection and intervention, effects of testing, effects of experimental arrangements, and multiple treatment effects.[23] There is always a risk that participants may behave differently when they know that they are in a study. Multi-center studies that recruit patients based on criteria rather than self-selection and incorporate an appropriate sample size aid in improving external validity. The dabigatran study was a multi-center study conducted in 228 sites in 29 countries. The patient recruitment from multiple centers would strengthen the likelihood that similar results may be applied to a broader population and minimize interaction of selection and intervention; however, most patients (95%) were Caucasian and few had cancer (5%).

Patients from both arms were treated similarly; however, one aspect from this study to additionally compare to what occurs in practice is the low rate of patients in the warfarin arm being maintained in a therapeutic INR range. Time within therapeutic INR range was reported less than 60% of the time, which is a low percent of time compared to the general goal (100% of time) and to other studies evaluating warfarin efficacy. If patients were not well controlled in the warfarin group in this study, then there may have been a decreased difference found between the groups compared with what may actually be seen in practice. This may then have implications regarding the generalizability of the results due to this experimental arrangement.[21] Inclusion and exclusion criteria, characteristics of the participants and experimenters, the setting in which the study was conducted, and time of interventions, including the effects of multiple interventions and external events, should be assessed when evaluating potential for decreased external validity. A study with decreased external validity results in a limited ability to generalize the findings to a larger population.[23]

CRITICALLY EVALUATING RANDOMIZED CONTROLLED TRIALS

Although randomized trials are designed to provide the strongest evidence for clinical care, trial findings should not be accepted without critical evaluation of study design and implementation. Critical evaluation of a randomized trial requires assessment of the following major issues of study design and implementation:

- Study sample
- Randomization and blinding
- Intervention and control group

- Clinical endpoints
- Trial findings
- Limitations and implications

The article, "Dabigatran versus Warfarin in the Treatment of Acute Venous Thromboembolism," is used to identify and apply the knowledge of critical issues in randomized controlled trials.[21] **Table 18–3** summarizes the key factors evaluated in this trial.

TABLE 18-3 Example of Application of Literature Evaluation to a Randomized Controlled Trial[21]	
Major Areas for Evaluation	**Application to the Study**
Study Sample	
Recruitment strategies	This was a multi-center trial occurring in 228 sites in 29 countries with a detailed description of recruitment strategies.
Inclusion & exclusion criteria	The inclusion and exclusion criteria were appropriate to assess treatment efficacy and ensure patient safety.
Baseline characteristics	The age range was appropriate for patients with venous thromboembolism (VTE). Most patients were Caucasian and more had a DVT than a PE. Only 5% had cancer. The time within therapeutic INR for patients on warfarin in this study was only 60%.
Sample size calculation	A sample size calculation was present and was based appropriately on previous studies. The non-inferiority margin was defined *a priori*. A superiority margin was not defined in the article. The treatment effect size outlined was clinically appropriate.
Randomization	This was a randomized controlled trial, which is an effective study design to minimize bias. Blocked randomization with stratification was used. The blocks were computer-generated with variable block sizes.
Blinding	This was a double-blind, double-dummy study that used sham INRs for patients assigned to the dabigatran group. An event adjudication committee was also blinded to treatment assignments.
Intervention & control group	Warfarin is an active control that is standard treatment for VTE. The characteristics of the two treatment groups were similar to each other and patients were treated similarly in the study in terms of clinic visits and evaluations. Overall adherence to treatment was high (98%). The number of drop outs was small in both groups.
Clinical endpoints	The study used a composite of VTE events or death as the primary outcome and additionally reported the percent of events for the individual outcomes. The events were adjudicated by a blinded committee. Surrogate endpoints were not used.
Trial findings	
Accounting for all data	A modified intent-to-treat analysis was used. Adverse events were reported in the article and in the supplementary appendix.
Statistical tests	Statistical tests used were appropriate and confidence intervals were reported. Subgroup analyses were limited.
Conclusions	Conclusions focused on the primary outcome and were appropriate for the non-inferiority study design.
Limitations & implications	Study findings were compared to previous studies comparing dabigatran to warfarin.
Application to clinical practice	Dabigatran may be an appropriate alternative to warfarin in the treatment of VTE in some patients. Patient-specific risk factors and preferences and overall costs of the medications and monitoring should be considerations when applying the results of this study to clinical practice.

Study Sample

Investigators should clearly delineate recruitment strategies and eligibility criteria that allow for a representative sample to be studied, as this strongly affects the internal and external validity of the findings. Specific areas of an article to focus on when evaluating the study sample include recruitment strategies, inclusion and exclusion criteria, the baseline characteristics of the study population, and sample size calculations. A description of the recruitment strategies used may be helpful to determine similarities and differences between the population studied and the population that the clinician will be treating. It may be difficult to determine generalizability of results to the entire population when a convenience sample in a single center is used because it would be difficult to be sure that the general population would respond the same as those selected to participate in the study.[25] The dabigatran study was a multi-center study conducted in 228 sites in 29 countries with a detailed description of recruitment strategies.

Inclusion and exclusion criteria and baseline characteristics should be reviewed to determine appropriateness and ability to produce a similar population as the clinician's patient population. Inclusion criteria are important to ensure the appropriate patients with the disease state are evaluated and to create a homogenous group likely to respond to the treatment, while exclusion criteria are necessary to exclude patients for whom the treatment may be unsafe or who may have inconsistent responses. If inclusion criteria are not specific enough, it may be difficult to determine which population of patients may benefit most from the treatment. If exclusion criteria are extensive, it may be difficult to extrapolate findings to the general population. Each of the criteria should be valid and should have a reason for being listed.[26] Baseline characteristics of each individual group and the entire study sample should be reviewed to determine similarities between the groups as well as overall generalizability of the findings beyond the study.[16] In the dabigatran study, the inclusion and exclusion criteria were appropriate to assess treatment efficacy and ensure patient safety. Furthermore, the age range was appropriate for patients with venous thromboembolism (VTE). Most patients were Caucasian and more had a DVT than a PE. Only 5% had cancer.

Sample size and power calculation for the primary endpoint should be conducted on an *a priori* basis to aid in determining a clinically significant difference between the groups. This is especially important in studies that do not find statistically significant differences between groups to be able to determine if there truly was no difference between the groups or if no difference was found only because the study was underpowered. When statistically significant findings are missed due to inadequate power, this may have direct implications regarding overlooking possibly effective therapies.[24] Both the sample size and the treatment effect size or event rate are important to define *a priori* and in an assessment of the possibility of a type II error occurring. The number of patients actually evaluated in the study in relation to what was calculated is important. Additionally, the treatment effect size must be evaluated to determine clinical agreement with the defined definition of when a difference would be found between the groups.

In the dabigatran study, 2,550 patients (1,275 patients in each group and an expected total of 46 events) were determined to be necessary to have 90% power to exclude a hazard ratio of 2.75 and an absolute risk increase of 3.6% for the primary outcome. The study actually enrolled and evaluated a total of 2,539 patients and found 30 and 27 events in the dabigatran and warfarin groups respectively. This was close to what was anticipated. With the definition of non-inferiority in this trial, the investigators are stating that dabigatran would be considered to be no worse than warfarin if 2.75 was not included in the hazard ratio confidence interval for the primary endpoint and that the absolute increase in risk was not above 3.6%. This would mean that when comparing the agents, the total number of primary events occurring between the groups could not exceed 3.6% and that the confidence interval for the hazard ratio of the primary endpoint could not include 2.75. This appears to be a clinically acceptable definition.[21]

RANDOMIZATION AND BLINDING

Randomization helps to ensure that the baseline characteristics of the groups being compared are similar to each other. Investigators should describe the methodology used for randomization, including how sequences were generated and how allocation was concealed to ensure randomization. Blocked randomization is a common form of restricted randomization used to ensure similar sample sizes of the treatment groups. Stratification further allows for balanced assignment to groups based on one or more specific characteristics. Often, studies will state that patients were randomized to groups, but will not provide an additional description of the process. It is important to know if randomization is used and how sequence generation and allocation was concealed to assess for bias and determine true estimates of effects. This can be seen by a detailed description of randomization and blinding provided by the investigators and also by assessing similarities in reported baseline characteristics of the groups to determine if randomization was successful. Often, any difference in baseline characteristic after randomization can be attributed to sampling error and is statistically controlled to explore for effects on the outcome.[16] Successful randomization helps to ensure internal validity of the study. In the dabigatran study, patients were randomized by "a computer-generated randomization scheme with variable block sizes, stratified according to presentation (pulmonary embolism or deep-vein thrombosis without symptomatic pulmonary embolism) and the presence or absence of active cancer." Further it is stated that patients were assigned in a 1:1 ratio to the treatment groups and that patient group assignments were concealed from investigators and their staff.[21]

Many studies state that they use double blinding, but do not further specify which groups, in addition to the patients, are blinded and which methods are used to ensure blinding. Reports should specify whether investigators, biostatisticians, or both are blinded and how concealment of assignments is ensured.[16] Using and adhering to a strict protocol may be helpful in cases in which blinding is not possible. The dabigatran study used an assignment system external to the study center and variable block sizes to assign patients to treatment groups, which help to ensure blinding of treatment assignment. Additionally, a double-dummy format (multiple placebos) was used, including identical looking tablets and sham INRs for patients assigned to treatments. Investigators and the event adjudication committee were blinded to treatment assignment.[21]

INTERVENTION AND CONTROL GROUP

An appropriate comparator or control group is essential in randomized controlled trials. A placebo control group may be unethical to use when there is a well-established standard treatment. If an active control group is used, the treatment must have known efficacy for the disease state and an appropriate dosage regimen should be used. If the active control group has not been clearly shown to be effective, the basis for efficacy of the comparison group is then unknown.[27] The study protocol should fully describe how outcomes are defined, how safety is monitored, and when the trial may be stopped if necessary. A clearly defined protocol may improve internal validity of the study by guiding investigators to follow the same methods.[8] Treatment adherence should be objectively assessed and reported. If treatment adherence is low, it is difficult to determine true efficacy of the intervention; however, decreased adherence from significant side effects or a difficult regimen may also have clinical ramifications. Differences in adherence between the groups should be evaluated to determine if a difference in efficacy is actually due to the treatment benefits versus a significant number of patients discontinuing therapy in the opposite group. Discontinuation of therapy due to adverse effects or difficult regimens may be beneficial to be aware of in evaluating overall risk versus benefit of the new treatment.[27] The dabigatran trial compared the new agent to the standard therapy, warfarin. Warfarin is clearly recommended in standard practice guidelines for the population studied.[28] The protocol was adequately described with additional information available in a supplementary appendix. Adherence was assessed and most patients (98%) were found to be adherent to their assigned treatment.[21]

CLINICAL ENDPOINTS

The primary outcomes of the study should be measures that actually assess the true clinical outcome. The primary endpoints of randomized trials are often measures of efficacy; these include symptoms, clinical response rate, clinical cure rate, quality of life, morbidity, and mortality. These should be measured by validated instruments that have been shown to evaluate the outcome studied.[8] **Construct validity** refers to the extent to which the measurement process truly captures the disease outcome. If clinically appropriate endpoints are not used to measure overall effects of the treatment groups or if they are measured at inappropriate times, then there is little meaning to the study. Outcome variables and measures to assess the variables should be clearly defined to determine reproducibility and clinical acceptability of the endpoints. Various aspects of clinical outcomes are usually evaluated including whether they are objective or subjective, surrogate, or composite. Objective outcomes, such as clinical laboratory measures, are generally preferred as there is decreased subjectivity in assessment as long as they are measured at an appropriate time. If a surrogate outcome is used, then it must have a strong and consistent association with the clinical endpoint and conclusions should only relate to the endpoint used in the study.

One of the most cited examples of a study that has contradicted practice based on surrogate endpoint evidence is that of the Cardiac Arrhythmia Suppression Trial (CAST). The antiarrhythmic agents, encainide and flecainide, were routinely used in practice to treat ventricular arrhythmia following myocardial infarction (which is a risk factor for mortality) based on their antiarrhythmic properties (a surrogate endpoint). However, when the CAST study compared these agents to placebo to investigate effects on mortality (the true endpoint), the antiarrhythmic agent group was found to nearly triple the rate of death compared to the placebo group.[29] When surrogate markers are used in clinical trials, only validated surrogate markers should be used. Ideally, the trials using surrogate markers should continue to further measure the true endpoint. A **composite endpoint** is when multiple single endpoints are combined and reported together. If composite endpoints are used, the frequency of events for each of the factors within the composite should be reported. Scales used to describe outcomes should be clearly defined and have clinical and biologic significance. Finally, if co-primary endpoints are used, appropriate statistical tests should be used to account for the multiple endpoints. A composite of venous thromboembolism (VTE) or death was used as the primary endpoint in the dabigatran study. Each of these were clearly defined and appropriately measured. Data for all DVTs, PEs, and deaths were reported individually and in composite. A committee adjudicated reports of VTE and death. These were objective, true (vs. surrogate) clinical endpoints.[21]

TRIAL FINDINGS

Intention-to-treat analysis is the only method of evaluating data that preserves randomization. If only patients who comply with the treatment protocol and finish the study are included in the analysis (per-protocol), there is a risk of creating an imbalance between the groups based on potential confounding variables.[26] Investigators may report using intention-to-treat to analyze the data; however, when looking closely at the results reported, the sample size may not account for all patients. Data should account for all patients, including the number of patients who withdrew or were lost to follow-up and a description of how the missing data was handled. If multiple patients withdraw or drop out of the study, this may have implications on the similarity of the treatment groups and decrease the beneficial effects of randomization resulting in significant changes from the study beginning. If a "modified" intention-to-treat analysis is reportedly used, this process should be adequately defined. Overall adherence to the protocol by investigators and patient adherence with treatment regimens should be reported.

Reporting of appropriate external factors, such as use of concomitant medications, may also be important in assessing overall impacts on outcomes. Additionally, adverse effects are often not well described in reports of clinical trials. An intention-to-treat analysis should be used to analyze and describe harms, and general statements, such as, "few side effects were reported," should be avoided.[26] In the dabigatran article, the difference between the number of patients enrolled ($N = 2,564$) and analyzed for efficacy ($N = 2,539$) was described, including reasons for each specific patient withdrawal from the study. A modified intention-to-treat principle is described to have been used, but was not fully defined. Most patients were adherent to the treatment assignments as assessed by capsule counts. Adverse effects were reported either in the article or the supplementary appendix.[21]

Investigators should report if the assumptions of the statistical test are met in addition to naming the statistical test used. Using inappropriate statistical tests may result in type I or type II error or may overestimate or underestimate the significance of effects.[24] The dabigatran study appropriately used a Kaplan–Meier analysis and Cox proportional hazards model to assess the time to the first occurrence of the composite endpoint and to assess the effects of confounding variables on the outcome.[21] Probability values indicate if the result was likely to have occurred due to chance or not. The lower the p-value, the more confident you are in rejecting the null hypothesis, but the value does not indicate the size of the overall effect. Additional information such as the estimated effect size and confidence interval related to the result provide greater evidence regarding the magnitude and precision of results as well as overall clinical importance of the result.

Some investigators focus on the size and trend of the p-value when the focus should be on the actual results. When the variance of data is reported, confidence intervals and standard deviation are preferred to reporting standard error of the mean. Compared to standard error of the mean, standard deviation is a descriptive statistic that describes the variability of the sample. Standard error of the mean is calculated to describe the expected variation of mean values rather than individual values.[23] The variables included in a confidence interval and the overall width should be evaluated when assessing clinical significance. A confidence interval is generally more precise (less variable) with a larger sample size. In the dabigatran article, 30 VTEs or deaths occurred in the dabigatran group versus 27 in the warfarin group. This resulted in a hazard ratio of 1.10 (95% CI 0.65–1.84). The upper bound of this confidence interval is less than the predefined margin of 2.75. Thus, compared to warfarin, dabigatran is non-inferior with respect to the primary endpoint. Including the confidence interval provides more details regarding the variability of the data and also provides a better picture regarding the precision of the estimate of the treatment effect.

Investigators should determine *a priori* and report the margin at which they will determine the intervention to be either non-inferior or superior to the control, or the minimum and maximum allowable differences to be detected (treatment effect size). This definition is important for practitioners to assess whether or not the margin encompasses a clinically meaningful difference.[10] The dabigatran article defined non-inferiority as meeting the upper bound of the 95% confidence interval of 2.75 for the hazard ratio and the upper bound of the 95% confidence interval of 3.6% for overall absolute risk. The authors stated that superiority would be evaluated if non-inferiority was established.[21] Non-inferiority analyses allow only conclusions that the treatment is or is not "no worse than" the comparator. If superiority is claimed, then the margin of superiority must be predefined and clearly met by the treatment. Dabigatran was found to be non-inferior to warfarin in the Schulman et al. study. Superiority was not demonstrated, so conclusions could not state that dabigatran was more effective than warfarin even if the data may have visually looked better.[21]

Conclusions should be made that are appropriately based on the methods used and the results found. For example, long-term safety and efficacy cannot be implied when a trial is conducted over only a few weeks. When interpreting the results of a clinical trial, variance noted by the standard deviation and confidence intervals may be useful in determining if the likely magnitude of difference is clinically meaningful. The focus of the conclusions should be on the primary outcome of the study. If no statistically significant difference was found with the primary outcome but a subgroup analysis or other secondary outcome produced a significant result, conclusions should be made that suggest further study of the secondary outcome. The study is designed and powered for the primary outcome; therefore, findings from secondary outcomes may be influenced to a greater degree by effects of error.[30]

Analysis of subgroups, such as investigating differences in responses to treatment between males and females, should be planned *a priori* based on hypothesized effects on outcomes. When multiple subgroup analyses are conducted, groups become smaller and the likelihood of a type I error increases. Investigators should avoid conducting statistical tests on each piece of data collected just because it is there. There should be a reason behind investigating relationships.[30] Subgroup analyses may be at risk of the same limitations that observational analyses are prone to because the subgroup is no longer randomized for this assessment. Before further evaluating results from subgroup analyses, there should be adequate justification for investigating the subgroup. If a subgroup analysis finds a statistically significant difference, further confirmatory studies should be conducted on the subgroups.[16]

LIMITATIONS AND IMPLICATIONS

Randomized controlled trials are potentially stronger than other trial designs in terms of decreasing bias; however, it is almost impossible to avoid bias completely in any study. Individuals evaluating studies often must balance the degree of bias possibly included in a study with the ability to generalize the results.[25] Some bias may be completely avoidable with use of techniques such as stratified randomization, blinding, and objective measures. However, bias may be unavoidable in other cases, such as in the case of open-label trials comparing effects on an outcome from major surgery versus medication therapy. Blinding patients and having medication therapy patients undergo a sham major surgery would be unethical in this case and treatment by physicians following surgery would be different for patients assigned to surgery compared to those assigned to medication therapy. Methods that use more objective rather than subjective measures of outcomes may be used to decrease possible effects from bias in this case. Ideally, any potential sources of bias and study limitations should be recognized and described by the authors in the discussion of the study. Clinicians need to recognize that authors do not always recognize all potential study limitations.

In the dabigatran versus warfarin study, which was a multi-center study conducted in 29 countries, double-dummy methods and sham INR for patients in the dabigatran group were used to ensure double-blinding, and objective primary outcome measures were used that were evaluated by a central adjudication committee unaware of treatment assignment.[21] These factors help decrease risk of potential biases and errors. However, manufacturer support of the trial and subjective adverse event reporting of minor bleeding events may have been factors that could increase potential for bias. Therefore, the results have to be weighed in light of strengths and limitations of study design. Additionally, noting overall if there may be an explanation of the findings, especially if they were unexpected, and how the results compare to results found in similar studies may be helpful. If the results are inconsistent with other studies, then it should be determined if there are any differences that may have led to the dissimilar findings and if these differences could affect the conclusions in any way. When looking at the dabigatran study, the authors include a comparison to previous studies comparing dabigatran and warfarin and studies evaluating other oral direct thrombin inhibitors. Similar findings were noted with previous dabigatran studies.[21]

Because clinical trials can only incorporate a sample population with specific inclusion and exclusion criteria, clinicians can infer the potential implications for the broader population. The dabigatran trial included mostly Caucasian patients and further study including a more diverse population would be preferred; however, given what is known about the medications and the disease state, the study results could likely be extrapolated to patients of other races until further studies are conducted.[21] The degree of effect on outcomes varies by the type of bias but also by the type of study conducted, how outcomes are measured, and population studied. Both the magnitude and direction must be considered when assessing the potential for bias and overall impact on results. Overall, do the potential effects of bias and error matter?[16]

APPLICATION TO CLINICAL PRACTICE

When determining how this study should be applied to practice, clinicians should think about what is currently known about the topic, what this study adds that was previously unknown or unclear, what questions remain regarding long-term efficacy and safety or the exact place in therapy related to other current treatment options, and how these results translate to specific patient care. Related to the dabigatran trial, it was previously known that warfarin has been the standard treatment for patients with venous thromboembolism. Dabigatran is a new antithrombotic agent that may have a benefit over warfarin therapy in that it may not require regular INR monitoring. This study found that dabigatran was not worse than warfarin in safety and efficacy when treating venous thromboembolism.[21] This study does not answer clearly what are the characteristics of patients most likely to benefit from dabigatran therapy over warfarin therapy, what is the long-term safety of dabigatran, and what is the cost effectiveness of dabigatran versus warfarin in the treatment of venous thromboembolism?

To assess how this study may be applied to specific patient care, the patient should be compared to the patients included in the study to identify similarities and differences and ability to generalize the findings, overall risk of the outcome should be weighed against potential risks of the therapy and patient-specific concerns and beliefs should be considered. Considerations of generalizability of the results to the patient have been described in the external validity discussion. Risk reduction may be used in clinical trials to draw conclusions. Conclusions based on relative risk reduction rather than absolute risk reduction should be used cautiously. Relative risk reduction provides the degree of difference in risk between the groups; however, it does not account for the overall incidence of the events. Absolute risk reduction takes into account the rate of events in determining reduction of risk between the groups. Therefore, relative risk reduction may appear to be great, but if the overall incidence of the event is low, this may not be clinically significant. Absolute risk reduction could assist in determining clinical significance, taking into account the rate of events and the value can then be used further to calculate the number needed to treat which is also helpful in interpreting clinical significance of the findings.[31] In the dabigatran study, 1.6% of patients in the dabigatran group and 1.9% of patients in the warfarin group had a major bleeding event. This would translate to a relative risk reduction of 16% and an absolute risk reduction of 0.3%. The relative risk reduction makes the risk of bleeding look much better for dabigatran than the absolute risk reduction does. Overall, the incidence of major bleeds in the study was low and, therefore, the absolute risk difference of major bleeds is low. The corresponding number needed to treat is 333, meaning that 333 patients would need to be treated with dabigatran for 60 days to prevent one major bleed.[21]

Other factors that may influence translating research into practice include cost to the patient or acceptability of the intervention and should be included in an overall analysis as well. Factors of cost should include cost of the treatment and cost of necessary monitoring and follow-up and potential costs of adverse events or harms. Acceptability of the intervention may include issues that influence adherence. All costs and consequences of the intervention should be incorporated into an overall conclusion. In the dabigatran trial, factors such as the decreased need for routine INR monitoring with dabigatran should be weighed with the greater cost of dabigatran and the fact that there is no reliable reversal agent in the event of bleeds. All of these factors should be considered when determining how to incorporate the intervention into practice.

SUMMARY AND CONCLUSIONS

Biomedical journals have adopted evidence-based recommendations for improvement of reporting of clinical trials; however, bias and error are impossible to avoid completely. Bias in clinical trials must be minimized to be able to determine the true estimates of effects. Numerous scales and checklists are available to assist in assessing randomized trials. These tools vary considerably. Clinicians should be able to identify and evaluate potential flaws and bias especially in the areas of: the study sample, randomization, blinding, intervention and control groups, clinical endpoints, trial findings, and overall study limitations and implications. It is the responsibility of the clinician to fully evaluate the magnitude and impact of bias in randomized trials to determine effects on outcomes and ultimately on patient care. Applications to patient care should include considerations of how the new information adds to current practice as well as a thorough risk and benefit analysis for the specific patient. Randomization decreases the potential for multiple types of bias in clinical trials, but careful and critical evaluation of the findings are necessary to assess for potential flaws and generalizability of the results.

REVIEW QUESTIONS

1. There are multiple checklists and scales that have been developed to evaluate randomized controlled trials that vary in content; however, they all share three common themes. What are the three themes that the checklists and scales described have in common and why are these items important in evaluating clinical trials?
2. What are common factors that should be considered when evaluating clinical trials for internal and external validity?
3. Describe the common concerns when evaluating randomized controlled trials.
4. What are five key factors that should be considered when evaluating the conclusions of a clinical trial?

ONLINE RESOURCES

CONSORT statement website: http://www.consort-statement.org/home

Critical Appraisal for Randomized Controlled Trials, Centre for Evidence-Based Medicine: http://www.cebm.net/index.aspx?o=1157

International Committee of Medical Journal Editors: http://www.icmje.org/index.html

Methods for Development of NICE Public Health Guidance, National Institute for Health and Clinical Excellence: http://www.nice.org.uk/nicemedia/pdf/CPHEMethodsManual.pdf

SIGN 50: A Guideline Developer's Handbook, Scottish Intercollegiate Guidelines Network: http://www.sign.ac.uk/guidelines/fulltext/50/checklist2.html

REFERENCES

1. Moher D, Hopewell S, Schulz KF, Montori V, Gøtzsche PC, Devereaux PJ, Elbourne D, Egger M, Altman DG, for the CONSORT Group. CONSORT 2010 Explanation and Elaboration: updated guidelines for reporting parallel group randomised trial. *BMJ*. 2010;340:c869.
2. Chan AW, Altman DG. Epidemiology and reporting of randomised trials 16 published in PubMed journals. *Lancet*. 2005;365:1159–1162.
3. Hopewell S, Dutton S, Yu LM, Chan AW, Altman DG. The quality of reports of randomised trials in 2000 and 2006: comparative study of articles indexed in PubMed. *BMJ*. 2010;340:c723.
4. Lai TY, Wong VW, Lam RF, Cheng AC, Lam DS, Leung GM. Quality of 19 reporting of key methodological items of randomized controlled trials in clinical ophthalmic journals. *Ophthalmic Epidemiol*. 2007;14:390–398.
5. Santaguida P, Oremus M, Walker K, Wishart LR, Siegel KL, Raina P. Systematic reviews identify important methodological flaws in stroke rehabilitation therapy primary studies: review of reviews. *J Clin Epidemiol*. 2012;65(4):358–367.
6. Strech D, Soltmann B, Weikert B, Bauer M, Pfennig A. Quality of reporting of randomized controlled trials of pharmacologic treatment of bipolar disorders: a systematic review. *J Clin Psychiatry*. 2011;72(9):1214–1221.
7. Uniform Requirements for Manuscripts Submitted to Biomedical Journals. International Committee of Medical Journal Editors. Available at http://www.icmje.org/urm_main.html. Accessed December 3, 2012.
8. Schulz KF, Altman DG, Moher D, for the CONSORT Group. CONSORT 2010 Statement: updated guidelines for reporting parallel group randomised trials. *Ann Int Med*. 2010;152.
9. CONSORT statement website. Available at: http://www.consort-statement.org/home. Accessed July 2, 2012.
10. Piaggio G, Elbourne DR, Altman DG, Pocock SJ, Evans SJW. Reporting of noninferiority and equivalence randomized trials: An extension of the CONSORT statement. *JAMA*. 2006; 295:1152–1160.

11. Moher D, Jadad AR, Nichol G, Penman M, Tugwell P, Walsh S. Assessing the Quality of Randomized Controlled Trials: An Annotated Bibliography of Scales and Checklists. *Control Clin Trials*. 1995;16:62–73.

12. Jadad AR, Moore Ra, Carroll D, Jenkinson C, Reynolds DJM, Gavaghan DJ, McQuay HJ. Assessing the quality of reports of randomized clinical trials: Is blinding necessary? *Controlled Clin Trials*. 1996;17:1–12.

13. Chalmers TC, Smith H Jr, Blackburn B. A method for assessing the quality of a randomized control trial. *Controlled Clin Trials*. 1981;2:31–49.

14. Verhagen AP, de Vet HC, de Bie RA, et al. The Delphi list: a criteria list for quality assessment of randomized clinical trials for conducting systematic reviews developed by Delphi consensus. *J Clin Epidemiol*. 1998;51:1235–1241.

15. van Tulder MW, Assendelft WJ, Koes BW, Bouter LM. Method guidelines for systematic reviews in the Cochrane Collaboration Back Review Group for Spinal Disorders. *Spine*. 1997;22:2323–2330.

16. Higgins JPT, Green S, eds. *Cochrane Handbook for Systematic Reviews of Interventions*. Version 5.0.0 [updated February 2008]. The Cochrane Collaboration, 2008. Available at www.cochrane-handbook.org. Accessed July 10, 2012.

17. Critical Appraisal for Randomized Controlled Trials. Centre for Evidence-Based Medicine. Available at http://www.cebm.net/index.aspx?o=1157. Accessed September 15, 2012.

18. Methods for Development of NICE Public Health Guidance. National Institute for Health and Clinical Excellence. Available at http://www.nice.org.uk/nicemedia/pdf/CPHEMethodsManual.pdf. Accessed September 15, 2012.

19. SIGN 50: A Guideline Developer's Handbook. Scottish Intercollegiate Guidelines Network. Available at http://www.sign.ac.uk/guidelines/fulltext/50/checklist2.html. Accessed September 15, 2012.

20. Polit DF, Hungler BP. *Nursing Research: Principles and Methods*. 5th ed. Philadelphia, PA: Lippincott Williams & Wilkins; 1995

21. Schulman S, Kearon C, Kakkar AK, et al. Dabigatran versus warfarin in the treatment of acute venous thromboembolism. *New Engl J Med*. 2009;361:2342–2352.

22. Campbell DT, Stanley JC. *Experimental and Quasi-Experimental Designs for Research*. Boston, MA: Houghton Mifflin Company; 1963.

23. Bracht GH, Glass GV. The external validity of experiments. *Am Educ Res J*. 1968;5:437–474.

24. Cook TD, Campbell DT. *Quasi-Experimentation: Design & Analysis Issues for Field Settings*. Boston, MA: Houghton Mifflin Company; 1979.

25. Sica GT. Bias in research studies. *Radiology*. 2006;238(3):780–789.

26. Glasser SP, Howard G. Clinical trial design issues: at least 10 things you should look for in clinical trials. *J Clin Pharmacol*. 2006;46:1106–1115.

27. Bigby M, Gadeene AS. Understanding and evaluating clinical trials. *J Am Acad Dermatol*. 1996;34:555–90.

28. Guyatt GH, et al. Executive summary: Antithrombotic therapy and prevention of thrombosis, 9th ed. American College of Chest Physicians evidence-based clinical practice guidelines. *Chest*. 2012;141:Suppl:7S.

29. Fleming TR. Evaluating therapeutic interventions: some issues and experiences. *Stat Sci*. 1992;7:428–456.

30. Lang TA, Secic M. *How to Report Statistics in Medicine: Annotated Guidelines for Authors, Editors and Reviewers*. 2nd ed. Philadelphia, PA: American College of Physicians; 2006.

31. Shaughnessy AF. Evaluating and understanding articles about treatment. *Am Fam Physician*. 2009;78(8):668–670.

EVALUATING OBSERVATIONAL STUDIES

CHENGHUI LI, PhD

CHAPTER OBJECTIVES

▸ Explain the extent of biases in observational studies

▸ Understand the need for critical appraisal of observational studies

▸ Understand formal criteria to assess observational studies

▸ Appraise design, methods, and analytical approaches in observational studies

▸ Evaluate the results of observational studies with randomized controlled trials

KEY TERMINOLOGY

Bias
Confounding factor
Information bias

Instrumental variable
Measurement bias
Selection bias

Strengthening the Reporting
of Observational studies in
Epidemiology (STROBE)

INTRODUCTION

Observational studies have played an important role in medical literature. Although well-designed and conducted randomized controlled trials (RCT) are the gold standard, they may not be feasible in many situations. For instance, rare events or events that take long time to develop are often examined by observational studies because of the constraints of time and resources needed to conduct an RCT to evaluate such events. Observational studies also have a unique role in research into the harms of medical interventions. For those events, conducting RCTs would not be ethical because it is unethical to impose a known harm on anyone. In recent years, observational studies have played an increasingly important role in comparative effectiveness research, with the additional benefit of providing more "realistic" effects in daily medical practice.

Despite their wide application in medical literature, the quality of observational studies can vary largely, affecting both internal and external validity of these studies. Consequently, it is important to be able to critically review findings from observational studies instead of blindly accepting and interpreting the finding as evidence. This requires familiarity with observational study designs, their inherent limitations, and critical evaluation of the findings. This chapter will first provide a brief review of the biases and confounding arising from observational studies that may threaten the internal validity of their findings. Next, it will introduce formal criteria for critical assessment of various aspects of an observational study, which include the study design, methods, and analytical approaches. The chapter ends with suggestions on how to compare results of observational studies with RCTs when discordance in findings is encountered.

BIAS AND CONFOUNDING

Like clinical trials, observational studies are "susceptible to error, bias, and confounding that may lead to erroneous finding(s) and/or conclusion(s) in the study."[1] Because observational studies are not randomized, bias caused by confounding factors is a particularly important threat to the integrity of observational studies and should be carefully controlled for and/or examined in the study. The following discussion briefly reiterates different types of biases and confounding encountered in observational studies.

BIAS

Bias results from systematic errors in the way study subjects are selected, measured, and analyzed. Systematic errors will result in inaccurate estimates that lead to invalid conclusions. Similar to clinical trials, bias can be introduced at every stage of an observational study and it would be impossible to discuss in detail all potential biases. The following two common types of biases is based on the stage of the research when the bias may occur.[2]

Selection bias refers to systematic error in the estimate of effect due to procedures used to select subjects, or factors that influence study participation or follow-up. There are many sources of selection bias. For instance, admission rate bias occurs in case–control studies, when exposed patients may be more likely to die before being admitted to the hospital and, therefore, less likely to be identified among hospitalized patients ("cases"); nonresponse bias occurs when individuals who experienced an outcome are more likely to participate in a study.[3,4] Selection bias is particularly problematic in observational studies because the treatment assigned is not randomized; this can lead to differences in observable and unobservable baseline demographic and clinical characteristics between the study groups, which may lead to inaccurate findings and conclusions if not properly statistically adjusted.

Measurement bias, also called **information bias**, occurs at data collection stage when there are systematic differences between study groups regarding how the exposures and outcomes are measured or reported by study participants, caregivers, or researchers.[1,5,6] Recall bias is one example of measurement bias when study participants who experienced an outcome event are more likely to report an exposure. Measurement bias can also arise from inaccuracy in measurement instruments that bias the detection of an outcome towards certain group. For instance, a new diagnosis tool may be able to detect cancer at earlier stages and therefore appears to extend patients' survival more than an existing tool.[4] This issue could be reduced in prospective studies but can be problematic in a retrospective study as the researchers may not have control over the measurement process or when researchers are relying on existing data.

CONFOUNDING

A **confounding factor** is associated with both the outcome and the treatment, but is not a consequence of the treatment. An example of this is age as a confounding factor in the association between antidepressants use and mortality. Older people are more likely to be prescribed antidepressants but mortality risk also increases with age; however, aging is not a consequence of antidepressants use. Confounding factors, if unbalanced between treatment and comparison groups, can lead to selection bias. In well-executed randomized trials, all confounding factors are balanced across groups such that they will not result in biased estimates. However, in observational settings, without proper control of confounding factors, the true relationship between exposure and outcome may be attenuated and a spurious association can result.

Known confounders such as age can be controlled through stratification by the confounders (if there are only a few of them) or multivariate statistical adjustment methods such as propensity score matching or adjustment.[7,8] However, unknown confounders may still exist that will lead to biased estimates. Several approaches such as the instrumental variable method[9–11] or the Heckman selection model[12,13] are available to control for selection bias resulting from latent or hidden confounders. Drawbacks of these statistical methods are that they rely on specific assumptions which may not be applicable to the data at hand and can also be difficult to implement.[14]

GENERAL CRITERIA FOR EVALUATING OBSERVATIONAL STUDIES

When appraising observational studies for evidence-based medicine, two broad issues should be considered: 1) Are the study results valid? 2) Will the results be generalized to local practice? The first issue deals with the internal validity of the study and should be assessed by careful examination of the study design, conduct, and analysis. The second issue deals with the external validity of the study, which involves comparison of the study population described in the study with the patient population encountered locally. The following discussion introduces some general criteria for evaluating observational studies. The **Strengthening the Reporting of Observational studies in Epidemiology (STROBE) Statement**[15,16] and other published studies[1,5,17] were used to develop these criteria. The most widely used STROBE Statement is a checklist of items for reporting of research based on observational study designs—cross-sectional, case-control, and cohort studies. Although the STROBE Statement is intended for reporting of an observational study, it can also "help readers when critically appraising published articles."[16] **Table 19-1** summarizes the list of items for consideration and questions that should be asked when evaluating published observational studies.

TABLE 19-1 Checklist for Critical Assessment of Observational Studies	
Item	**Question to Ask**
Research question	Were the research questions, including any pre-specified hypotheses, clearly stated?
	Were the scientific background and rationale for investigating the research questions provided?
Study design	Was the observational study design clearly stated?
	Was the choice of observational study design appropriate for the research question(s) under investigation?
Study population	What was the source population and how does it compare to the target population underlying the research questions?
	How were the participants selected and were the inclusion and exclusion criteria appropriate?
	Have the characteristics of the study population been sufficiently described and how do these characteristics compare to those of the patients encountered at my clinical practice?
	Was an appropriate comparison group used in the study? If yes,
	• Was justification for selecting the particular comparison group provided?
	• Is the comparison group appropriate to address the research questions under investigation?
	• Is the comparison group comparable to the treatment group?
	• Are there standing differences at baseline between the treatment and comparison groups that may lead to biased outcomes?
	For primary data collection:
	• Has the response rate been clearly reported and were efforts made to maximize participation rate?
	• Have the investigators reported the characteristics between the respondents and non-respondents and whether any standing differences may lead to biased results?
	• Has attrition rate over time been clearly reported and have reasons for attrition and impact of attrition been discussed?
Exposure and outcome	How are the exposure and outcome measured?
	Are the tools used to measure exposure and outcome accurate?
	In a cohort study, is the follow-up period sufficient to identify the outcome?
	In case-control studies, is the look-back period appropriate to identify exposure?
Data analysis and confounding	Were the statistical methods appropriate for the study design and measurement of the outcome variable?
	Were the statistical analyses appropriately adjusted for observed confounding?
	Were residual confounding discussed and assessed?
Presentation of results and interpretation	Are the interpretation and conclusion supported by the study findings?
Practice and policy implications	What is the impact of the findings on practice or policy?

The following discussion provides details of key issues such as research question, study design, subject selection, measurement of exposure and outcomes, data analyses, results, and implications. As an example, these criteria are applied to the study by Grodstein et al. (1996), which examined the effect of estrogen-progestin combination use on risk of cardiovascular disease (CVD) in postmenopausal women using the Nurses' Health Study (NHS).[18]

RESEARCH QUESTION

- Were the research questions, including any pre-specified hypotheses, clearly stated?
- Were the scientific background and rationale for investigating the research questions provided?

A good research study should clearly state the research questions under investigation and any pre-specified hypotheses tested. Research questions may be formulated as objectives or aims of the study. In a research paper, statements of hypotheses or study aims often appear at the end of the introduction section. Well-articulated objective statements should make clear to the readers the patient population to whom the findings are generalized to, the outcome(s) under consideration, and the risk factors or interventions studied.

Given that spurious association may be identified in observational studies in the absence of adequate control for confounding, it is important that stated hypotheses be clinically and biologically plausible. Prior to the statements of research questions, the scientific background and rationale should have been provided to justify the investigation carried out in the study. These may include previous clinical findings and/or theoretical pathological evidence to support the proposed hypothesis of an association and evidence of a gap in the literature that suggests a need of such investigation.

BOX 19-1	Research Question Application[18-19]

In Grodstein et al. (1996),[18] the research question is clearly indicated by the title "postmenopausal estrogen and progestin use and the risk of cardiovascular disease" and is explicitly stated on page 453. This study is a follow-up of an earlier report by the investigators,[19] which have looked at the relationship between postmenopausal estrogen therapy and CVD using data from NHS. The current study included additional 6 years of follow-up from NHS and more data on estrogen-progestin combination use, which has since become more popular. In the introduction, the authors clearly articulated the rationale for this study: (1) previous evidence from experimental studies and a randomized controlled trial suggested that progestin use may increase the risk of CVD by elevating the low-density lipoprotein (LDL) cholesterol levels and lowering high-density lipoprotein (HDL) cholesterol levels, and reducing the beneficial effect of estrogen on arterial dilation and blood flow; (2) there is insufficient information on the effect of estrogen-progestin combination use on CVD (page 453).

STUDY DESIGN

- Was the observational study design clearly stated?
- Was the choice of observational study design appropriate for the research question(s) under investigation?

Observational studies have many different study designs and each has its own advantages and limitations. Overall, there are four general observational study designs often used in clinical research: (1) cohort studies; (2) case–control studies; (3) cross-sectional studies, including surveys; and (4) case-series studies or case reports.[4] In addition, there exist many variations of these designs. When examining the appropriateness of the chosen observational study design, a clinician should consider whether the choice of study design is reasonable in relation to the stated research questions. In particular, a clinician should ask whether the chosen design is the best to answer the research question proposed.

BOX 19-2	Study Design Application[18]

In Grodstein et al. (1996),[18] the goal is to be able to infer a causal relationship between HRT and CVD. The study used a prospective cohort study design, which is the strongest design to examine causality in observational studies. One disadvantage of such a design is that, if the occurrence of an outcome is rare or takes long time to develop, a large sample size and/or longer follow-up time would be needed to observe sufficient incidences. The paper did not report the rate of CVD in this population from previous studies, nor did it conduct sample size calculation (which is common for observational studies). Thus, rarity of the outcome events was unknown. Nonetheless, even though the study employed a large number of postmenopausal women ($n = 59,337$) and a long follow-up period (up to 16 years), only 8 cases of major coronary diseases and 17 cases of stroke were found over 27,161 person years in the estrogen-progestin arm (Table 2, page 456), suggesting the sample size and follow-up period, although large, may have been insufficient to assess the CVD risk of estrogen-progestin combination therapy. This limitation is acknowledged by the authors on page 455.

SUBJECT SELECTION

Understanding the subject selection process, including the selection of both the treatment group and appropriate comparison groups, is crucial for evaluating the validity and generalizability of the findings. The following questions should be asked when critically evaluating the subject selection process.

- What was the source population and how does it compare to the target population underlying the research questions?
- How were the participants selected and were the inclusion and exclusion criteria appropriate?
- Have the characteristics of the study population been sufficiently described and how do these characteristics compare to those of the patients encountered at my clinical practice?
- Was an appropriate comparison group used in the study? If yes,
  - Was justification for selecting the particular comparison group provided?
  - Is the comparison group appropriate to address the research questions under investigation?
  - Is the comparison group comparable to the treatment group?
  - Are there standing differences at baseline between the treatment and comparison groups that may lead to biased outcomes?
- For primary data collection:
  - Has the response rate been clearly reported and were efforts made to maximize participation rate?
  - Have the investigators reported the characteristics between the respondents and non-respondents and whether any standing differences may lead to biased results?
  - Has attrition rate over time been clearly reported and have reasons for attrition and impact of attrition been discussed?

Understanding the source from which the study population was selected is important. When subjects are selected from certain sources such as inpatients, outpatients, health registry, referral registry, or individuals with certain public insurance or certain professional groups (e.g., physicians, nurses), the study sample may not possess characteristics that are representative of patients in clinical practice, thereby limiting its applicability to other patient groups. Also, the inclusion and exclusion criteria used to select subjects should be carefully examined. While stringent restrictions may help select homogenous samples and reduce the chance of confounding, they could also limit the generalizability of the findings by selecting a study population that is not comparable to patients generally encountered in everyday clinical practice. If detailed baseline characteristics of study subjects are provided, clinicians should compare them to the patient population encountered in clinical practice for determination of applicability to their daily practice.

For causal inferences, a comparison group should always be employed. In case-control studies, a comparison group is required by design. These are subjects who did not experience the outcome events ("controls"). To increase comparability, control subjects may be identified from the same family (e.g., spouses, sibling), treated by the same provider and/or in the same geographic location, or taken from patients hospitalized at the same time as the case subjects. At other times, case subjects may function as their own controls in a cross-over design to "tease out" the effect of a subject's individual characteristics that may affect the risk of outcome. Comparison groups are also used in the cohort studies to control for common trend change over time in similar individuals (e.g., policy analysis of changes in prior authorization procedure in a Medicaid program may use another state's Medicaid program without such a change as a comparison to examine the change in drug costs over time).

In both cohort and case-control studies, comparison groups may be matched to treatment groups by key socio-demographic or clinical characteristics to increase comparability. It is important to be aware that choice of the comparison group may affect the interpretation of the findings. For instance, a comparison of mortality between subjects treated with an antidepressant drug and a placebo group tests the mortality risk of this drug. But comparison of this antidepressant with another antidepressant drug tests the differences in mortality risk between the two antidepressants. Non-significant finding in the latter does not mean that this antidepressant drug is not associated with mortality risk; rather, both drugs have the same mortality risks. Comparisons in baseline characteristics across treatment groups should be reported to help clinicians assess their comparability and identify any existing confounding due to observed variables that could bias the results. This is particularly important in small studies when statistical tests may indicate no statistically significant differences, but large measured differences in baseline characteristics may exist.

If primary data collection is conducted, then clinicians should carefully evaluate the response rates. A low response rate may reduce the generalizability of the study findings to the source population. Clinicians can assess this if investigators reported the characteristics of both the respondents and non-respondents, or provided information regarding such comparisons. If large differences are present, then clinicians should consider whether any standing differences may lead to biased results. If subjects are followed over time, then clinicians should also carefully examine the attrition rate and reasons for attrition (if reported) to determine whether patterns of attrition are related to the outcome and if there are any differences in attrition between treatment and comparison groups. If true, then this will lead to biased findings. Studies using only subjects with complete information are not appropriate. Intention-to-treat analysis where subjects are analyzed in the group to which they are initially assigned may be used. While doing so may generate more conservative findings on a beneficial effect, it reduces the chance of detecting a true harmful effect and should be cautioned in safety studies.

BOX 19-3	Subject Selection Application[18-21]

In Grodstein et al. (1996),[18] subjects are selected from the NHS, which has been used in previous studies by the authors to study CVD risk of HRT (page 453). A brief description of NHS is provided on page 454: NHS employed a large cohort of female nurses aged 30–55 years ($n = 121,700$), who were surveyed biennially since 1976. The paper did not provide detailed information on how the nurses were selected and it is therefore unclear, based on the information reported in the paper, whether the participating nurses could represent all female nurses or all women in the United Sates. The NHS website[19] states that the participating nurses were selected from the 11 most populous states. This suggests that the findings may not be generalizable to female nurses in less populated states. According to the NHS website,[20] nurses were specifically selected to increase accuracy of self-reported medical information and long-term survey retention due to their nursing training. Because of this, the results may not generalize to all females as nurses may be more adherent to medications, more likely to take preventive measures of CVDs, and better able to identify the pre-symptoms of CVDs. In the study, current estrogen-progestin combination users are compared to never users, past users, and current users of estrogen-alone, with evolving group assignments at each 2-year survey (i.e., never users in 1976 may be classified as current users if initiated HRT after 1976). This prevalence users approach (i.e., current users) allows the researchers to maximize their use of the data set, but may underestimate the risk if CVD develops quickly after initiation because those who experienced adverse events are more likely to discontinue the use and therefore less likely to be included. To "tease out" the influence of pre-existing CVD or cancer on HRT use, the investigators restricted the sample to women without these conditions at the time of each survey (page 454). Given the study design of NHS, this appears to be the best way to reduce the confounding by pre-existing conditions. However, this restriction may further exacerbate the chance of underestimating the risk because those who initiated HRT use between surveys (2-year period) but developed CVD before the following survey will be excluded. As shown in the clinical trials,[21] CVD risk increases in the first year of use but decreases over time, which has been suspected to be a reason for discordant findings between the observational studies and randomized trials.[21] Given this design, these comparison groups are appropriate because not only could one infer whether the current combination use is associated with changed CVD risk (compared with never-users), but also whether combination use attenuates the effect of estrogen (compared with estrogen-alone users). Table 1 (page 454) compared the age-standardized distribution of eligible subjects' characteristics in these groups defined at the 1990 NHS survey. Both groups of estrogen users appear to be in general younger, healthier, more likely to take multivitamin, vitamin E, and aspirin, but consume more alcohol and saturated fat than never or past users. No statistical significance tests of the differences are reported, but these characteristics were adjusted later in multivariate analysis (page 454). Response rates are not reported in this paper, but reported on the NHS website to be 70% for the initial survey and 90% at each 2-year follow-up survey, although no comparison of responders and non-responders was reported.[20]

EXPOSURE AND OUTCOME MEASURES

- How are the exposure and outcome measured?
- Are the tools used to measure exposure and outcome accurate?
- In a cohort study, is the follow-up period sufficient to identify the outcome?
- In case-control studies, is the look-back period appropriate to identify exposure?

The appropriateness of exposure and outcome measures should be critically evaluated. Prescription or non-prescription medication exposures in pharmacoepidemiology research are often measured using patient reports, medical records, or pharmacy claims data. Exposure to a drug may be measured as any exposure, and/or by the level of exposure such as dosage, duration, strength, and route of administration, which may result in varying estimated drug effect. Moreover, combination drugs may have different effects than the drugs alone. This is particularly important for comparison of multiple studies of the "same" drug. In case-control studies, the look-back period is crucial for determining the exposure. If an outcome event takes a long time to develop (e.g., cancer), a short look-back period may underestimate the exposure; however, a long look-back period may overestimate the exposure if the drug is expected to have a more immediate effect on the outcome. If drugs are prescribed to treat the symptoms associated with a disease before a clinical diagnosis, then look-back windows that include the period immediately before the diagnosis may falsely attribute the risk of the disease to the drug use. For instance, gabapentin is often prescribed for cancer-related pain or worsening of neuropathic or non-neuropathic pain before clinical cancer diagnosis.[22] This will make gabapentin appear to cause cancer, resulting in "protopathic bias." To alleviate such bias, a researcher should exclude sufficient time before a diagnosis to check for prior drug exposure. With increasing availability of large databases for pharmacoepidemiology studies, prescription drug exposure is often defined using prescription claim records. While pharmacy claims capture the fills of prescription drugs, it could not inform of their actual use and may misclassify some users and nonusers.

Outcomes in pharmacoepidemiology research often include safety and effectiveness measures. Ideally, the outcome measure should be an objective measure to eliminate potential bias in collection due to subjective factors. However, even with objective measures, the collection procedure may introduce variations that lead to bias. For instance, blood pressures taken by different persons, using different tools, at various time during the day may affect the reliability of the outcome. Sufficient details regarding the measurement process should be provided for readers to judge the reliability of measured outcomes and these differences should be explicitly adjusted for in the study. When outcome of interest can only be measured subjectively (e.g., measurement of pain, appetite, satisfaction, attitude and belief, quality of life), validated standardized instruments should be used so that the findings may be easily tested by other researchers and can be readily compared with other studies using the standardized tools.[1] Clinicians should carefully examine the differences between the populations for which the instrument has been validated and their own patient population to see if it could result in significant differences in reported outcome. Additionally, the outcome measure chosen should be appropriate for the study purpose. In prospective studies, study duration should be sufficient to observe the outcome of interest. If delayed side effects are expected based on current knowledge, then a minimum follow-up period sufficient to observe these events should be allocated. On the other hand, an excessively long follow-up period may increase the chance of additional confounding by other factors which are also changing over time, thereby making it hard to attribute the observed change in outcome to a drug exposure or intervention that occurred a long time ago. Moreover, patients who better tolerated a drug and/or experienced a beneficial effect are more likely to stay on the drug longer and, therefore, make the drug appear more effective over time.

For safety studies, either insufficient or excessive follow-up period may bias the results towards null and thereby increase the chance of a false negative conclusion of drug safety. In addition, patients who have a higher risk of experiencing a harmful event or could not tolerate the side effects will drop out earlier, creating the false impression that treatment safety profile improves over time. If data were from secondary sources, then clinicians should be aware of the limitations associated with these data sources. In addition to self-reporting, many observational studies use electronic medical records or claims databases and outcomes events are often identified by International Classification of Diseases 9 or 10 codes. Claims data are created for purposes other than research (i.e., for reimbursement). Therefore, their quality of reporting may be affected by insurance reimbursement incentives. Diagnosis and procedure codes may be incompletely coded (e.g., a limitation on the number of diagnoses or procedures codes per record) or differentially coded (e.g., less severe conditions such as hypertension are less likely to be coded in patients with many comorbidities).[17] In addition, administrative databases have limited ability to differentiate the severity of a condition and distinguish between complications (adverse outcome) and pre-existing conditions (risk factors).[17] Detection of outcomes could also be affected by differences in coding practice over time and across institutions if studies are restricted to a few institutions and/or within a specific geographic area.

BOX 19-4	Exposure and Outcome Measures: Application[18]

In Grodstein et al. (1996),[18] HRT exposure was ascertained through self-report by the participants. Since the participants are all registered nurses, the information was considered reliable by the investigators (page 457). The exposure was measured as *current estrogen-progestin combination use*, *current estrogen-alone use*, *past use*, or *never use*. Current dose of estrogen was further stratified at 4 levels (0.3, 0.625, 1.25, ≥1.25mg) to examine the CVD risk by dose (Table 4, page 458). Stratified analysis by duration of use among current users were also conducted (<2 years and ≥10 years, page 456). In addition, effects by time since last use (0 (current user), <3, 3–4.9, 5–9.9, or >10 years) were also compared (Figure 7, page 457). Nonfatal CVD events were identified first by participants' self-report. Fatal CVD events were reported by deceased participants' family and supplemented by search of the National Death Index data. With permissions from the participants or their families, both fatal and nonfatal cases were further confirmed by medical records review (page 454).

Data Analysis and Confounding

- Were statistical methods appropriate for the study design and measurement of the outcome variables?
- Were the statistical analyses appropriately adjusted for observed confounding?
- Were residual confounding discussed and assessed?

Data analysis is crucial for making correct inferences from observational data. Clinicians should carefully examine the appropriateness of the statistical tests. This depends on how the data are collected and measured. In addition, each statistical test implicitly makes a specific assumption regarding the distribution of outcomes in the target population (e.g., normal distribution), which should be examined for its appropriateness against data. Sample size affects the power of a statistical test. With rare events or exposure, insufficient sample size may lead to erroneous conclusions. Clinicians should carefully examine if sample size and the number of events across the treatment and comparison groups are clearly reported in the study and whether insignificant findings could have resulted from insufficient sample size. A back-of-envelope type of power analysis may be conducted using observed effect to determine if under-power is indeed an issue. In addition, non-response and attrition may further reduce usable observations in prospective studies.

Confounding is an important threat to the internal validity of observational studies and should be carefully adjusted. Statistical adjustment for multiple confounders is usually accomplished through multivariable regression analysis. The choice of a regression model depends on how the outcome variable is measured. For instance, data measured in continuous forms can be analyzed using linear regression model. The logistic regression model is used for analysis of outcomes that are measured as binary variables.

When the time-to-event is the outcome of interest, survival analysis should be conducted and a Cox proportional hazards regression model is often used for statistical adjustment of confounding effects of other factors.

While standard statistical adjustments can adjust for confounders observed and measured in the data, clinicians should be aware of residual confounding bias resulting from unobservable or unmeasured confounders. When evaluating a study, clinicians should carefully consider the factors adjusted in the regression model and whether any clinically-relevant confounding factors have been excluded from the model. For instance, in studies using large insurance claim databases, many important confounders are not measured. One such factor is smoking, which has been shown to be associated with the risk for many diseases and health outcomes including death, and may also interact with many drugs. If smoking prevalence is also imbalanced between patients who use a drug and those who do not, then biased estimates will be obtained even with intensive statistical adjustment of observed confounders.

Clinicians should examine if this potential bias is acknowledged by the investigators. In most cases, investigators may provide a qualitative discussion recognizing this limitation and may list several important unobserved confounders not included in the study. Those statements should be carefully examined to see if any efforts have been made by the investigators to reduce or assess the impact of these confounders using sensitivity analysis. For instance, if information on a critical unobserved confounder is available for a subset of patients in the study, a subgroup analysis of these patients may offer some insights on the potential impact of the unobserved factor. However, one drawback of such analysis is that there may be systematic differences between patients in the subgroup with observed information and those without, such that the effect of the unobserved confounder may not be generalized to the population represented by the whole sample. More sophisticated analysis to account for unobserved confounding is to use **instrumental variable** approach, in which an "instrument" acts like a randomizer. Instruments such as physician preference are often used as they are strongly associated with the drug exposure but are not directly associated with the outcome. Sometimes, investigators may not conduct any sensitivity analysis, but provide discussions on the potential direction of residual confounding bias. Clinicians should critically evaluate such statements for consistency with existing knowledge and identify any additional unobserved confounders not discussed by the investigators (e.g., severity of disease) that may attenuate the drug effect.

BOX 19-5	Data Analysis and Confounding: Application[18]

In Grodstein et al. (1996),[18] sample size estimation is not conducted. For some subcategories of stroke, it appears that the sample size may have been insufficient. Only 3 cases of hemorrhagic stroke were identified in the estrogen-progestin combination arm (p. 455), despite the large person years observed (27,161). Although the estimated relative risk (RR) indicates a large decrease in risk (RR: 0.53), it fails to reach statistical significance. The study compared characteristics of current, past, and never users, but did not report any statistical significance tests; nonetheless, these characteristics were adjusted in multivariate analysis (page 454). Both age-adjusted and multivariate-adjusted RR ratios are estimated. A large number of subgroup analyses were conducted to test the robustness of the finding (Table 5, page 459). In addition, several other potential confounding factors not adjusted in the regression model, such as frequency of physician visits and socioeconomic factors, were explored (page 458). Given the large RR ratio, possibility of residual confounding is discussed but not explicitly examined. It is suspected by the investigators that only very significant unobserved confounders could change the direction of the estimated protective effect (page 458).

PRESENTATION OF RESULTS AND INTERPRETATION

- Are the interpretation and conclusion supported by the study findings?

The findings in observational studies are often reported as risk ratio, odds ratio, or hazard ratios. These ratios provide the strength and direction of the relationship between exposure and outcome. However, because they are estimates of relative risk between the treatment groups, they may exaggerate the actual risk/benefit of a treatment when outcome events are rare. To better understand the risk reduction, two clinically more meaningful concepts can be used: numbers needed to treat (NNT) and numbers needed to harm (NNH). NNT is the number needed to treat to avoid one adverse event, which is calculated as 1 over the absolute risk reduction. If a treatment increases the risk of an adverse event outcome, then one could calculate the NNH, which is similarly estimated as 1 over the absolute risk increase. Statistical significance of the estimated effect can be assessed using either p-values or confidence intervals. While p-values can be used to determine the statistical significance at a certain significance level (usually 0.05), confidence intervals additionally could indicate the precision of the estimated effects. Since p-values use a single threshold to determine the statistical significance, it can be rather arbitrary when p-values are near the significance level. For instance, suppose two drugs both estimated an odds ratio of experiencing a beneficial outcome to be 3 against placebo; one has a p-value = 0.049 and the other has a p-value = 0.051. At a significance level of 0.05, the first drug will be interpreted as having a positive effect while the latter will be regarded as having no effect. Such an interpretation could be misleading.

BOX 19-6   **Presentation of Results: Application[18]**

In Grodstein et al. (1996),[18] the relationship between HRT and risk of CVD are presented as relative risk ratio. Both the point estimate and 95% confidence intervals of the relative risks are reported in the text and the tables. In addition, the investigators also reported the total person years and the number of cases for each relative risk calculation, enabling calculation of absolute risk. For instance, the age adjusted relative risk of major coronary disease is estimated to be 0.45 between postmenopausal women who used estrogen alone and those who never used HRT, suggesting a 55% reduction in risk (Table 2, page 456). However, the unadjusted rates in the two groups are 0.6 and 1.4 per 1000 persons per year respectively, suggesting an absolute risk reduction of only 0.08%. In this example, NNT = 1/0.0008 = 1183, which indicates that 1183 patients will be needed to receive estrogen alone in order to prevent one major coronary disease.

APPLICATION TO PRACTICE AND POLICY

- What is the impact of the findings on practice or policy?

Although well-designed and conducted RCTs are still the gold standard for assessing efficacy and safety of a drug, they often lack representations of the diversity and complexity of patients seen in clinical practice. Using data from real-world settings, well-designed and conducted observational studies can complement the findings from RCTs for clinical decision making in practice.[17] As RCTs are seldom conducted after drug approval, observational studies play an important role in post-market drug safety surveillance. Many black-box warnings issued by the Food and Drug Agency (FDA) were based on evidence from observational studies. One example is the black-box warning of conventional antipsychotics issued in 2008 for increased mortality risk in elderly patients treated for dementia-related psychosis, which was based on two large, well-conducted observational studies.[23] These warnings were instrumental in optimizing antipsychotic use in the elderly. Increasingly, findings from observational studies are being used to inform comparative drug safety and effectiveness. In general, no study should be considered alone for its implication on practice and policy; existing evidence from RCTs and observational studies should be carefully considered after critical evaluation of study design, conduct, and analysis.

BOX 19-7	Practice and Policy: Application[1, 18, 24, 25]

In Grodstein et al. (1996),[18] the authors concluded that "the addition of progestin to estrogen does not appear to attenuate the cardioprotective effects" (page 460). At the time of this publication, no large RCTs were available on this issue.[1] This finding is consistent with existing but limited epidemiology evidence at that time (page 460). The overall evidence on cardioprotective effect of HRT, including this study, has led to wide use of HRTs in women prior to the negative findings from RCTs.[1] However, as has been discussed in this section, the choice of female nurses may limit its generalizability to clinical practice. Also, although large relative risk was estimated in this study, the absolute risk reduction was relatively small, which, in joint consideration of increased risk of breast cancer, particularly for estrogen-progestin combination use,[24,25] cautions the use of HRT for primary prevention of heart disease.

COMPARISON OF RESULTS FROM OBSERVATIONAL STUDIES AND RANDOMIZED TRIALS

Both RCTs and observational studies have been used to make causal inferences. While consistency is generally found,[26–28] occasionally inconsistent findings may result. The highly debated recent example is the risk of coronary heart disease (CHD) associated with HRT in postmenopausal women. While observational studies generally found reduced risk of heart disease,[19] two RCTs, Heart and Estrogen/progestin Replacement Study (HERS) and Women's Health Initiative (WHI) trials,[28–30] found no or increased risk for both primary and secondary preventions. In the presence of apparent inconsistency, one easy mistake is to disregard findings from observational studies because of their non-randomized study design. This practice is particularly dangerous if there are only a few small RCTs but large observational studies are available. Randomization does not guarantee absence of biases in actual implementation. Besides randomization, many differences may exist in how RCTs and observational studies are conducted and analyzed. Before comparing RCTs and observational studies, clinicians should first determine their validity. If the studies are by themselves sound but report seemingly inconsistent findings, how should the results be reconciled? The following discussion provides some possible explanations for discordant findings from RCTs and observational studies using HRT studies as illustrations.

Study Population: Trial populations could differ in significant ways from populations included in observational studies.[31] In general, in an effort to increase homogeneity across comparison groups and also for ethical and practical reasons, trial subjects are often healthier, with fewer/no comorbidities, and/or have fewer/no concurrently used medications than patients in typical clinical practice. Observational studies are more likely reflect common clinical practice. In the HRT studies, differences in subjects' age and time since menopause for initiation of HRT are suggested as a potential explanation for the discordant findings between RCTs and observational studies.[31,32] It has been suggested[17] and shown[33–35] that if the inclusion and exclusion criteria used in RCTs were applied in observational studies, similar findings could result.

Exposure and Outcome: RCTs and observational studies may differ in exposure measurements by the timing (e.g., initial exposure vs. any exposure), duration, or extent (e.g., cumulative or maximum dose) of exposure. RCTs by design use incident users and assess outcomes resulting from a "new" exposure. Observational studies can include prevalent users and assess the outcomes of "ever" exposure. In a reanalysis of NHS restricting to incident users, comparable findings with RCTs were generated.[36] For causal inference of an intervention, it is recommended that observational studies should always use an incident-user approach.[37] Differential adherence to treatment could also lead to different exposure measurements. Subjects in RCTs are generally more adherent due to close monitoring, more eager to be compliant because they volunteered for the study, and use fewer drugs concurrently because of stringent inclusion and exclusion criteria. In the HERS trial, potential recruits were pre-screened with a trial of placebo before the study and only adherent subjects were recruited.[21] Outcomes may be detected at different rates in RCTs and observational studies. RCTs are conducted under strictly controlled environments with close monitoring of outcomes at pre-defined intervals. Detection of outcomes in observational studies is often dictated by how frequently a person visits a provider and may be affected by barriers to health care providers and/ or patients' decision to seek medical attention based on symptom.[17] Additionally, more rigorous methods to detect outcomes are often used in RCTs than observational studies.[18,30] Also, if an intervention requires significant skill and/or a long learning curve to master (e.g., robotic surgeries), findings from RCTs may be dictated by the skills of the clinicians in the trials and can be hard to reproduce in a "real world" clinical setting.[17] However, clinicians' skill levels are rarely measured or are imperfectly measured (e.g., clinicians' age, years' since starting practice, or number of similar procedures performed in the past as surrogates) in observational studies, which may partially explain the discordant findings on these medical interventions.

SUMMARY AND CONCLUSIONS

Observational studies are increasingly being used to evaluate important issues relevant for practice and policy. Consequently, it is imperative to critically assess an observational study for evidence-based medicine, which include careful evaluation of its study design as well the conduct and analysis of the study. Since observational studies are prone to biases and confounding, these methodological issues should be carefully evaluated. Critical assessment requires detailed evaluation of study reporting and presentation, which may be lacking in many published studies. This could be due to either intentional or unintentional overlooking of details by the researchers for practical reasons, such as data source limitations. As both consumers and contributors of the medical literature, clinicians are encouraged to follow the consensus guidelines, such as the STROBE Statement, to appropriately report research findings and general criteria for sound scientific evaluation, such as those discussed in this chapter, to translate research into practice. When there is discordance in findings between observational studies and RCTs, it is necessary to reconcile such inconsistencies.

REVIEW QUESTIONS

1. How can selection bias influence study findings in observational research?
2. How can confounding factors influence study findings in observational research?
3. How are exposures and outcomes usually measured in pharmacoepidemiology research?
4. What are the limitations of observational studies using data from claim databases?
5. A recent large observational study found reduced risk of prostate cancer associated with multivitamin use in male physicians. Could this finding be generalized to all males and why?
6. Why are multivariate analyses critical in analyzing data from observational research?

ONLINE RESOURCES

Agency for Healthcare Research and Quality: Effective Health Care Program-Helping You Make Better Treatment Choices: http://effectivehealthcare.ahrq.gov/search-for-guides-reviews-and-reports/?pageaction=displayproduct&mp=1&productID=318

The Canadian Partnership Against Cancer Guideline Resource Center: Critical Appraisal for Observational Studies: http://www.cancerview.ca/cv/portal/Home/TreatmentAndSupport/TSProfessionals/ClinicalGuidelines/GRCMain/GRCGD/GRCGDCriticalAppraisalOf Evidence/GRCGDObservationalStudies;jsessionid=SwwvRcmDJp84L8Zy88VpxXrPz DgPnQwL8YmF156L4k3F2rR01mHQ!1540376534?_afrLoop=927651287776000&_afrWindowMode=0&_adf.ctrl-state=fpt52qo6n_4

Scottish Intercollegiate Guidelines Network (SIGN) Critical Appraisal Notes and Checklists: http://www.sign.ac.uk/methodology/checklists.html

REFERENCES

1. Shields KM, DiPietro NA, Kier KL. Principles of drug literature evaluation for observational study design. *Pharmacother*. 2011;31(2):115–227.
2. Yamamoto ME. Analytic nutrition epidemiology. In: Monsen ER, Horn LV, eds. *Research: Successful Approaches*. 3rd ed. Chicago, IL: American Diabetic Association; 2008: 81–89.
3. Sachett DL. Bias in analytic research. *J Chron Dis*. 1979;32:51–63.
4. Dawson B, Trapp R. *Basic & Clinical Biostatistics*. 4th ed. New York, NY: McGraw-Hill Companies; 2004.
5. Zaccai JH. How to assess epidemiological studies. *Postgrad Med J*. 2004;80:140–147.
6. Page LA, Henderson M. Appraising the evidence: what is measurement bias? *Evid- Based Ment Health*. 2008;11:36–37.
7. Rosenbaum PR, Rubin DB. The central role of the propensity score in observational studies for causal effects. *Biometrika*. 1983;70:41–55.
8. Cochran W, Rubin DB. Controlling bias in observational studies. *Sankyha*. 1973;35:417–446.
9. Angrist JD, Imbens GW, Rubin DB. Identification of causal effects using instrumental variables. *J Am Statistical Assoc*. 1996;91(434):444–455.
10. Newhouse J, McClellan M. Econometrics in outcomes research: the use of instrumental variables. *Ann Rev Pub Health*. 1998;19:17–34.
11. Angrist JD, Krueger AB. Instrumental variables and the search for identification: from supply and demand to natural experiments. *J Econ Perspect*. 2001;15:69–85.
12. Heckman JJ. The common structure of statistical models of truncation, sample selection, and limited dependent variables and simple estimator for such models. *Ann Econ Social Measure*. 1976;5:475–492.
13. Heckman JJ. Sample selection bias as a specification error. *Econometrica*. 1979;47:153–161.
14. Staiger D, Stock J. Instrumental variables regression with weak instruments. *Econometrica*. 1997;65:557–586.

15. Vandenbroucke JP, von Elm E, Altman DG, Gøtzsche PC, Mulrow CD, et al. Strengthening the Reporting of Observational Studies in Epidemiology (STROBE): explanation and elaboration. *PLoS Med.* 2007;4(10):e297. doi:10.1371/journal.pmed.0040297

16. von Elm E, Altman DG, Egger M, et al. The Strengthening the Reporting of Observational Studies in Epidemiology (STROBE): guidelines for reporting observational studies. *PLoS Med.* 2007;4(10):1623–1627.

17. Hannan EL. Randomized clinical trials and observational studies. *JACC: Cardiovasc Int.* 2008;1(3):211–217.

18. Grodstein F, Stampfer MJ, Manson JE, et al. Postmenopausal estrogen and progestin use and the risk of cardiovascular disease. *N Engl J Med.* 1996;335(7):453–461.

19. Stampler MJ, Colditz GA, Willet WC, et al. Postmenopausal estrogen therapy and cardiovascular disease: ten year follow-up from the Nurses' Health Study. *N Engl J Med.* 1991;325:757–762.

20. The Nurses' Health Study. Harvard University. Accessed on December 14, 2012. Available at: http://www.channing.harvard.edu/nhs/?page_id=70.

21. Blakely JA. The Heart and Estrogen/Progestin Replacement Study revised: hormone replacement therapy produced net harm, consistent with the observational data. *Arch Intern Med.* 2000;160:2897–2900.

22. Irizarry MC, Webb DJ, Boudiaf N, et al. Risk of cancer in patients exposed to gabapentin in two electronic medical record systems. *Pharmacoepidemiol Drug Saf.* 2012;21:214–225.

23. Information for healthcare professionals: conventional antipsychotics. U.S. Food and Drug Administration. Accessed on December 14, 2012. Available at: http://www.fda.gov/Drugs/DrugSafety/PostmarketDrugSafetyInformationforPatientsandProviders/ucm124830.htm.

24. Barrette-Connor E, Grady D. Hormone replacement therapy, heart disease, and other considerations. *Annu Rev Public Health.* 1998;19:55–72.

25. Beral V, Million Women Study Collaborators. Breast cancer and hormone-replacement therapy in the Million Women Study. *Lancet.* 2003;362(9382):419–427.

26. Benson K, Hartz AJ. A comparison of observational studies and randomized, controlled trials. N Engl J Med, 2000; 342: 1878–1886.

27. Concato J, Shah N, Horwitz RI. Randomized, controlled trials, observational studies, and the hierarchy of research designs. *N Engl J Med.* 2000;342:1887–1892.

28. Ioannidis JP, Haudich AB, Pappa M, et al. Comparison of evidence of treatment effects in randomized and nonrandomized studies. *JAMA.* 2001;286(7):821–830.

29. Grady D, Applegate W, Bush T, et al. Heart and Estrogen/Progestin Replacement Study (HERS): design, methods and baseline characteristics. *Control Clin Trials.* 1998:19:314–315.

30. Hulley S, Grady D, Bush T, et al. for the Heath and Estrogen/Progestin Replacement Study (HERS) Research Group. Randomized trial of estrogen plus progestin for secondary prevention of coronary heart disease in postmenopausal women. *JAMA.* 1998;280:605–613.

31. Rossouw JE, Anderson GL, Prentice RL, et al. Risks and benefits of estrogen plus progestin in healthy postmenopausal women: principal results from the Women's Health Initiative randomized controlled trial. *JAMA.* 2002;288:321–333.

32. Barrett-Connor E. Commentary: Observation versus intervention—what's different? *Int J Epidemiol* 2004;33:457–459.

33. Stampfer M. Commentary: Hormones and heart disease: do trials and observational studies address different questions? *Int J Epidemiol.* 2004;33:457–459.

34. Hernan MA, Alonson A, Logan R, et al. Observational studies analyzed like randomized experiments an application to postmenopausal hormone therapy and coronary heart disease. *Epidemiology.* 2008;19:766–779.

35. Lawlor DA, Smith GD, Ebrahim S. Commentary: the hormone replacement–coronary heart disease conundrum: is this the death of observational epidemiology? *Intl J Epidemiol* 2004;33:457–459.

36. Grodstein F, Manson JE, Stampfer MJ. Postmenopausal hormone use and secondary prevention of coronary events in the Nurses' Health Study. *Ann Intern Med.* 2001;135(1):1–8.

37. Danaei G, Tavakkoli M, Hernan MA. Bias in observational studies of prevalent users: lessons for comparative. *Am J Epidemio.* 2012;175(4):250–262.

38. Ray WA. Evaluating medication effects outside of clinical trials: new-user designs. *Am J Epidemiol.* 2003;158:915–920.

APPLYING DRUG LITERATURE TO PATIENT CARE

Katy E. Trinkley, PharmD

Steven M. Smith, PharmD, MPH

CHAPTER OBJECTIVES

▸ Understand the general principles of applying evidence to patient care

▸ Discuss application of randomized trial results to patient care

▸ Discuss application of practice guidelines to patient care

▸ Determine appropriateness of applying evidence to patient care

▸ Develop a system to keep up-to-date with drug information

KEY TERMINOLOGY

Clinical practice
 guidelines

Foraging tool
Patient-centered care

Patient-Oriented Evidence that
 Matters (POEM)

INTRODUCTION

Evidence-based medicine (EBM) is considered the best method of caring for patients.[1] Although this concept appears relatively straightforward—that is, employing the best available evidence to guide clinical decisions for patients—the actual practice of EBM is complicated by a variety of factors. Included in these factors are patient-specific values and circumstances, clinician-specific judgment and expertise, and the availability and appropriate assessment of evidence on which a decision can be based. For a clinician, incorporating these factors into healthcare decisions for a given patient is integral to ensuring optimal treatment outcomes. For example, many Jehovah's Witnesses believe it a gross sin to receive blood products. In situations where Jehovah's Witnesses are volume depleted due to significant blood loss, the best option based on the evidence is to give them blood products, but for many Jehovah's Witnesses, this is unacceptable and they refuse blood products based on their beliefs. As per EBM, the next best treatment plan is implemented, giving them non-blood fluid products.

Developing a systematic approach to EBM can promote efficiency and ensure that all relevant aspects of healthcare decisions are being considered. However, no two patients, clinicians, or situations are the same; thus, clinicians must remember that EBM is a process by which various intervention options can be assessed and, ultimately, individualized decisions can be made. This chapter will review the general principles of applying evidence to patient care. Specifically, it will focus on incorporation of evidence from clinical trials and recommendations from clinical practice guidelines using examples. In addition, this chapter will discuss methods of staying up-to-date with the rapidly expanding body of drug information using the framework of Patient-Oriented Evidence that Matters (POEM) and foraging tools.

GENERAL PRINCIPLES OF APPLYING EVIDENCE TO PATIENT CARE

The practice of EBM is guided by two underlying principles: (1) care should be patient-centered, and (2) decisions should be based on the most applicable and highest-quality evidence available.[1] The first principle, **patient-centered care**, includes understanding the impact of the problem and various interventions on the patient's quality of life, recognizing and incorporating the patient's values and preferences, and collaborating with the patient on managing the problem.[2] While patient values and preferences are often synonymous, values may be more reflective of a person's belief system, whereas preference may be more reflective of a person's wants or desires. The second principle requires the clinician to obtain relevant evidence that is applicable to the clinical scenario. The clinician is responsible for expertly assessing the evidence on intervention options, synthesizing this information for the patient, and then collaborating with the patient to determine the management plan. These aspects must be considered from the beginning because they help frame the clinical question and organize the evidence review process necessary for EBM. In addition, some patients may actively participate in their own healthcare decisions, whereas others may prefer the clinician make decisions on their behalf. In the latter cases, clinicians must be responsible for incorporating, to the extent possible, patient values in the decision-making process. Previous chapters discussed at length searching and assessing relevant literature to obtain the best possible evidence. The following discussion will focus on integrating best evidence into patient care.

Just as EBM cannot be driven solely by patient preferences, neither can it be driven only by evidence. In other words, few clinicians would recommend treatment with a non-steroidal inflammatory drug in a patient with an active gastrointestinal bleed, even if the patient requested that drug for pain control, because the evidence suggests a high risk of worsening the bleeding. Likewise, few clinicians would recommend life-saving measures in a terminal patient who has specifically requested not to be resuscitated, even though the evidence clearly shows that such life-saving measures are effective. However, for a patient with moderate chronic kidney disease and hypertension who places a high value on not progressing to end-stage renal disease and dialysis, an angiotensin-converting-enzyme inhibitor would be clearly indicated by the evidence and, in this case, would be consistent with patient values. Thus, for EBM, the principles of patient-centered care and decisions are based on applicable, high-quality data, and are necessarily intertwined.

The management plan must account for what the patient is willing to and can do, which includes how much they are willing to pay for a given treatment. In practice, the best treatment choice may not be the best for a given patient because the cost is more than that patient is willing to spend. Similarly, other factors such as complexity of a treatment regimen and adherence are important considerations when choosing a treatment plan. Adherence barriers may be resource limitations, lack of understanding of the correct regimen, or religious views that only a higher power has the ability to control one's fate; thus, socioeconomic, health literacy, and cultural factors all influence compliance. Consequently, it is important that clinicians have an understanding of the factors that could influence a patient's adherence, and systematically screen them for adherence and barriers to adherence to achieve better health outcomes.

Other factors to consider when choosing a treatment option for patients are biological factors that can influence the effectiveness of a given medication regimen. For example, African Americans respond differently to certain classes of antihypertensives than other races because of a biological difference in sodium retention. African Americans being treated for hypertension with diuretics are likely to see a significant drop in their blood pressure, whereas when treated with a beta-blocker or angiotensin-converting enzyme inhibitor monotherapy, they may not see any change in their blood pressure.[3] When considering a treatment option for a given patient, their biologic differences must be considered, because some drugs work differently in persons with different biological makeup.[4] Drug therapy management is not always black and white and is often gray when the patient's values, preferences, and biologic and cultural characteristics are integrated into the plan.

APPLICATION OF RANDOMIZED TRIAL RESULTS TO PATIENT CARE

Many clinical decisions are based on the findings from one or more clinical trials. Clinical trial research generates evidence about a given health situation and informs practitioner treatment decisions. However, clinical research encompasses a broad range of study designs, ranging from randomized controlled trials to observational studies. The quality of evidence produced from a given trial depends largely on the study design. Randomized controlled trials are considered to be the most robust study designs; however, other methodological factors must be considered beyond study design before applying a trial's findings to patient care. First and foremost, the study findings should only be considered further after careful evaluation of the quality of the study, including

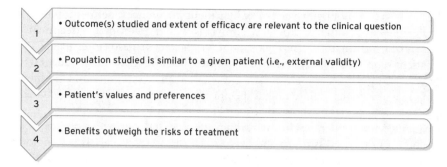

1 • Outcome(s) studied and extent of efficacy are relevant to the clinical question

2 • Population studied is similar to a given patient (i.e., external validity)

3 • Patient's values and preferences

4 • Benefits outweigh the risks of treatment

FIGURE 20-1 Steps in the application of randomized trials data.

methodology and design, as discussed in previous chapters. When deciding whether to apply randomized trial results to a given patient (application), consider (1) whether the outcome(s) studied and extent of efficacy are relevant to the clinical question(s), (2) whether the population studied is similar to a given patient (i.e., external validity), (3) the patient's values and preferences, and the measures the patient and provider are willing and able to take, and (4) whether the benefits outweigh the risks of treatment (i.e., interpreting results). **Figure 20-1** describes the steps to take when deciding whether to apply randomized trial results to a given patient.

When considering the outcome of a trial and the extent of efficacy, the outcome must align with the given situation and demonstrate such a degree of efficacy that the benefit outweighs the risk for a given patient. For example, when considering whether lubiprostone is beneficial for a female patient with chronic, idiopathic constipation, whose main complaint is stool hardness, ideally the study will have stool consistency as an outcome measure. If the study did not consider stool consistency, yet considered stool frequency, then the needs of the patient, which is improved stool consistency, may not be addressed if lubiprostone is started. Further, if the patient complaining of stool hardness states that she does not want anything that causes her nausea, the risk vs. benefit ratio needs to be considered. If a given study demonstrates lubiprostone improved stool consistency satisfactorily in all 259 patients studied, but caused nausea in 3%, then the benefit may outweigh the undesired nausea for this patient, depending on her personal preferences.

The ability to generalize a clinical trial's results to a given patient requires a thorough understanding of whether a given patient is similar to the patients studied (e.g., race, age, medical history, current medications), whether there are certain factors that could preclude your patient from the results of a given trial, and the patient's values and preferences. There are many factors to consider beyond demographics (e.g., race, age, medical history, current medications), such as adherence, ability to pay for treatment, and dexterity or cognitive status to administer medication. For example, a trial demonstrating that a series of Botox injections are highly effective for persons with severe, refractory migraines may not be an option for everyone with severe, refractory migraines, such as may be the case for a patient and provider who are in a rural setting. In such a setting, the provider may not be able to obtain the injections and/ or the patient may not have the means to travel back and forth to the provider to get the invasive injections. For many treatment options, the ability (e.g., laboratory measurements, imagining equipment) or clinical expertise to monitor treatment safety and efficacy may not be sufficient or available and thus prevent the implementation of such treatments.

BOX 20-1	Case Scenario 1

RJ is a 26-year-old obese man with newly diagnosed type II diabetes who wants to get his glucose controlled. The physician wants to start him on a medication for diabetes and asks the clinical pharmacist for advice on whether to start metformin or exenatide. After carefully reviewing the clinical trials, the pharmacist found that metformin has demonstrated improved glucose control and mortality and decreased diabetes-related comorbidities in well-designed clinical trials. In contrast, exenatide, a newer drug, has been shown to improve glucose control and decrease weight in many smaller, but well-designed studies, but it has not been shown to improve mortality or decrease diabetes-related comorbidities. What are the best recommendations and rationale for treating RJ's diabetes?

Solution

Start metformin because the benefits are greater and reflective of patient values. Metformin is the only antihyperglycemic agent that has been found to reproducibly improve morbidity and mortality in persons with type II diabetes. Metformin has been found to reduce the risk of any diabetes-related endpoint (e.g., sudden death, angina, heart failure, stroke, renal failure, amputation, or death from uncontrolled glycemia), myocardial infarction, and all-cause mortality. Exenatide has only been on the market for a short time compared with metformin and has not demonstrated benefits in morbidity and mortality. The robust evidence supporting metformin is why it is considered first-line therapy for type II diabetes and the reason it is the best option for this patient who wants to get his diabetes under control.

References

UK Prospective Diabetes Study (UKPDS) Group. Effective of intensive blood-glucose control with metformin on complications in overweight patients with type II diabetes (UKPDS 34). *Lancet*. 1998;352:854–865.
Qaseem AI, Humphrey LL, Sweet DE, Starkey M, Shekelle P. Oral pharmacologic treatment of type II diabetes mellitus: A clinical practice guideline from the American College of Physicians. *Ann Intern Med*. 2012;156:218–231.

Other patient-specific considerations that may limit the generalizability of findings include biological reasons, such as differences in race, that can lead to differences in efficacy. For example, African Americans respond better to diuretic therapy than angiotensin converting enzyme inhibitors for high blood pressure. Genetic reasons, such as presence or absence of certain polymorphisms that are contingent upon a treatment's success (e.g., the BRCA polymorphism in breast cancer), should be carefully considered. Treatment decisions must be individualized for every patient (incorporating patient values/preferences), the benefits must outweigh the risks, and the evidence must support the treatment decision. If any of the aforementioned are not met, then the treatment decision may not be a good option for a given patient.

APPLICATION OF PRACTICE GUIDELINES TO PATIENT CARE

Clinical practice guidelines are evidence-based statements that serve to assist practitioners and patients about appropriate healthcare decisions for specific healthcare situations.[3] Ideally, clinical practice guidelines review all issues relevant to a given clinical decision or scenario, including alternative treatment options. Therefore, clinicians reference guidelines with primary objectives that are consistent with the given patient care situation or clinical question. Because clinical practice guidelines generally provide a comprehensive review of available treatment options, they are considered to provide higher quality recommendations than those that are not based on a systematic process.

Similar to applying evidence from clinical trials, important considerations with clinical practice guidelines beyond the quality of evidence include ensuring the outcomes align with the clinical situation, and the results are generalizable to a given patient. One such example is the recommendation by the American Diabetes Association that metformin is first line therapy for most people with type II diabetes; however, for someone who has stage four chronic kidney disease, the recommendations do not apply, because metformin in combination with severe chronic kidney disease increases the risk of lactic acidosis.[5] Before accepting a guideline recommendation, the generalizability to a given patient must be thoroughly considered and should not be taken at face value.

The recommendations made by clinical practice guidelines are typically made by the consensus of a panel of experts in the given field or area. Sometimes, the recommendations made are not based merely on the evidence, but are also influenced by the opinions of the experts on the panel. The opinions of the expert panel members are especially helpful when there is limited evidence available to support one decision over another. Recommendations from a group of experts are very helpful in making clinical decisions; however, care must be taken to understand what is evidence-based and what is merely expert opinion. Further, the quality of the evidence supporting recommendations and the process of arriving at a given recommendation must be understood to ensure you are making the best clinical decision for your patients. Rather than simply taking the recommendation and implementing it in practice, it is important to review the evidence supporting the recommendation to ensure it is of high quality and determine whether the recommendation is based on a systematic process to support the recommendations. Clinical practice guidelines compile evidence, making it easy to review the evidence supporting a given recommendation. Often, the evidence supporting a given recommendation is limited and, after reviewing the evidence, the clinician may decide that an alternate treatment option is better than that recommended by the guidelines. Clinicians must understand the degree of uncertainty and level of evidence supporting a given recommendation, which includes understanding whether the recommendation is expert opinion or based on evidence, as well as understanding the limitation in the evidence that supports the recommendation.

Recommendations from practice guidelines are recommendations, not rules, and they do not apply to all scenarios, nor are they always up-to-date. Clinical guidelines consider the best available evidence up to a given time point, so it is important to identify the time period the guidelines are based on and determine whether there is more up-to-date information since that time. Thorough understanding of the guidelines, including the evidence they are based on, as well as their limitations, will assist in achieving optimal patient health outcomes. Although not implemented by all practice guidelines, grading systems that quantify the level of evidence that recommendations are based on are helpful in determining the strength of evidence supporting a given recommendation. There is no standard method of grading the evidence supporting clinical practice guidelines, but the GRADE criteria, or adaptations of the GRADE, have been used by many guidelines.[6]

When considering whether to apply guideline recommendations, the clinician must also consider that each recommendation made in a clinical practice guideline is based on certain value judgments. Value judgments are decisions about the relative importance of certain health outcomes in a given situation.[7] Value judgments can be from the perspective of the patient, society, or others. Sometimes there is evidence from the literature that is used to determine a judgment decision. However, evidence is often lacking; therefore, the value judgment is determined by the expert panel members. Further, the values applied to a given outcome vary between each person and group of persons. The value judgments should be made with the one who is most impacted in mind, the patient. Therefore, the outcomes addressed in the guidelines should also be made with the patient in mind. Those recommendations that are based on patient–centered value judgments are more clinically significant than those that are not patient–centered.

Value judgments and outcomes are ideally patient–centered; however, this is not possible for all situations, such as controlling blood pressure. For instance, persons with hypertension may not feel any different when their blood pressure is high or low, but the evidence indicates that attaining certain blood pressure goals improves mortality and prevents complications; therefore, clinical practice guidelines may value blood pressure goals, which is not a value judgment that impacts the patient directly. In addition to blood pressure goals as a value judgment, practice guidelines may also determine mortality and other hypertension complications to be value judgments, which do directly impact the patient. It is important for practice guidelines to clearly state value judgments, so that the clinician can determine whether those values are aligned with the patient's values.

Before applying guideline recommendations to practice, it is important to review the strength of evidence supporting the recommendation and determine whether the recommendations are generally patient–centered, ensure that the primary objective of the guideline is consistent with the given patient care situation, and assess whether the recommendation is aligned with a given patient's values and preferences

---

BOX 20-2	Case Scenario 2

PC is a 57-year-old woman with reflux who has tried antacids, but they only provide minimal relief for a short period of time. PC has already implemented lifestyle modifications. She is requesting something to help alleviate her reflux. Her nurse practitioner consults you because she isn't sure if she should initiate an H2RA or proton pump inhibitor (PPI). She is considering adding a PPI because she read that H2RAs are not as effective at persistently elevating the pH; however, she read the gastroesophageal reflux disease (GERD) guidelines and saw they recommend either an H2RA or PPI for persons with mild GERD symptoms. How would you explain to the nurse practitioner that either an H2RA or PPI are reasonable treatment options for PC at this time, despite the fact the H2RAs are not as effective at elevating the pH over time?

Solution

Although H2RAs are not as effective at persistently elevating pH, they are comparable in their ability to improve reflux symptoms and these symptoms are what the PC is most concerned with, not pH. The clinical practice guidelines for GERD address the outcome of symptom resolution (e.g., reflux, heartburn), rather than the surrogate marker of pH from endoscopy. Patients generally place a higher value on symptom resolution than changes in pH. The GERD guideline recommendations are not only based on patient-centered value judgments, but the objectives of the guidelines align with the patient's needs.

References

AGA Institute. American Gastroenterological Association medical position statement on the management of gastroesophageal reflux disease. *Gastroenterol.* 2008;135:1383–1391.

BOX 20-3	Case Scenario 3

A new practice guideline recommends that a direct thrombin inhibitor should be given for stroke prevention for persons with atrial fibrillation and a CHADS score of 2 or greater because it is superior to warfarin for stroke prevention. The thrombin inhibitor was compared with warfarin because warfarin was considered the standard of care for preventing stroke in persons with atrial fibrillation. SJ has atrial fibrillation with a CHADS score of 2, but cannot use the thrombin inhibitor because he needs to use a pill box for his medications and the thrombin inhibitor must be stored in the original container to maintain the potency of the medication. In the past, SJ had very poor medication adherence, likely due to dementia, but is doing well now with his pill box. What is the best recommendation for SJ?

Solution

Start warfarin because although it is not as effective as the thrombin inhibitor, it is still effective and is the best option for SJ. The study that found the thrombin inhibitor was superior to warfarin did not include patients that required the use of a pill box; thus, the results are not generalizable to SJ. In fact, SJ would be at increased risk of stroke if he was started on a thrombin inhibitor, because the effectiveness of the drug would be compromised if he was non-adherent. The atrial fibrillation guidelines made a general recommendation, but did not consider patient-specific factors such as the need for a pill box to avoid poor adherence. In fact, the guidelines do not mention anywhere that the new thrombin inhibitor cannot be stored outside the original packaging. While some guidelines provide more detail about practice considerations when using a particular medication, some do not; therefore, it is up to the clinician to be aware of these other considerations and then decide whether the recommendation treatment option is the best for a given patient.

References

You JJ, Singer DE, et al. Antithrombotic therapy for atrial fibrillation: Antithrombotic therapy and prevention of thrombosis, 9th ed: American College of Chest Physicians evidence-based clinical practice guidelines. *Chest.* 2012;141:e531S–575S.

STAYING UP WITH DRUG INFORMATION

The enormous wealth of drug information literature is increasing exponentially, making efforts to stay up-to-date more challenging. However, a proactive and systematic approach to reviewing literature can make this process manageable. Clinicians have varied strategies and methods of staying up-to-date with pertinent literature to ensure optimal patient care. Therefore, what works for one clinician may differ from strategies that work for other clinicians.

Every clinician must ask (and continually reassess) three important questions:

1. What is the scope in which I need to focus?
2. In what way(s) do I learn most efficiently?
3. How can I incorporate this learning process into my usual routine?

Determining the scope of what one will stay up-to-date on is crucial given the current volume of drug literature (over 22 million citations in MEDLINE alone). Fortunately, most of these citations are of little value to clinicians because they do not focus on patient care or because they do not provide sufficient evidence to warrant a substantial change in practice. Consequently, an important skill for information mastery is learning to filter this literature and focus solely on that information which is applicable to patient care—that is, **Patient-Oriented Evidence that Matters** (POEM).

A POEM is new clinical approach that meets three criteria.[8] First, POEMs evaluate the effect of a test, drug, procedure, or intervention on an outcome that patients care about. For example, a patient may care little about how effectively a drug reduces fasting blood glucose levels, but may place a high value on preventing diabetic retinopathy. Thus, a study that examines only glucose levels or A1c as the primary (surrogate) end-point would not qualify as a POEM, whereas a study assessing a drug's effect on reduction in the incidence of retinopathy would. Secondly, POEMs must study a "common" medical problem where the intervention is feasible in a given setting. A study in which a treatment is shown to be very effective is unlikely to be useful to a clinician if the intervention is cumbersome and not likely to be adhered to by patients. Lastly, POEMs must supply information that has the potential to induce a practice change among clinicians. Applying these three criteria as a litmus test allows the clinician to drastically reduce the volume of literature requiring review.

The process of identifying POEMs was developed in the 1990s, initially for primary care, but can be applicable to any specialty medical scope. Consequently, identification of POEMs will largely be driven by one's job responsibilities. For example, a clinician practicing in oncology may need to stay abreast on all new research surrounding oncology and may not need to focus their limited time on all new research in the area of dyslipidemia. Conversely, a primary care practitioner may decide that a more general approach is appropriate, focusing on major research in common acute and chronic diseases rather than the nuances of a specific disease state or therapeutic area.

Once the scope has been determined, the clinician should give careful thought to the method(s) that will effectively and efficiently allow them to learn new information. One of the most common methods involves reviewing journal articles. However, for most clinicians, it is not possible to read all journal articles in a field, nor is it feasible to search PubMed (http://www.pubmed.gov) regularly for new articles.

Instead, many clinicians rely on summaries of the important literature within a given field. These summaries are often referred to as foraging tools. **Foraging tools** browse the available literature for new and important information, which is different than searching for an answer to a specific question.[9] Foraging is helpful, not only because it helps the clinician stay up-to-date with topics that they would otherwise not be aware of, but also because it can unlock answers to questions that the clinician had not yet identified as a problem. A good foraging tool identifies valid POEMs and selects evidence that is clinically important, based on outcomes that matter to the patient. To be helpful, a good foraging tool pulls information relevant to your interest or practice area and is comprehensive. Ideally, you will know how the foraging tool appraises and filters the literature. Further, a good foraging tool puts new information into the context of previous information and is searchable. **Table 20-1** describes some foraging tools. In addition, many clinicians subscribe to the table of contents for relevant journals. Importantly, this process removes the burden of actively seeking new articles (which may or may not have been published) from the clinician, and instead places that burden on the foraging tool to alert the clinician to newly published literature. Most biomedical journals provide, free-of-charge, an electronic notification (usually by e-mail) of new publications. The journal contents can then be quickly scanned for relevance and articles of interest can be accessed via imbedded links within the notification. Similarly, PubMed allows registered users to set up automatic updates. These regular e-mail updates contain new articles that meet the user's predefined search criteria. Other similar services offer variations on these themes (Table 20-1).

Some clinicians may also prefer a briefer summary of important literature rather than reading numerous full journal articles. Various services are available that meet this need, including both electronic and print services. Examples include ACP Journal Club, or Journal Watch, as seen in Table 20-1. A common theme among these services is that

TABLE 20-1   Selected Foraging Tools for Staying Up with Medical Literature

Name	Description	Cost	Sponsor/Publisher
Journals			
ACP Journal Club (http://www.acpjc.org)	Subscription-based one-page summaries of recently-published research; published monthly	Annual subscription *Annals of Internal Medicine*	American College of Physicians
American Family Physician (http://www.aafp.org/afp)	Twice-monthly print and online publication	Annual subscription to journal (free to qualified primary care physicians)	American Academy of Family Physicians
The Journal of Family Practice (http://www.jfponline.com)	Monthly clinical reviews of evidence-based medicine; includes an online archive of POEMs	Annual subscription to journal (freely available to family physicians)	Quadrant HealthCom Inc.
Journal Watch (http://www.jwatch.org)	Brief, clinically-oriented reviews of recently-published literature; available on-line and in print format	Annual subscription	Massachusetts Medical Society (publishers of *New England Journal of Medicine*)
Evidence Summaries			
AHRQ Effective Health Care Program (http://www.effectivehealthcare.ahrq.gov/)	Clearinghouse of comparative-effectiveness systematic reviews by various academic institutions funded by AHRQ	Free	Agency for Healthcare Research and Quality
Clinical Evidence (http://clinicalevidence.bmj.com)	Compendium of systematic reviews on various topics	Annual subscription	BMJ Publishing Group
The Cochrane Database of Systematic Reviews (http://www.cochrane.org)	Warehouse of extensive collection of systematic reviews	Free abstracts; annual subscription for full-text	The Cochrane Collaboration
DynaMed (http://www.dynamicmedical.com)	Database of evidence summaries incorporating various primary and secondary literature sources	Annual subscription	DynaMed
Up-To-Date (http://www.uptodate.com)	Database of evidence summaries incorporating various primary and secondary literature sources	Annual subscription	Up-To-Date
FIRSTConsult (http://www.firstconsult.com)	Database of evidence summaries from various sources	Annual subscription	Elsevier
Essential Evidence Plus (http://www.essentialevidenceplus.com)	Search engine for various evidence-based sources; also provides daily POEMs (summaries) via e-mail	Annual subscription	Wiley-Blackwell
SUMSearch (http://sumsearch.org)	Search engine that gathers original research, systematic reviews, and practice guidelines from various sources	Free	University of Kansas

Name	Description	Cost	Sponsor/Publisher
TRIP Database (http://www.tripdatabase.com)	Searchable database that gathers evidence-based clinical information from various sources and rates them according to strength of evidence, date, and applicability to search query	Free	Gwent, Wales
Clinical Guidelines			
Institute for Clinical Systems Improvement (http://www.icsi.org/guidelines__more/)	Guidelines for preventive services and disease management developed by ICSI; also includes various protocols and order sets for clinical use	Free	Institute for Clinical Systems Improvement
National Guideline Clearinghouse (http://www.guidelines.gov)	Database of evidence-based clinical practice guidelines based on systematic reviews of the literature; contains only English language guidelines	Free	Agency for Healthcare Research and Quality
U.S. Preventive Services Task Force Recommendations (http://www.uspreventiveservicestaskforce.org/)	Database of recommendations for preventive services; based on systematic reviews by the USPSTF	Free	USPSTF
Other			
Amedeo (http://www.amedeo.com)	Service that allows clinicians to specify therapeutic areas and journals to be searched for relevant publications; the service sends an e-mail with citations and links to PubMed abstracts.	Free	Flying Publisher (supported by educational grants from various pharmaceutical companies)
MedScape (http://www.medscape.com)	Service that offers tailored news, medical information, and continuing education programs for a variety of subspecialties	Free	WebMD, LLC
TheHeart (http://www.theheart.org)	Service that offers tailored news and medical information, and continuing education programs tailored to cardiovascular medicine	Free	WebMD, LLC
Pharmacist's/Prescriber's Letter (or similar) (http://www.pharmacistsletter.com)	Monthly newsletter providing concise evidence-based updates and recommendations on approximately 10 topics per issue; includes continuing education	Annual subscription	Therapeutic Research Center

the literature is reviewed for importance (and sometimes for methodologic quality) and summarized for the busy clinician. An advantage to many of the electronic services is that they are often free-of-charge or involve a relatively small subscription fee.

OTHER APPROACHES

Other common methods include continuing education activities, journal clubs, and precepting students. Many national and state organizations and associations offer continuing education, which ranges in format from readings followed by an assessment to live seminars or conferences. All of these formats provide valuable information, usually regarding timely and new drug information. Journal clubs, as discussed in Chapter 21, can provide a mechanism for critical evaluation of research articles and can be a tool for life-long learning. Moreover, journal clubs can serve to keep clinicians abreast of important literature outside of their own specialty beause they are often conducted with clinicians from multiple specialties or therapeutic expertise.

Teaching is the best form of learning; many clinicians find that precepting students forces them to be aware of the current research so that they are able to guide students. Precepting students is challenging in that students question what is done and how it is done and bring fresh perspectives and information to practice. Students push clinicians to think outside of the way they have been practicing and bring their new knowledge to practice. For clinicians not employed in academia, precepting students also provides an indirect link to the "big picture" themes that are being taught didactically at the student's institution. Other techniques for learning should also be explored, such as developing an educational newsletter or seminar series where colleagues discuss important themes related to their area of expertise.

Additionally, within the practice of pharmacy, each state has a pharmacy association and there are many national organizations, including the American College of Clinical Pharmacy (ACCP), American Pharmacists Association (APhA), and the American Society of Health Systems Pharmacists (ASHP), all of which offer continuing education opportunities.

SUMMARY AND CONCLUSIONS

Practicing evidence-based medicine requires clinicians to stay up-to-date and be able to determine how to apply evidence to a given health situation. Identifying and implementing a system of staying up-to-date and a system of assessing whether evidence should be applied to patient care is important to ensure optimal health outcomes. There are many methods to choose from in developing a system to stay up-to-date, including subscribing to summaries of recently published literature, journal tables of contents, journal clubs, and continuing education. Further, strategies to stay up-to-date, such as POEM, must be implemented to ensure optimal patient care. Whatever the system employed, the clinician must filter the vast body of medical literature to identify patient-oriented evidence likely to have a significant impact on practice. Moreover, all systems used to determine whether to apply evidence to patient care should include careful consideration of patient-specific factors and applicability of the evidence. When deciding whether to apply evidence to a given patient, key considerations include clinical relevance of outcomes, external validity of findings, patient's values and preferences, practical patient and provider factors, and specific benefits and risks of treatment.

REVIEW QUESTIONS

1. What are the necessary considerations when applying evidence to patient care?
2. What are important considerations when assessing the results of a randomized trial to patient care?
3. How can you determine whether the practice guideline recommendations are patient-centered?
4. What is an efficient method of staying up-to-date with drug information in your area of interest?
5. What are ideal characteristics of a good foraging tool?

ONLINE RESOURCES

Journal Watch: Medicine that Matters: http://www.jwatch.org/. Accessed December 20, 2012.
Pharmacists Letter: http://www.pharmacistsletter.com/. Accessed December 20, 2012.
Prescribers Letter: http://www.prescribersletter.com/. Accessed December 20, 2012.

REFERENCES

1. Guyatt GH, Haynes RB, Jaeschke RZ, et al. users' guides to the medical literature: XXV. Evidence-based medicine: principles for applying the users' guides to patient care. Evidence-Based Medicine Working Group. *JAMA*. 2000;284:1290–1296.
2. Stewart M, Brown JB, Donner A, et al. The impact of patient-centered care on outcomes. *J Fam Pract*. 2000;49:796–804.
3. American Heart Association. Seventh report of the Joint National Committee on prevention, detection, evaluation, and treatment of high blood pressure. *Hypertension*. 2003;42:1206–1252.
4. Dans AL, Dans LF, et al. Users' guides to the medical literature XIV. How to decide on the applicability of clinical trial results to your patient. *JAMA*. 1998;279:545–549.
5. American Diabetes Association. Standards of medical care in diabetes—2013. *Diabetes Care*. 2013;36:S11–S66.
6. Guyatt G, Oxman AD, Akl EA, et al. GRADE guidelines: 1. Introduction-GRADE evidence profiles and summary of findings tables. *J Clin Epidemiol*. 2011;64:383–394.
7. Hayward RS, Wilson MC, Tunis SR, Bass EB, Guyatt G. Users' guides to the medical literature. VIII. How to use clinical practice guidelines. A. Are the recommendations valid? Evidence-Based Medicine Working Group. *JAMA*. 1995;274:570–574.
8. Slawson DC, Shaughnessy AF, Bennett JH. Becoming a medical information master: Feeling good about not knowing everything. *J Fam Pract*. 1994;38:505–513.
9. Maughan K, Gazewood J, et al. Foraging tolls: Patient-oriented evidence that matters bulletin boards. In: Rosser WW, Slawson DC, Shaughnessy AF, eds. *Information Mastery: Evidence-based family medicine*. 2nd ed. People's Medical Publishing House, 2004.

BASICS OF JOURNAL CLUB

Catherine L. Hatfield, PharmD

CHAPTER OBJECTIVES

▸ Explain the purpose of journal clubs

▸ Describe the general format of a journal club

▸ Examine characteristics of an effective journal club

▸ Discuss common evaluation tools used in journal clubs

KEY TERMINOLOGY

CATmaker software

Critical appraisal

Critical appraisal tools

Journal club

INTRODUCTION

Journal clubs are valuable to clinicians to keep up with medical literature, especially with the advent of evidenced-based practices. Although journal clubs have become popular in pharmacy education in the last 15 years, they have been in practice for more than a century. Historical accounts give credit to Sir William Osler for the origin of journal clubs in 1875.[1,2] He established the first journal club at McGill University in Montreal, Canada, due to economic restraints that prohibited many physicians from purchasing books and periodicals for their personal use. However, it has also been documented that the phrase "journal club" may have been coined earlier by Sir James Paget while at St. Bartholomew's Hospital in London in 1835–1854.[1,3] Sir James noted that medical pupils would meet in a room over a baker's shop to read journals and formed a group, or club, in doing so. Some early goals of journal clubs included introducing junior staff to a systematic process of using medical literature and allowing more senior staff to survey the literature. In 1966, Mattingly published an article discussing journal clubs and wrote about the various formats and logistics that surround journal clubs, such as the benefit of providing food, meeting frequency, and number of articles to review.[4]

Today journal clubs are common in medical and health education training programs. In pharmacy, journal clubs are used in the academic and practice environments to develop and enhance critical skills for patient care. Pharmacists are often asked for recommendations regarding medications. To make sound and unbiased suggestions, knowing the literature and properly interpreting it is a necessary skill. When making these recommendations, pharmacists need to not only know how the drugs differ in efficacy, but also how they differ in dosing, adverse effects, and pharmacokinetics to make the best recommendation for an individual patient. This chapter will explore the function and types of journal clubs, the preparation and format of journal clubs, and the characteristics of effective journal clubs.

DEFINITION AND PURPOSE OF JOURNAL CLUBS

In a **journal club**, a group of participants who have common practice or research interests meet regularly for a defined pedagogical purpose. The club often discusses current research articles and the appropriateness of the study design, the data analysis, the conclusions drawn, and the potential applications or implications of the research to practice and patient care. In pharmacy, these clubs allow pharmacists to know and understand the current drug research to help make knowledgeable recommendations. The goals of journal clubs in education and practice include keeping up with the literature, teaching critical appraisal skills, promoting evidence-based medicine, providing continuing education, and promoting social interaction.[5]

Journal clubs are used for multiple purposes in the education and practice arena (**Table 21-1**).[6] Most journal clubs incorporate the education of critical appraisal skills as one of their reasons for having the club.[7] **Critical appraisal** is defined as the systematic analytical evaluation of research to determine its value and relevance for a given situation. These skills can be learned from a book, but it is difficult to become truly proficient without practice. Journal clubs allow clinicians with minimal critical appraisal skills to learn how to use and improve their skills by critically evaluating an article in a group setting for the mutual benefit of all in attendance. For pharmacists, these skills are needed to make knowledgeable drug recommendations based on the evidence.

TABLE 21-1 Advantages of Journal Clubs[6]	
Learn critical appraisal skills	Promote research skills
Encourage evidence-based medicine	Encourage use of research
Stay up-to-date with the literature	Promote social contact
Provide continuing education	Stimulate debate
Improve understanding of current topics	

When choosing to recommend one drug over another, the recommendation needs to be based on studies that compare medications on several levels (e.g., efficacy, adverse effects, dosing regimen) and proper interpretation of the study results is a necessary skill.

It has been documented that journal clubs can improve critical appraisal knowledge, improve ability to appraise original research, and increase the amount of time reading by residents.[8] Critical appraisal can help clinicians determine if and how the article should be used in practice, thus developing skills that are necessary when trying to incorporate evidence-based medicine into practice. For this reason, journal clubs are considered to link the realm of research to that of clinical practice and can be instrumental in translating research to practice.

Staying current with the literature is another commonly cited reason for journal clubs. New treatment guidelines are based on the literature, and it is important for pharmacists to understand why treatment guidelines change and what research was done to warrant that change. Finding time to read the vast array of articles in a given discipline is a difficult task. Having a journal club in place allows clinicians to have a set schedule that incorporates reading and discussion of the current literature at a defined time in their busy schedule. Additionally, the benefits of social contact and professionalism should not be underrated. Interprofessional journal clubs can improve relations among different healthcare professions by allowing club members to work together and learn to appreciate the differing expertise each profession has to offer.

FORMAT OF JOURNAL CLUBS

There are many different ways to organize a journal club, and there is not one way that stands out as being the best way. The setting, interests, and needs of the target participants will all need to be taken into account to determine the best format for any given situation (**Table 21-2**). The following sections describe in detail the development and implementation of journal clubs in education and practice areas.

TYPES

Some common types of journal clubs include unit-based, hospital-based, clinic-based, and academic-based journal clubs. Unit-based clubs are usually very specific to topics that occur in the unit. These clubs are often much smaller in size than other clubs because of their specialized focus. One example might be a pediatric intensive care unit (PICU) journal club where all healthcare professionals in the PICU might benefit from articles relating to human touch for the neonate, but this topic would not be very beneficial for healthcare professionals in other units of the institution. However, the articles presented at unit-based clubs are usually relevant to all members.

The hospital and clinic-based clubs are usually much larger and are more likely to include professionals with different backgrounds. These types of journal clubs can be

TABLE 21-2 Journal Club Format Highlights
Types—The type of journal club used will help define the purpose and focus
Focus—May vary based on the needs of the participants
Article selection—Generally original research based on the focus area(s)
Preparation—Expectations for preparation should be set up front
Timing—Always end the journal club on time
Presentation—Critical appraisal tools help with timing and format
Leadership—Having a designated leader improves journal club effectiveness
Presenter—It is most common to have a single presenter at each journal club
Environment—Rooms of adequate size that promote eye contact improve participation
Audience—Participants with similar clinical interests is beneficial
Feedback—Periodic feedback on the logistics and format of the journal club should be gathered from the members

beneficial to participants, but the larger group often comes with larger obstacles such as scheduling and leadership. It is more difficult in this environment to find articles that will benefit the entire group. However, the interactions and discussions of members who might not otherwise work together can stimulate discussion and improve communication among different services at the institution. For example, having professionals with expertise in nutrition support present at a hospital-based journal club could allow an extensive discussion to occur on the benefits of beginning nutrition support in a timely manner. The social interaction created in this type of environment forms personal connections across the disciplines, which can improve communication when needed for a patient encounter. Academic-based journal clubs usually incorporate one or more academic training programs; participation for the students, residents, and/or fellows is often mandatory. Thus, attendance is not an issue, but participation and discussion by an audience that is not present by choice can be minimal if plans to engage the audience are not implemented.

FOCUS

Within each of the types of journal clubs mentioned above, the focus of the clubs can vary depending on the needs of the participants. Some documented focus areas for journal clubs include a critical appraisal focus, an evidence-based focus, and a leadership focus.[5,6,9]

Critical appraisal journal clubs have the primary purpose of educating the audience on critical appraisal through a systematic process of interpretation and evidence. In clubs with this focus, usually only one article is reviewed at a time. This type of club is more likely to review landmark articles that are frequently referred to in the literature, such as the antihypertensive and lipid lowering treatment to prevent heart attack trial (ALLHAT) published in *JAMA* in 2002.[10] While this study is several years old, it is considered a landmark trial because it was a long-term, multicenter trial with a large group of participants comparing medications for the treatment of hypertension. It is important to vary the study design and put the randomized controlled trial aside for critical appraisal clubs, so that all study designs are analyzed. Critical appraisal tools can be very beneficial for this form of journal club. **Critical appraisal tools** are checklists or rubrics that provide a systematic approach to appraise an article to easily discover methodological flaws. The framework for critical appraisal of common pharmacy literature discussed in other chapters of this book can be helpful.

Journal clubs with an evidence-based medicine approach differ in purpose from that of critical appraisal clubs because there is a shift to using the evidence to help with clinical decisions surrounding individual patients. For example, when a question arises on how to treat a patient, the club members may be asked to perform independent literature searches and bring articles to the journal club meeting. Clubs with this focus have four key elements: asking questions, searching the literature, selecting relevant articles, and critically appraising those articles.[5] This type of journal club has a larger scope than critical appraisal journal clubs because it focuses on a topic that may require analyzing multiple articles, rather than a single article. These clubs are more appealing to senior clinicians and are more likely to change practice. It has been documented that of the four key elements of an evidence-based medicine journal club, searching the literature seems to be the weakest link.[11] To help with this, a real-time internet search during meetings lead by a skilled clinician or health research librarian can be beneficial in developing searching strategies and skills. Since most clubs are one hour in length, it may take a couple of meetings to fully discuss the topic and answer any patient-related questions.

A leadership-focused journal club takes on a completely different approach to those previously mentioned. Wombwell and colleagues developed a club that was structurally similar to critical appraisal journal clubs, but the focus was to discuss articles on leadership.[11] They discussed the incorporation of leadership concepts and principles into the daily lives of the students, residents, and practitioners who participated. Eighteen articles were chosen from six key leadership concepts: managerial development, resident-specific learning, defining leadership, leadership development, compassionate leading, and creating change. The authors state that this can be an effective way to increase exposure to leadership principles and practices.

ARTICLE SELECTION

The type of article selected for journal club is based on the focus of the journal club. In general, journal clubs should select original research, and often reviews should be excluded. When selecting an article, it is best to consider the audience. Interesting, engaging, and beneficial articles are more likely to elicit audience participation and discussion. This can be done by choosing articles that were used for a recent patient encounter or by choosing an article that discusses a common problem found in practice, such as medication errors. Articles that cover controversial topics or change current practice can also be engaging. The articles chosen should be relevant to all participants, and align with the purpose of the journal club.

Articles with valid results have the potential to be more beneficial to the audience. These articles are more likely to be used in practice and are more likely to change practice. However, articles with invalid results should be incorporated into the journal club periodically. This will help incorporate education and critical appraisal skills into the discussion.

Most journal clubs present two articles per meeting.[7] Articles should be distributed to all audience members; often this is done at least one week before the journal club meets.[7] Distribution via email as an attached document is the easiest way to distribute the articles, though many times the articles sit in the inboxes of participants. One advantage of email is that one can send inivitations to the participants so that the date/time/location of the journal club can be placed on their calendar and less easily forgotten. However, by copying and distributing the articles by hand, one can ensure everyone has a copy to read, and can obtain a verbal commitment to come to journal club as articles are distributed. A combination of both distribution methods might also prove to be beneficial.

PREPARATION

Time, effort, and resources are needed to prepare for journal club. Clinicians should get extra copies of the article as some may have forgotten to bring it with them. There may be others who haven't read the article, but will want to follow along and read as the discussion ensues. In a systematic review of journal clubs, it was found that the expected preparation of participants prior to journal club varied considerably.[7] Some clubs documented required reading, attendance, and training, while other clubs had no expectation for attendance or preparation. Additionally, preparation for journal clubs has varying definitions. Setting these expectations up front and reviewing as needed may be necessary for a successful journal club.

TIMING

Journal clubs are scheduled for specific time period; most journal clubs are one hour in length.[7] It is important to end the journal club on time, even if the discussion is still ongoing. This allows participants to budget their time accurately and they will be more likely to return to future journal clubs. Journal clubs that are shorter in duration may find it beneficial to distribute an article summary prepared by the presenter using a one- to two-page appraisal tool at the beginning of the journal club.

PRESENTATION

The presentation of content in journal club can vary based on the purpose of the journal club. Presentation slides can help to structure the content and discussion and can be beneficial in shorter journal clubs. However, in a longer journal club where discussion is promoted, the use of slides can inhibit the audience and the discussion because it is perceived that the discussion has already been predetermined by the slides. Critical appraisal tools have been shown to allow for efficient presentation of an article and allow more time for discussion.[12] These tools, either in the form of checklists or software, have the advantage of consistency in presentation format and timing. Clinicians with unpolished critical appraisal skills quickly learn how to report the results from an article, but struggle with learning to report the items that have been omitted or are incorrect. For this reason, the systematic process that these tools establish can also be beneficial in alerting new readers to potential flaws.

LEADERSHIP

Effective journal clubs have a leader responsible for identifying, or helping the presenters to identify, articles for discussion.[7] A designated leader who takes responsibility for the club has been shown to improve effectiveness.[13] In pharmacy, the leader in an academic environment is usually a faculty member and in an institutional environment the leader is usually the pharmacy educator, clinical coordinator/manager, or the chief pharmacy resident. Presenters should rotate to allow different audience members the chance to build presentation and leadership skills. There is data that suggests that senior trainees should be journal club leaders because attendance is improved when the clubs are run independent of faculty.[14,15]

PRESENTER

Presenters have an important role to play as they initiate the content discussion. A presenter should always keep the audience involved as much as possible. This can be done by asking questions to the audience, by referring to tables and figures, and by incorporating clinical questions into the presentation. If a couple members are dominating the discussion, then it is acceptable to ask others for their input. If some audience members seem to be quietly discussing the article among themselves, then they can be asked to share with the group.

While having a single presenter for a given journal club meeting is the most common, there have been reports that small group discussions can be effective as well. Sackett and colleagues divided their audience members into small groups to increase audience participation.[16] After the presenter's introduction to the article, each group was assigned questions to discuss and answer. After correctly answering the questions, the group adjourned. Another presentation format used in journal clubs is a facilitated group discussion. In this scenario, the article is presented by the facilitator, but all questions regarding critical appraisal and clinical importance are directed to the audience for discussion. The role of the facilitator is simply to move the group forward and keep the club running on time. A debate among audience members can also be an effective presentation format. This particular format works best with evidence-based medicine journal clubs that are discussing a controversial topic. The two groups would pick differing opinions on the topic, find supportive literature and then present their findings in a moderated debate. The moderator in this situation is responsible for keeping the time and tone on track.

ENVIRONMENT

The environment for running a journal club can be very important and should not be overlooked. This includes room specifications, seating, and food arrangements. Journal clubs should be conducted in rooms of adequate size; if the room is too small, then it may discourage attendance and if the room is too large, then it may encourage passivity and discourage discussion.[5] Rooms that allow participants to sit in a circle or horseshoe are preferable because they increase eye contact and promote participation. Monthly, one-hour journal clubs over lunch seems to be the most commonly used time for journal clubs.[7,14] To encourage attendance, providing food may be helpful.[14,17,18]

AUDIENCE

There can be considerable variability in the number of participants in journal club. It can range from as small as 12 to a large group of 135.[7] It is recommended that all journal club participants be either of the same discipline or have similar clinical interests, such as cardiology or nephrology. When students or trainees are the primary audience members, attendance is usually mandatory. This has its advantages and disadvantages. When the audience is there by mandate, it may be difficult for them to see the values and benefits that the journal club can offer. On the flip side, mandatory attendance has been associated with successful journal clubs because it promotes a core group of members, which helps with continuity.[14] Another mechanism that has been shown to improve attendance without a mandate is the support of the program director. If the residency program director rates the educational value of journal clubs as vital to the training of residents, then attendance improves. Attendance is lowest if the program director rates the journal clubs as having no educational value.[19]

FEEDBACK

Success of a journal club has been defined as having high attendance and being in existence longer than two years.[14] To achieve both of these goals, periodic evaluation and feedback of club members is necessary.[20] Feedback should be sought on the logistics (timing, location, etc.) and on the topics and on the format (tools, slides, presenters, etc.). Members should also be asked what they found to be most beneficial, what they found to be least beneficial, and what improvements would make the club more beneficial on a regular basis. Academic journal clubs also involve evaluating the delivery and organization of the presentation by peers and/or faculty. Having the club moderated by a faculty member improves attendance and the presence of subspecialty staff at the journal club enhances learning.[12,19]

CHARACTERISTICS OF EFFECTIVE JOURNAL CLUBS

Successful journal clubs have several common features with respect to leadership, attendance, and support. Swift found that successful journal clubs have a single person responsible for the club, provide food, have mandatory attendance, and have support from the program director.[5] Sidorov reviewed the literature regarding internal medicine residency journal clubs in an effort to define what makes some clubs successful.[14] Success was defined as having high attendance or a long existence (>2 years). According to the research, successful resident journal clubs have mandatory attendance, are independent of faculty, have food available, focus on original research, formally teach critical appraisal skills, and are associated with smaller residency programs.

Deenadayalan and colleagues performed a systematic review of the literature on how to run effective journal clubs.[7] They identified multiple characteristics of effective journal clubs, outlined in **Table 21-3**.

Hartzell and colleagues developed a successful resident run journal club based on the adult learning theory.[12] For their club, they developed a journal club committee consisting of residents and a faculty mentor. This committee was responsible for setting the journal club goals, selecting articles, and running the meetings. The journal club met monthly for one hour and discussed two articles at each meeting. The CATmaker software was used to help residents with reviewing and presenting the articles.[21] The study found that of the 87% of eligible internal medicine residents who responded to a questionnaire, 88% felt journal club increased their medical knowledge, 85% felt the journal club was applicable to their practice, 82% learned appraisal techniques that they were using when reviewing articles outside of journal club, and 89% believed that emailing the articles prior to the club aided in learning.

TABLE 21-3   Characteristics of Effective Journal Clubs[7]
Regular and anticipated meetings
Mandatory attendance
Clear long- and short-term purpose
Appropriate meeting time
Appropriate incentives
A leader to choose papers and lead discussion
Circulation of articles before the meeting
Internet usage for dissemination and data storage
Use of established critical appraisal tools
Summarizing journal club findings

TABLE 21-4 Commonly Available Journal Club Tools	
Users' guides to the medical literature	http://jamaevidence.com/resource/520
CATmaker software	http://www.cebm.net/index.aspx?o=1216
Centre for Evidence-Based Medicine	http://www.cebm.net/index.aspx?o=1157

CRITICAL APPRAISAL TOOLS FOR JOURNAL CLUBS

Using checklists and tools for developing critical appraisal skills has been effective in journal clubs, and a few commonly available tools can be found in **Table 21-4**.[12,22–25] Some of the first tools were developed by the Department of Clinical Epidemiology and Biostatistics at McMaster University in Canada.[26–29] They developed a framework for critical appraisal, which was later expanded on in the *Journal of the American Medical Association* as users' guides to the medical literature.[30] These checklist/tools help the learner develop a systematic process of analyzing the literature by posing several questions and then helping the reader answer those questions by providing information and examples. The three primary questions for an article about therapy are, "Are the results of the study valid?," "What were the results?," and "Will the results help me in caring for my patients?" Each of these primary questions has sub-questions that guide the reader through the critical appraisal process.

There are many online resources available that provide education on and tools for critical appraisal of the literature. The Centre for Evidence-Based Medicine at the University of Oxford focuses on teaching and promoting evidence-based medicine (EBM) and provides some tools on its website. They provide resources to guide the clinicians through every step of the EBM process, including critical appraisal and applying the results in practice.

One of the appraisal tools available is the **CATmaker software**.[21] This CAT (critically appraised topics) software is a free download and helps guide the reader through the critical appraisal process of several different types of articles, such as therapy, harm, diagnosis, and prognosis. This CATmaker software was used in a study looking at resident run journal clubs.[12] This study determined that only 39% of residents found the software to be useful and the authors suggest that having designated people available to help first-time users of the CATmaker software would be beneficial. The study also found that the CATmaker software streamlined presentations in a more organized fashion that allowed more time for discussion.

SUMMARY AND CONCLUSIONS

Journal clubs have deep roots in the healthcare education and training programs. Successful journal clubs have high numbers of consistent attendees, which can be achieved by creating an environment where all members benefit from the time spent at the club meeting. The most successful clubs have one leader who organizes the club; lunchtime monthly meetings lasting one hour; an effective way to disseminate information before the club meeting; mandatory attendance; and appropriate incentives, such as lunch. There are many different formats of journal clubs that have been used, and the format chosen should fit the needs of the audience. The use of checklists and tools has been shown to help members with weak critical appraisal skills develop a systematic process to approach the literature and enhance their knowledge. Journal clubs can have a wide range of characteristics and formats, which can lead to stimulating discussions and enhanced knowledge of its members. With increasing emphasis on life-long learning, journal clubs can be instrumental in keeping with evidence-based practices.

REVIEW QUESTIONS

1. What are the advantages of having a journal club?
2. Describe different journal club formats.
3. What are the characteristics of successful journal clubs?
4. Discuss commonly available journal club tools.

ONLINE RESOURCES

McMaster University. Critical appraisal resources: http://fhswedge.csu.mcmaster.ca/cepftp/qasite/CriticalAppraisal.html

National University of Health Sciences. Critical appraisal for research papers. Appraisal checklist and guide questions: http://www.nuhs.edu/media/25485/studyguide-criticalappraisalforresearchpapers.pdf

University of Oxford. Centre for evidence-based medicine (CEBM): http://www.cebm.net/.

University of South Australia. Sansom Institute for Health Research. Critical appraisal tools: http://www.unisa.edu.au/Research/Sansom-Institute-for-Health-Research/Research-at-the-Sansom/Research-Concentrations/Allied-Health-Evidence/Resources/CAT/

REFERENCES

1. Linzer M. The journal club and medical education: over one hundred years of unrecorded history. *Postgraduate Medical Education.* 1987;63:475–478.
2. Cushing H. The Life of Sir William Olser. Volume 1. Oxford: Oxford University Press; 1926:132–133,154.
3. Paget S. *Memoirs and letters of Sir James Paget.* London: Longmans, Green and Co; 1901: 42.
4. Mattingly D. Journal clubs. *Postgrad Med J.* 1966;42:120–122.
5. Swift G. How to make journal clubs interesting. *Adv Psychiatr Treatment.* 2004;10:67–72.
6. Esisi M. Journal clubs. *BMJ Careers.* 2007.
7. Deenadayalan Y, Grimmer-Sommers K, Prior M, Kumar S. How to run an effective journal club: a systematic review. *J Eval Clin Prac.* 2008;14:898–911.
8. Seelig CB. Affecting residents' literature reading attitudes, behaviors and knowledge through a journal club intervention. *J Gen Intern Med.* 1991;6:330–334.
9. Wombwell E, Murray C, Davis SJ, Palmer K, Nayar M, Konkol J. Leadership journal club: new practitioners forum. *Am J Health-Syst Pharm.* 2011;68:2026–2027.
10. The ALLHAT Officers and Coordinators for the ALLHAT Collaborative Research Group. Major Outcomes in High-Risk Hypertensive Patients Randomized to Angiotensin-Converting Enzyme Inhibitor or Calcium Channel Blocker vs Diuretic: The Antihypertensive and Lipid-Lowering Treatment to Prevent Heart Attack Trial (ALLHAT). *JAMA.* 2002;288(23):2981–2997.
11. Coomarasamy A, Latthe P, Papaioannou S, Publicover M, Gee H, Hkan KS. Critical appraisal in clinical practice: sometimes irrelevant, occasionally invalid. *J Royal Soc Med.* 2001;94:573–577.
12. Hartzell JD, Veerappan GR, Posley K, Shumway NM, Durning SJ. Resident run journal club: a model based on the adult learning theory. *Medical Teacher.* 2009;31:e156–e161.
13. Heiligman PM, Wollitzer OW. A survey of journal clubs in US family practice residencies. *J Med Educ.* 1987;62:928–931.
14. Sidorov J. How are internal medicine residency journals organized, and what makes the successful? *Arch Intern Med.* 1995;155:1193–1197.

15. Linzer M, DeLong ER, Hupart KH. A comparison of two formats for teaching critical reading skills in a medical journal club. *J Med Educ.* 1987;62:690–692.

16. Sackett DL, Straus SE, Richardson WS, Rosenberg W, Haynes RB. Evidence-based medicine: how to practice and teach EBM. 2nd ed. London: Churchill Livingstone; 1999.

17. Langkamp DL, Pascoe JM, Nelson DB. The effect of a medical journal club on residents' knowledge of clinical epidemiology and biostatistics. *Family Medicine.* 1992;24:528.

18. Bazarian JJ, Davis CO, Spillane LL, Blumstein H, Schneider SM. Teaching emergency medicine residents evidence-based critical appraisal skills: a controlled trial. *Ann Emerg Med.* 1999;34:148.

19. Van Derwood JG, Tietze PE, Nagy MC. Journal clubs in family practice residency programs in the southeast. *South Med J.* 1991;84:483–487.

20. Kleinpell RM. Rediscovering the value of the journal club. *American J Crit Care.* 2002;11(5):412–414.

21. Center for Evidence-Based Medicine. CATmaker software 2007. Available from: http://cebmh .warne.ox.ac.uk/cebmh/education_catmaker.htm

22. Markert RJ. A research methods and statistics journal club for residents. *Acad Med.* 1989;64:223–224.

23. Woods JR Jr, Winkel CE. Journal club format emphasizing techniques of critical reading. *J Med Educ.* 1982;57:799–801.

24. Krogh Cl. A checklist system for critical review of the medical literature. *Med Educ.* 1985;19:392–395.

25. Alguire PC, Massa MD, Lienhart KW, Henry RC. A packaged workshop for teaching critical reading of the medical literature. *Med Teach.* 1988;10:85–90.

26. Department of Clinical Epidemiology and Biostatistics, McMaster University. How to read clinical journals, II: to learn about a diagnostic test. *Can Med Assoc J.* 1981;124:703–710.

27. Department of Clinical Epidemiology and Biostatistics, McMaster University. How to read clinical journals, III: to learn about the clinical course and prognosis of disease. *Can Med Assoc J.* 1981;124:869–872.

28. Department of Clinical Epidemiology and Biostatistics, McMaster University. How to read clinical journals, IV: to determine etiology or causation. *Can Med Assoc J.* 1981;124:985–990.

29. Department of Clinical Epidemiology and Biostatistics, McMaster University. How to read clinical journals, V: to distinguish useful from useless or even harmful therapy. *Can Med Assoc J.* 1981;124:1156–1162.

30. Guyatt G, Rennie D, Meade M, Cook D. *Users' Guides to the Medical Literature: Essentials of Evidence-Based Clinical Practice.* 2nd ed. New York: McGraw-Hill Professional; 2008.

Journal	Description	Internet Address
ACP Journal Club	Publishes articles according to explicit criteria and to abstract those studies that warrant immediate attention by physicians attempting to keep pace with important advances in the treatment, prevention, diagnosis, cause, prognosis, or economics of the disorders managed by internists.	http://www.acpjc.org
American Journal of Health-System Pharmacy (AJHP)	Publishes peer reviewed scientific papers on contemporary drug therapy and pharmacy practice innovations in hospitals and health systems.	http://www.ajhp.org
American Journal of Pharmacy Benefits (AJPB)	Publishes research that examines the impact of formulary management strategies on the use, cost, and quality of pharmacy services.	http://www.ajmc.com/publications/ajpb
Clinical Therapeutics	Publishes evidence derived from clinical pharmacology and other therapeutic approaches for research, academic, and clinical practice settings.	http://www.clinicaltherapeutics.com
Current Medical Research and Opinion (CMRO)	Publishes research on new and existing drugs and therapies, phase II–IV studies, and post-marketing investigations.	http://informahealthcare.com/loi/cmo
Evidence-Based Mental Health	Informs clinicians regarding important advances in treatment, diagnosis, etiology, prognosis, continuing education, economic evaluation, and qualitative research in mental health.	http://ebmh.bmj.com

(continues)

Journal	Description	Internet Address
Evidence-Based Nursing	Selects from the health-related literature research studies and reviews that report important advances relevant to best nursing practice. The clinical relevance and rigor of the studies is assessed to identify research that is relevant to nursing.	http://ebn.bmj.com
Evidence-Based Medicine	Systematically searches a wide range of international medical journals applying strict criteria for the validity of research.	http://ebm.bmj.com
Formulary	Publishes research aimed at evaluating drugs for formularies and developing policies and procedures to guide the appropriate, rational, safe, and cost-effective use of drugs.	http://formularyjournal.modernmedicine.com
Journal of Evaluation in Clinical Practice (JECP)	Publishes research related to evaluating and developing clinical practice across medicine, nursing, and the allied health professions	http://www.wiley.com/bw/journal.asp?ref=1356-1294
International Journal of Evidence-Based Health Care	Publishes original scholarly work relating to the synthesis (translation), transfer (distribution), and use (implementation and evaluation) of evidence to inform multidisciplinary health care practice.	http://www.wiley.com/bw/journal.asp?ref=1744-1595
Journal of Managed Care Pharmacy (JMCP)	Publishes original research, subject reviews, and other content intended to advance the use of the scientific method, including the interpretation of research findings in managed care pharmacy.	http://www.amcp.org/jmcp
Journal of Pharmaceutical Health Services Research (JPHSR)	Publishes all aspects of research within the field of health services research that relate to pharmaceuticals.	http://onlinelibrary.wiley.com/journal/10.1111/(ISSN)1759-8893
Journal of the American Pharmacists Association (JAPhA)	Publishes papers on pharmaceutical care, drug therapy, diseases and other health issues, trends in pharmacy practice and therapeutics, informed opinion, and original research; the journal publishes papers that link science to contemporary pharmacy practice to improve patient care.	http://www.japha.org
PharmacoEconomics	Publishes articles on applying pharmacoeconomics and quality-of-life assessment to optimum drug therapy and health outcomes.	http://www.springer.com/adis/journal/40273

Journal	Description	Internet Address
Pharmacoepidemiology and Drug Safety (PDS)	Publishes original research, invited reviews, and commentaries embracing scientific, medical, statistical, legal, and economic aspects of pharmacoepidemiology and postmarketing surveillance of drug safety.	http://www3.interscience.wiley.com/journal/5669/home
Pharmacotherapy	Publishes research and review articles about all aspects of human pharmacology and drug therapy.	http://www.accp.com/bookstore/th_journal.aspx
Research in Social & Administrative Pharmacy (RSAP)	Publishes original scientific reports and comprehensive review articles in the social and administrative pharmaceutical sciences.	http://journals.elsevierhealth.com/periodicals/rsap
The Annals of Pharmacotherapy	Publishes research reports, reviews, commentaries, case reports, and other articles that will advance patient care and clinical pharmacy practice.	http://www.theannals.com
Therapeutic Innovation & Regulatory Science	This is a new branding of The Drug Information Journal and covers areas beyond pharmaceuticals and their research and development to include innovations in drugs, devices, diagnostics, and global regulatory issues.	http://www.sagepub.com/journalsProdDesc.nav?prodId=Journal202090
Value in Health	Publishes original research articles in the areas of economic evaluation, outcomes research, and conceptual, methodological, and health policy articles.	http://www.ispor.org/valueinhealth_index.asp

GLOSSARY

Abstract A structured research summary at the beginning of a research report or journal article that enables readers to quickly and easily obtain information about an investigation.

Active control The group in a study that receives a known or accepted standard of care or treatment in a randomized controlled trial.

Adaptive design A clinical trial design that involves changing the conditions of the study or analysis plan over time based on the results of preliminary analysis at interim points of time.

Adaptive randomization The process of assigning patients to a treatment group generally based on previous success of the treatment as the trial progresses.

α (alpha) The probability of a type I error or the probability of rejecting the null hypothesis when it is true. Sometimes called the level of significance or the significance level.

Alternate hypothesis The complement of the null hypothesis that typically states there is a relationship between two variables.

Analysis of variance (ANOVA) A statistical method that can be used for testing the differences among the means of two or more groups (the t-test is often used for testing the differences in the means of two groups, but ANOVA can be used for this purpose as well).

Analytical studies or research Research studies that are aimed at understanding the relationship and/or causal mechanism that may exist between two or more variables.

Applied research Systematic study to gain the knowledge or understanding necessary to determine the means by which a recognized and specific need may be met.

Arithmetic mean A measure of central tendency that is calculated as the sum of all of the values of a variable divided by the total number of observations. More commonly referred to as simply the average of a set of values.

Ascertainment bias Bias that occurs due to differences in assessing or analyzing outcomes by the researcher due to awareness of which participants received the active versus control interventions.

Attributable fraction in the exposed An expression of the risk difference relative to the risk in the exposed group in a cohort study.

Attributable risk The difference in risk for the outcome between an exposed and unexposed group in a cohort study. Also called risk difference.

Attributable risk percent Percentage of the incidence of disease in the exposed group due to the exposure in a cohort study.

Attrition Withdrawal or loss of subjects over time from study groups.

Attrition bias Bias caused by differential drop out of patients in treatment and control groups in randomized control trial.

Bar chart A chart format used to display discrete, categorical data. Most are aligned horizontally.

Base population The population at risk for the outcome who, if they were to have the disease or event, would be selected to be a case in a case–control study.

Basic research Systematic study directed toward fuller knowledge or understanding of the fundamental aspects of phenomena and of observable facts without specific applications toward processes or products in mind.

Belmont Report Report that articulates the fundamental ethical principles that underpin all research with human subjects.

Beneficence Ethical principle of doing or producing good. In scientific research involving human subjects, actions are taken to protect the public from harm and to maximize possible benefits and minimize possible harms.

β (beta) The probability of a type II error or the probability of failing to reject the null hypothesis when it is false.

Bias A systematic error in a study design or in the way study subjects are selected, measured, and analyzed that can lead incorrect findings.

Biased In statistical estimation, when an estimate is generated that on average is fundamentally different than the population parameter that one is trying to estimate.

Binary logistic regression A regression model commonly used to describe and evaluate the relationship between a single dichotomous (or binary) dependent variable and one or more independent variables.

Biochemical methods Laboratory methods used to measure chemical constituents in bodily fluids such as blood or urine.

Biological assessments Assessments that are made using biophysical, biochemical, and/or microbiological methods.

Biomedical research Broad area of research that includes the biological and medical sciences that seeks to understand and improve the health of patients and populations.

Biophysical assessments Assessments that measure physical characteristics, such as bone density, blood pressure, and forced expiratory volume.

Bivariate analyses Methods for analyzing just two variables, such as when testing hypotheses about whether the mean response on a dependent variable is different for an experimental treatment group and a comparison group or when assessing the association between two variables.

Bivariate linear regression A regression model commonly used to describe and evaluate the relationship between a single continuous dependent variable and a single independent variable. Also referred to as simple linear regression or two-variable linear regression.

Blinding (masking) Technique that ensures that those involved (patients, investigators, or monitors) in a research investigation are unaware of which treatment group patients have been allocated to until the study has ended.

Block randomization The process of dividing potential study subjects into a specified number of "blocks" to be randomized at the beginning of a trial as a means to ensure that the number of subjects in each treatment group will be equal.

Boolean operators Literature search terms that are used to connect key words based on mathematical logic.

Box and whisker plot A visually meaningful way of presenting the range or spread of data that allows the researcher to pinpoint the minimum and maximum values in the data and highlight the interquartile range and median (and sometimes the mean). Also call a boxplot.

Carryover effect Outcomes that remain or linger after the first treatment phase in crossover designs.

Case-control study Research design that compares the frequency of exposure among cases that experience an outcome event and controls who do not have the outcome event.

Case report A brief report of clinical characteristics or course from a single clinical subject or event without a comparison.

Case series A descriptive study that consists of a group of patients who have been diagnosed with the same condition or are following similar procedures over a period of time.

CATmaker Critically appraised software that guides the reader through the critical appraisal process for several different types of articles, such as those on therapy, harm, diagnosis and prognosis.

Causality The presence of a cause-and-effect relationship between the treatment (cause) and clinical outcome (effect).

Censoring The situation that occurs when the time to event occurrence is not known exactly such that there is some information about survival time, but not complete information.

It may occur because participants drop out of the study before its conclusion or some participants may not experience the event over the time frame of the study.

Central limit theorem An underlying concept in inferential statistics related to the law of large numbers. It states that the mean of the sampling distribution of the mean will be equal to the mean of the underlying population (i.e., the mean of all the sample means will equal the population mean), the standard deviation of the sampled means is equal to the standard error of the mean, and the sampling distribution of the sample mean will approach a normal distribution as the sample size increases regardless of the underlying distribution of the variable.

Chalmers scale A 32-item scale used to assess descriptions of methodology, statistical analysis, and presentation of results of clinical research.

Chi-square test of homogeneity A statistical method that can be used for testing the differences between the proportions of two or more groups, where the groups are said to be independent; thus, it involves comparing the groups on a dichotomous outcome variable.

Clinical endpoint Direct measure of how a patient feels, functions, or survives.

Clinical expertise The use of clinical skills and previous experience to evaluate evidence and the patient's health status and preferences.

Clinical practice guidelines Systematically developed statements that can be used to assist practitioners and patients in making healthcare decisions for specific clinical circumstances.

Clinical research Research that directly involves a particular person or group of people or uses materials from humans, such as their behavior or samples of their tissue.

Clinical research protocol A standardized document that provides instructions to the investigators on all aspects of carrying out the clinical research.

Clinical significance The practical importance or relevance to practice of the findings from a study.

Clinic-based case-control studies Study design whereby cases with the relevant disease of interest at a clinic are selected and then controls without the disease are selected from the same clinic.

Closed cohort A study that starts start with a set group of individuals who are followed forward in time to determine if they develop the disease outcome.

Close-ended question A type of question format whereby respondents are presented with a specific set of response choices from which they have to choose an answer.

Cluster randomization design Research design that involves selection of a specific group of subjects for randomization, such as those enrolled in a clinic or hospital.

Coefficient estimates Estimates of the parameters from a regression analysis summarizing the relationship between a dependent variable and the independent variable(s). In simple linear regression, the coefficient estimate for the predictor variable (i.e., the slope estimate) provides information about the average amount of change in the dependent variable for each one-unit increase in the predictor variable, whereas in multiple linear regression the coefficient estimate for a certain predictor variable, X, provides information us about the average amount of change in the dependent variable for each one-unit increase in X, holding all other specified predictors in the model constant.

Coefficient of variation A measure of relative variation for visualizing the extent of variability in a set of data; it is calculated as the standard deviation divided by the mean and should only be used for ratio level data.

Cohen's *d* A standardized effect size that is calculated by dividing the difference between the two means by an estimate of the population standard deviation (e.g., the pooled standard deviation for the two groups).

Cohort study Observational study wherein two groups, exposed and unexposed, are followed over a period of time until the development of the outcome of interest.

Common Rule Refers to the Federal Policy for the Protection of Human Subjects in the Code of Federal Regulations at 45 CFR 46 that has been adopted by 15 federal agencies.

Comparative effectiveness research The generation and synthesis of evidence that compares the benefits and harms of alternative methods to prevent, diagnose, treat, and monitor a clinical condition or to improve delivery of care.

Compendium A summary of information on a particular subject, such as drug information.

Composite endpoint An endpoint that represents the combining of multiple single endpoints that are then reported together.

Concordant pair When the exposure status is the same for both the case and control within a pair in a matched case-control study.

Confidence interval The range of values denoted by the upper and lower limits that describe the plausible values of a calculated point estimate; this relates to the amount of uncertainty or precision in an estimate of the parameter.

Conflict of interest Situations in which a researcher's financial or other personal considerations may compromise, or appear to compromise, the investigator's professional judgment in conducting or reporting research.

Confounder A factor in a study that is associated with both the exposure (e.g., treatment) and the outcome. Also called a confounding factor.

Confounding effect The distortion of the relationship between an independent variable and a dependent variable due to another variable called a confounder.

Confounding factor A factor in a study that is associated with both the exposure (e.g., treatment) and the outcome. Also called a confounder.

Consolidated Standards of Reporting Trials (CONSORT) The minimum set of recommendations for preparing reports of randomized controlled trials.

Construct validity The extent to which an instrument measures the underlying construct that it purports to measure.

Content validity The extent to which a measurement contains the required domains or areas to accurately measure a concept.

Continuous variables Variables that may take an infinite number of values within a given range.

Control variables Variables that are related to the dependent variable that are typically included in research studies in an effort to hold external conditions constant; statistical methods can be used to assess the effect of the independent variable on the dependent variable while keeping the control variables constant.

Controls In a case-control study, those subjects who do not have the outcome event or disease.

Convenience sample A nonrandom sample of respondents that is available to a researcher at a given place or time.

Convergent validity The extent to which similar constructs are correlated with one another.

Cost-benefit analysis An evaluation of the monetary value assigned to the costs of therapy and the beneficial health outcomes.

Cost-effective analysis A measure of cost per unit health outcome in natural units.

Cost-minimization analysis An evaluation of the costs of comparable drug therapies.

Cost-utility analysis The assignment and analyses of utility weights to outcomes in relation to costs.

Cox proportional hazards regression model A regression model commonly used to describe and evaluate the relationship between a dependent variable that represents the occurrence and timing of an event with the possibility of censored data (i.e., time-until-event data with censoring) and one or more independent variables. It is a statistical model used in survival analysis.

Criterion validity The ability of an instrument to correlate well with a particular criterion or standard.

Critical appraisal Systematic analytical evaluation of research to determine its value and relevance for a given situation.

Critical-appraisal tools Checklists or rubrics that provide a systematic approach to appraise an article to easily discover methodological flaws.

Crossover design Research design that ensures that each subject receives all of the interventions based on a specified sequence of events.

Cross-sectional study Study that examines population characteristics at a cross-section (one point) in time.

Data and Safety Monitoring Board A committee of scientists who are not associated with the conduct of a study who evaluate adverse events at regularly scheduled intervals during the course of a study and provide feedback to the investigator and the Institutional Review Board (IRB) regarding continuation of a study as planned.

Dependent variable The presumed effect, outcome, or response in a study; it is the variable that is to be explained or predicted by the independent variables.

Descriptive statistics The branch of statistics devoted to summarizing, organizing, and presenting data through tables, plots, graphs, charts, and numerical summary measures.

Descriptive studies Studies that describe or summarize information about a disease or events without making any causal inferences.

Detection bias Bias caused by systematic differences between groups in how outcomes are determined.

Development Systematic application of knowledge or understanding that is directed toward the production of useful materials, devices, or systems or methods.

Diagnostic bias Bias that occurs when the exposure affects the diagnosis and hence the selection of cases in a case-control study.

Differential misclassification Occurs when the accurate measurement of a disease depends on the exposure and results in a biased estimate of effect.

Directional test A type of statistical hypothesis test where a direction is specified *a priori*; for example, stating that the effect in the treatment group is greater than the control group.

Discordant pair When the exposure status differs for the case and control within a pair in a matched case-control study.

Discrete variables Variables that usually take on only a few possible values and are characterized by gaps or interruptions in the values they can assume. Also called categorical variables.

Discriminant validity The extent to which an instrument purporting to measure a construct is different from theoretically unrelated constructs.

Discussion section The part of a research report or journal article that provides the interpretation and explanation of the research findings in the context of previous research or theory.

Double-blind trial A trial in which the participants (subjects) as well as those involved in the assessment (investigators and assessors) are unaware of the randomization schedule.

Dummy variables Variables that can be used to represent the categories of discrete independent variables in regression analysis.

Ecological fallacy Inappropriately making an inference about an individual based on aggregate data for the observed group.

Ecological studies Studies that compare groups of individuals rather than the individuals themselves.

Effect modification The finding that the relationship between the independent variable of interest and the dependent variable depends on the values of a third variable, called an effect modifier.

Effect modifier A variable that alters the strength and/or direction of the relationship between an independent variable and the dependent variable.

Effect size A measure to communicate the magnitude of a relation or an effect; in power analysis, it reflects a clinically (or scientifically) relevant treatment effect that the study should be able to detect. In the case of a two-group problem, it may be the difference between two means or proportions.

Effectiveness The effect of the treatment on disease outcomes in typical clinical settings.

Efficacy The effect of a treatment on disease outcomes in ideal settings.

Empirical distribution A type of distribution of a given variable based on the observed relative frequencies of the occurrence of the values in the data set.

Empiricism A theory of knowledge that states that knowledge comes primarily from human experience.

Ethical principles The principles of respect for persons, beneficence, and justice that must underpin all research with human subjects.

Evidence Findings from clinical research, especially from patient-centered research, that are relevant to patient care.

Evidence-based medicine The integration of the best research evidence with clinical expertise and patient values for provision of patient-centered care.

Exclusion criteria Factors that could confound or impair the ability to interpret a study's results.

Experimental design Research design whereby the researcher controls the treatment (independent variable) through randomization and determines its impact on the clinical outcome (dependent variable).

Exploding The use of all of all relevant subheadings for a term in a literature search in order to gather as many relevant search results as possible.

Exposed group Those subjects who are observed to have the exposure at baseline in a cohort study.

Exposure (or exposure status) An innate trait, contact, experience, intake, etc. that is potentially detrimental or protective and whose effect on the outcome is being examined in a cohort study.

External validity The extent to which the results of a study can be generalized to other populations or settings.

Face validity The extent to which a test appears to measure what it is supposed to measure.

Factorial randomized trials Trials that are designed to evaluate multiple interventions in a single experiment.

False negative rate The proportion of individuals with the disease who are incorrectly identified by the test as being negative for the disease (i.e., do not have the disease).

False positive rate The proportion of individuals without the disease who are incorrectly identified by the test as being positive for the disease (i.e., have the disease).

Fixed cohort Studies that incorporate closed cohorts with fixed follow-up times.

Focused search The use of a limited number of relevant subheadings for a term in order to limit the number of literature search results.

Foraging tool A tool used to browse the available clinical literature for new and important information.

Forest plot The primary mechanism for conveying the results of meta-analyses; such plots help to illustrate not only the pooled estimate, but also summarize the results of each study included in a meta-analysis and allow for an assessment of the contribution of each study.

Frequency table A simple form of visual representation of data that can be used to organize discrete or continuous data at any level of measurement; such tables are used to present counts or frequencies of each value category within a variable.

Funnel plot Scatterplot illustrating the relationship between treatment effect estimates from individual studies and precision (e.g., standard error or variance); such plots are one approach that can be used to assess the risk of publication bias.

Generalizability The extent to which observations in the study population can be extrapolated to the overall population of interest.

GRADE A framework that can be used to convey the strength of evidence when summarizing reviews. GRADE is an acronym that stands for **G**rading of **R**ecommendations **A**ssessment, **D**evelopment, and **E**valuation. The GRADE approach recommends evaluating the strength of evidence for each major outcome, and for each comparison made. The strength of evidence is evaluated for the body of evidence (rather than component studies) in terms of risk of bias, consistency, directness, and precision.

Hawthorne effect Modification in a study subject's behavior because of the fact that he or she is being studied or observed.

Hazard Can be thought of as the risk of event occurrence at time *t*. Technically, the hazard is a rate and takes the form of the number of events per interval of time.

Hazard function The collection of an individual's hazard for an event over time.

Hazard ratio (HR) Conceptually identical to a rate ratio (a ratio of two rates). The interpretation of the HR is similar to that of an odds ratio; an HR = 1.0 suggests no relationship between the predictor and the timing of event occurrence.

Heterogeneity Reflects the variation of results of studies included in a meta-analysis. Generally, lesser variability in study results and low heterogeneity is preferred.

Hierarchy of evidence A system to rank various types of evidence based on freedom from bias, scientific reliability, and clinical usefulness.

Histogram A way to graph continuous data that have been apportioned into discrete categories.

Historical control An external group of patients who were observed at a different time.

History Changes in the outcomes of a study due to the occurrence of external events during the course of the study.

Hospital case-control studies Study design whereby cases with the relevant disease of interest at a hospital are selected and then controls without the disease are selected from the same hospital.

Human subjects research Research on living individuals about whom an investigator conducting research obtains (1) data through intervention or interaction with the individuals, or (2) identifiable private information.

Hypothesis testing An approach to statistical inference where a null hypothesis is developed and data from a sample are used to generate test statistics to determine the strength of the evidence

against null hypothesis. Results in making a determination of whether the null hypothesis should be rejected.

Hypothesis A relationship that is being evaluated between an intervention/exposure and an outcome, or between two or more variables.

Incidence A measure of the number of new cases of a disease (or symptom or problem) that develop in a population during a given time period. It may be reported as a frequency count, proportion, or rate.

Incident cases Newly diagnosed cases.

Inclusion criteria The specific characteristics that the investigator is most interested in studying.

Independent groups *t*-test A statistical method that can be used for testing the differences between the means of two groups, where the groups are said to be independent (meaning that knowing the values of the observations in one group tells you nothing about the observations in the other group). Also called the unpaired or two-sample *t*-test.

Independent variable A variable that is hypothesized to explain an observed clinical phenomenon; thus, the independent (or explanatory) variables explain or predict the values of the dependent variable.

Induction period The time period between when a person is exposed and the disease or outcome is initiated.

Inefficient In statistical estimation, when the results in terms of variation of the parameter estimate (e.g., the estimated standard error) obtained without adjusting for certain variables are different than when adjusting for the variables. More generally, when the variation of estimator A is higher than the variation of estimator B, estimator A is said to be inefficient relative to estimator B.

Inferential statistics The branch of statistics concerned with analytic (e.g., estimation and hypothesis testing) and interpretation activities; its general purpose is to learn information about a population from a sample of the population.

Information bias Systematic differences in data collection between study groups regarding how the exposures and outcomes are measured or reported by study participants, care givers, or researchers. Also called measurement bias.

Informed consent The provision of sufficient information to individuals so that they can make an informed decision as to whether to participate in a research study.

Institutional review board (IRB) A board that is charged with protecting the rights and welfare of human subjects participating in research and ensuring that human subjects research is conducted in accordance with accepted ethical standards.

Instrumental variables Variables that act like randomizers; they are strongly associated with the drug exposure but are not directly associated with the outcome.

Instrumentation Changes in the outcomes due to instrumentation or technique used to measure the outcome.

Intent-to-treat analysis An analysis of patient outcomes as if all of the subjects completed the study in their originally assigned group.

Interaction The finding that the relationship between the independent variable of interest and the dependent variable depends on the values of a third variable. Effect modification is present when there is a statistical interaction between two independent variables. Although there is some debate, generally considered synonymous with effect modification.

Interim analysis Periodic analysis of study results while the study is ongoing.

Internal validity The extent to which the clinical outcome of interest (dependent variable) in a study is caused by the treatment (independent variable).

Interquartile range The middle 50% of a distribution (i.e., the middle 50% of the observations in a data set). It is equal to the upper quartile value minus the lower quartile value (i.e., the difference between the third and first quartiles).

Inter-rater reliability The extent to which results are consistent when the same measurement instrument is used by multiple raters (i.e., reproducibility).

Interval data Data where the numbers of a scale represent a rank order and equal differences between numbers represent equal differences on the variable being measured; however, a defined and meaningful zero point is lacking.

Intervention studies Studies where the researcher controls the treatment; this involves defining the treatment and provision of treatment randomly or nonrandomly.

Interview Technique for gathering information whereby researchers ask participants questions and then listen to their responses.

Introduction section The part of a research report or journal article that provides relevant background information and discusses existing literature on the subject of study.

Investigator bias Bias resulting from errors in study design, implementation, or analysis by the investigator.

Jadad scale A three-item scale used to assess descriptions of sequence generation, blinding methodology, and withdrawals and dropouts in clinical research.

Journal article A formal description of a scientific investigation that has been conducted that appears in a journal. It is often peer reviewed to ensure scientific discourse and scrutiny.

Journal club A group of participants who have common practice or research interests and who meet regularly for a defined pedagogical purpose.

Justice Ethical principle guiding human subjects research that refers to the moral requirement for fair procedures and outcomes in the selection of research subjects.

Kaplan–Meier method A method used for estimating survival functions from a sample; thus, a Kaplan–Meier survival curve summarizes the probability of survival over time estimated from a sample.

Kruskal–Wallis test A nonparametric statistical method that can be used for testing the differences between three or more independent groups. It extends the Wilcoxon–Mann–Whitney test to more than two groups, is a nonparametric alternative to ANOVA, and can be used to compare groups when the dependent variable consists of ordinal level data, or with continuous data when the assumption of normality is not tenable.

Latency period The time period between when the disease starts and the disease is detected.

Linear regression A regression model commonly used to describe and evaluate the relationship between a single continuous dependent variable and one or more independent variables.

Logit The natural log of the odds of success for Y_i (i.e., the odds of having the event of interest). The transformation of the probability of an event to the natural log of the odds is called the logit transformation, which is why logistic regression models are also called logit models.

Log-rank test A statistical test to compare the overall survival experience of two or more groups with respect to the study outcome; thus, it can be used to test the null hypothesis that two or more survival curves are equivalent.

Mail survey Technique for gathering information whereby selected participants from a population of interest are mailed a questionnaire along with a cover letter and postage-paid return envelope.

Matching Process of making the cases and controls similar (or balanced) with regard to a confounding factor in a case-control study.

Maturation Normal changes in study participants that occur over time.

Maximum likelihood estimation (MLE) An estimation method used in logistic regression (and other statistical methods) that focuses on maximizing the predictive capabilities of the regression, rather than minimizing its residuals, which is what is done by OLS estimation. MLE chooses values for the coefficient estimates that maximize the probability of obtaining the observed data.

Mean Most commonly refers to the arithmetic mean; there are other, less commonly used, measures of the mean, such as the geometric mean and the harmonic mean.

Measurement bias Systematic differences in data collection between study groups regarding how the exposures and outcomes are measured or reported by study participants, care givers, or researchers. Also called information bias.

Measures of association Measures such as risk ratios and rate ratios that estimate the effect of an exposure on a disease outcome.

Measures of central tendency Used to provide information about the center or "typical value" of a set of numbers; also called measures of central location. Examples include the mean, median, and mode.

Measures of dispersion Used to describe how data are spread and to provide information about the variability in a distribution of observations. Examples include the range, interquartile range, variance, and standard deviation.

Median A measure of central tendency that is calculated by listing the values of a variable in ascending or descending order and reporting the value that lies in the middle of this list. It is the middle value in a set of ranked values or the value such that half of the data points fall above it and half fall below it.

Mediating effect The finding that a primary independent variable leads to changes on another variable (i.e., the mediator), which, in turn, causes changes on the main dependent variable.

Mediator An intermediate or intervening variable in a causal chain relating an independent and a dependent variable. The most basic mediation model is one where an independent variable leads to changes on a mediator, which, in turn, causes changes on a dependent variable.

Meta-analysis Quantitative synthesis of data derived from individual studies (usually three or more) identified through a systematic review process.

Method section The part of a research report or journal article that provides a description of the research design, data collection methods, and statistical tests used in an investigation.

Microbiological methods Tools used to evaluate the presence of microorganisms in bodily fluids such as blood or urine.

Mode A measure of central tendency that is calculated by first counting the occurrence of each value of the variable and then selecting the value that appears most often; it is the most common (or frequent) value in a set of values.

Moderator A variable that alters the strength and/or direction of the relationship between an independent variable and the dependent variable. Synonymous with effect modifier.

Moderator effect The finding that the relationship between the independent variable of interest and the dependent variable depends on the values of a third variable, called a moderator. Synonymous with effect modification.

Multiple linear regression An extension of the bivariate (or simple) linear regression model (which involves only one independent variable) to the situation in which more than one independent variable is considered (in both cases, there is a single continuous dependent variable).

Negative predictive value The probability that a patient does not have the disease given that a negative test result was obtained.

Negative relationship A relationship between two variables such that as the value of one variable increases, the value of the second variable decreases, and vice versa.

Nested case-control A type of population-based case-control study where the study is nested within a cohort study.

Nominal data Data that can be placed into narrowly defined categories that are not in any particular order.

Non-differential misclassification A bias that occurs when the misclassification of the disease is the same for all categories of the exposure or the misclassification of the exposure is the same for all categories of the disease.

Non-directional test A type of statistical hypothesis test where no direction of effect is specified; for example, the effect in the treatment group is not the same as the effect in the control group.

Non-equivalent comparison group A group of individuals who are not subjected to the intervention in pre- and post-observational studies.

Non-inferiority trial Trial that seeks to determine whether a new therapy is no worse than a standard therapy by some prespecified margin.

Nonparametric methods Statistical methods that make few, if any, assumptions about the populations that generated the samples and/or focus on testing hypotheses that are not about specific population parameters.

Non-systematic review Tertiary resource that reviews a specific topic but differs from a systematic review in that the methodology is not based on a structured, predefined literature search strategy.

Normal distribution A type of statistical distribution with a graph that produces the familiar bell-shaped curve and has desirable statistical properties (e.g., the distribution is symmetrical around the mean; the mean, median, and mode are all equal). The normal distribution is completely determined by its mean (μ) and standard deviation (σ), and it plays a critical role in statistics.

Null hypothesis A type of statistical hypothesis that typically states there is no relationship between two variables. It is the hypothesis that is the focus of statistical hypothesis testing.

Number needed to harm (NNH) The number of patients that must receive the treatment in order for one patient to experience an adverse outcome.

Number needed to treat (NNT) The number of patients that must receive the treatment in order for one patient to experience the desired outcome.

Objectivity The absence of subjectivity or bias in any aspect of a research investigation, including definitions, measurement, design, and analysis.

Observational design Study design that involves observations by the researcher regarding the interplay of the independent variables (drug exposure) with the dependent variable (outcome of interest).

Observational technique The method by which the researcher watches, hears, or records a phenomenon of interest.

Obtrusive observation Observation technique in which the participant is aware that he or she is being observed.

Odds of exposure The ratio of the number of people with the exposure to those without the exposure in a case-control study.

Odds ratio (OR) A ratio of two odds; compares the odds of exposure for cases and controls in a case-control study.

Omitted variable A specific and observable factor that is omitted from the analysis. Failing to include (or omitting) a variable that is an important predictor of the dependent variable and is also correlated with any of the other predictors in a model can produce bias (this is referred to as omitted variable bias).

On-treatment analysis An analysis of patient outcomes based only on those subjects who completed all aspects of the protocol. Also called per-protocol analysis.

One-sided test A type of statistical hypothesis test where a direction is specified *a priori*; for example, stating that the effect in the treatment group is greater than the control group. Also referred to as a directional test or a one-tailed test.

Online (Internet) survey Technique for gathering information that involves the use of Web-based survey solution systems to administer a survey.

Open cohort Cohort in which subjects can enter and dropout over time and contribute variable follow-up time for the duration they are in the cohort.

Open-ended question A type of question format whereby respondents have the flexibility to provide responses in their own words.

Open label A study that involves unblinded participants, investigators, and assessors.

Ordinal data Data that consist of narrowly defined categories, but these categories have a rank order; the difference between the ordered categories cannot be considered to be equal.

Ordinary least squares (OLS) The simplest form of estimation for regression analysis. OLS estimation chooses values for the coefficient estimates of a linear regression equation to make the sum of the squared values of the residuals as small as possible.

Paired *t*-test A statistical method that can be used for testing the differences between the means of two groups, where the groups are said to be dependent or correlated (the sets of observations are said to be paired or dependent, such as when the same subjects are measured both before and after a treatment or at two different time points). Also called the dependent-groups or matched-groups *t*-test.

Parallel study design A study design that ensures that each subject is randomized to either a treatment group or a placebo group only.

Parameter A characteristic of the population of interest, usually represented by Greek letters (e.g., the mean of a population is called a parameter and is represented by μ).

Parametric methods Statistical analysis methods that attempt to test hypotheses that contain statements about population parameters (e.g., about populations means) and/or rely on assumptions about the specific nature of the sampled population (e.g., the variable on which the groups are being compared is normally distributed in each population). The distinction between nonparametric and parametric methods is not always clear-cut.

Patient-centered care Care that is focused on understanding the impact of the problem and various interventions on the patient's quality of life, recognizing and incorporating the patient's values and preferences, and collaborating with the patient on managing the problem.

Patient-centered outcomes research Research that is designed to incorporate patients' inputs into the research process and to provide relevant information to providers and patients to aid them in making healthcare decisions.

Patient-Oriented Evidence that Matters (POEMS) Research that (1) evaluates the effect of a test, drug, procedure, or intervention on an outcome that patients care about; (2) studies a "common" medical problem where the intervention is feasible in a given setting; and (3) supplies information that has the potential to induce a practice change among clinicians.

Patient values and preferences The collection of goals, expectations, predispositions, and beliefs that individuals have for certain decisions and their potential outcomes.

Pearson correlation coefficient A measure of how two variables are linearly related. It provides information about the strength and direction of the linear relationship between two continuous variables.

Peer review process Use of one or more independent reviewers to assess an article or research summary before acceptance for publication.

Performance bias Bias that occurs due to systematic differences in care between treatment groups or in exposure to factors other than the intervention being studied.

Per-protocol analysis An analysis of patient outcomes based only on those subjects who completed all aspects of the protocol. Also called on-treatment analysis.

Pharmaceutical practice and policy research Multidisciplinary field of scientific investigation that examines cost, access, and quality of pharmaceutical care from clinical, sociobehavioral, economic, organizational, and technological perspectives.

Pharmacoeconomic studies Studies that describe and analyze the costs and consequences of drug therapy.

Pharmacoepidemiology The application of principles of epidemiology to evaluate pharmaceutical products and services.

Phase I trial Experimental trial that involves the testing of a drug in humans with the intent of establishing the initial toxicity profile of the substance.

Phase II trial Experimental trial that involves the use of a drug with subjects with the disease in question. These trials are designed to give initial data on efficacy and continued safety/toxicity data on the drug.

Phase III trial Experimental trial that is designed to demonstrate efficacy in a statistically powered sample of subjects with the disease in question.

Phase IV trial (post-marketing trial) Study that is intended to generate longer-term safety/toxicity data on a particular drug.

PICO An acronym that stands for **P**atient, **I**ntervention, **C**omparison, and **O**utcome. The PICO question template is used to develop good questions for evidence-based medicine.

PICOTS A useful framework for thinking about clinical research questions, or key questions; PICOTS is an acronym that stands for **P**opulation, **I**ntervention, **C**omparator, **O**utcome, **T**iming, and **S**etting.

Pie chart A type of chart used to represent proportions or relative quantities of values; it is a circle with areas or slices used to represent proportions.

Placebo An inert substance that is identical in appearance to the active treatment.

Point estimate The single value that serves as an estimate of the statistical quantity of interest.

Population The general group of interest in a study; the target group to which inferences are made.

Population-based case-control study A type of case-control study that identifies cases and controls in a defined base population.

Positive predictive value The probability that a patient has the disease given that a positive test result was obtained.

Positive relationship A relationship between two variables such that as the value of one variable increases (decreases), the value of the second variable also increases (decreases).

Positivism Philosophy that states that all information derived from sensory experience is empirical evidence of science.

Poster A graphic/visual presentation of research for scientific conferences that usually employs the introduction, methods, results, and discussion format.

Power A measure of a study's capacity to detect a difference between or among study groups if a true difference exists. The probability of rejecting the null hypothesis given that the null hypothesis is actually false (i.e., making a correct conclusion); related to the probability of a type II error as $1-\beta$.

Power analysis A commonly used approach for sample size calculation for hypothesis-testing studies where a researcher uses a predetermined α and attempts to achieve a desired level of β (or conversely power) by choosing a sample size to detect some clinically or scientifically meaningful effect.

Practice-based research network A group of clinicians or practitioners involved in translational research who adopt best practices and conduct clinical research.

Pre- and post-observational designs Studies that examine the effect of an intervention by comparing observations occurring after the change to observations occurring before the change.

Precision analysis An approach to calculate sample size when the primary objective is estimation rather than hypothesis testing where a researcher is focused on determining a sample size necessary to achieve confidence intervals of a sufficiently narrow width at some fixed confidence level (i.e., $1 -$ some fixed probability of a type I error).

Prescribing information Compilation of information approved by the Food and Drug Administration (FDA) as submitted by the manufacturer as part of the New Drug Application (NDA).

Prevalence The proportion of individuals in a population with a disease or an attribute at a specified point in time; it reflects existing disease within a population.

Prevalent cases All persons with an existing disease.

Prevented fraction in the exposed The proportion of potential cases in the exposed group that were prevented by an exposure that is protective for a disease outcome in a cohort study.

Primary data Data collected directly from subjects for the purpose of a study.

Primary literature Original research; can be published or unpublished work.

Primary methods Data collected through techniques such as self-reported observations and biological assessments that are used to address a particular research question.

Primary outcome The main outcome of interest in a research study.

PRISMA A set of items designed to help authors improve the reporting of systematic reviews and meta-analyses. PRISMA is an acronym that stands for **P**referred **R**eporting **I**tems for **S**ystematic **R**eviews and **M**eta-**A**nalyses.

Proportion The number of observations with a given characteristic divided by the total number of observations in a given group.

Prospective cohort study A study design whereby groups of individuals (cohorts) that differ with respect to the factors being studied are recruited and followed over time to determine how these factors affect the occurrence of the outcome of interest in the groups.

Prospective study A study design whereby the researcher collects the data after the study onset by following individuals over a period of time.

Publication bias Bias that results from the likelihood that studies with positive findings are more likely to be published (at least in common, reputable journals), and these published findings are more likely to be identified and included in a systematic review and meta-analysis.

Purposive sample Sample of nonrandomly selected respondents who have the desired characteristics.

p-value The probability of finding a test statistic as extreme as or more extreme than the observed statistic given that the null hypothesis is true.

Qualitative data Meaningful information that is collected in words. Written observations or notes found in medical records are examples of qualitative data. Qualitative data may also refer to discrete or categorical variables.

Quality In health care, the degree to which health services for individuals and populations increase the likelihood of desired health outcomes and are consistent with current professional knowledge.

Quantitative data Data that are collected as numerical or countable information. Quantitative data may also refer to continuous variables.

Quasi-experimental studies Studies that look like experimental studies but that lack randomization.

Random sample A study population selected by a chance (random) process whereby every individual in the population has an equal chance of being selected.

Randomization The process of assigning patients to a treatment or control group randomly (i.e., by chance alone).

Range The most basic measure of how data are spread or dispersed; it is calculated by taking the difference between the largest and smallest values in the data.

Rate ratio Ratio that compares the rate of the outcome in the exposed group relative to that in the unexposed. Also called the relative risk.

Rates Similar to proportions, but they are computed over a specific time period (e.g., per year). They provide information on the frequency of occurrence of a phenomenon.

Ratio data Have all of the properties of interval data, but there is an absolute minimum or zero point to the scale; there is a defined and meaningful zero point that denotes "none of" the property being measured.

Recall bias Bias that occurs when cases are more likely to recall the true level of a previous exposure compared to controls in a case-control study.

Receiver operating characteristic (ROC) curve A graphical means to assess the ability of a diagnostic test to discriminate between patients with disease and those without disease; each point on the ROC curve represents the sensitivity and false positive rate at a different decision threshold (cutoff value). ROC curves help to illustrate the trade-offs between sensitivity (true positive rate) and the false positive rate (1 − specificity) and can be used to help determine the optimum cutoff point for a diagnostic test.

Regression to the mean Generally refers to shift in the initial extreme measures towards the mean or average in subsequent measures due to statistical variability.

Relative risk The ratio of the probability of an event occurring in an exposed group to the probability of the event occurring in a comparison, unexposed group (control).

Reliability The degree to which repeated measurements produce consistent results.

Research Systematic study directed toward fuller scientific knowledge or understanding of the subject studied.

Research and development Creative work undertaken on a systematic basis in order to increase the stock of knowledge, including knowledge of man, culture, and society, and the use of this stock of knowledge to devise new applications.

Research design The overall plan that enables researchers to gather answers to study questions and test hypotheses.

Research methodology The data collection and measurement techniques used in a study.

Research report A formal description of a scientific investigation that has been conducted. It is often peer reviewed to ensure scientific discourse and scrutiny.

Residual The difference between each individual observation and a regression (trend) line, or a measure of how far above or below the trend line each participant in the study is. It is the difference between an observed value and the value predicted by a regression equation. Also called the estimated error term.

Respect for persons Ethical principle that incorporates at least two ethical convictions: (1) that individuals should be treated as autonomous agents, and (2) that persons with diminished autonomy are entitled to protection.

Results section Part of a journal article or research report that describes the research findings based on the statistical analyses.

Retrospective cohort study A type of cohort study that involves the use of previously collected (historical) data to identify exposure status and occurrence of outcome in the study groups.

Retrospective power analysis The use of power analysis after a study has been conducted, in essence calculating power on the basis of the effect size observed in the sample and the final sample size achieved in the study. This attempt at sample size justification through power analysis generally should be avoided. Retrospective power is also referred to as observed power or post hoc power.

Retrospective study Study that involves the evaluation of data with regard to past events or existing data, such as medical records, to achieve the research objective.

Risk difference The difference in risk for the outcome between an exposed and unexposed group in a cohort study. Also called attributable risk.

Risk ratio Ratio that compares the risk of the outcome in the exposed group relative to that in the unexposed in a cohort study. Also called relative risk.

R-squared (R^2) The proportion of total variation in the dependent variable, y, that is explained by the independent variable(s).

Sample A portion of the larger population that is drawn in order to study some phenomenon of interest.

Sample size The number of participants enrolled in a study.

Sampling The selection of a subset of the population.

Scatterplot A plot of paired values on each of two variables on a traditional Cartesian coordinate plane (meaning the graph has both X- and Y-axes). Such plots are often helpful to display the relationship between the two variables.

Secondary data Data obtained from existing records or data sources.

Secondary literature Research that is intermediary between primary and tertiary literature in that it provides summary information on both original research articles and reviews. The most common format of secondary literature is an indexing/abstracting service.

Secondary methods Data collection methods that involve the use of data that were collected for a different purpose, such as patient care or reimbursement.

Selection bias Systematic error in the estimate of effect due to procedures used to select subjects or factors that influence study participation or follow-up.

Self-reports Collection of data through direct questioning of patients.

Semi-structured interview Use of structured and unstructured questions in an interview; they often include follow-up and/or clarifying questions.

Sensitivity The ability of a diagnostic test to correctly identify individuals with disease; it is the proportion of individuals with the disease who are correctly identified by the test as positive (i.e., have the disease). Also called the true positive rate.

Sign test A nonparametric statistical method that can be used for testing the differences between two dependent groups. It is a non-parametric alternative to the paired t-test when certain assumptions necessary for the paired t-test are not met or when the variable of interest cannot be considered continuous.

Simple linear regression A regression model commonly used to describe and evaluate the relationship between a single continuous dependent variable and a single independent variable. Also referred to as bivariate linear regression or two-variable linear regression.

Simple randomization The use of a random number generator to allocate participants to study groups.

Single-blind trial Study design whereby only one of the three categories of individuals (usually participants rather than the investigator or assessors) is unaware of the intervention assignment.

Skewness Indicates the degree to which data are not evenly distributed around the mean; in other words, more of the data are concentrated to either the right or the left of the mean value and the "tail" on the opposite side of the mean is longer.

Spearman rank correlation coefficient A measure of the degree to which the values on a reference variable increase or decrease relative to the values on the second variable. It is similar to the Pearson correlation coefficient, but it only considers whether the rank of the second variable is higher or lower than the rank of the reference variable.

Specificity The ability of a diagnostic test to correctly identify individuals without disease; it is the proportion of individuals without the disease who are correctly identified by the test as negative (i.e., do not have the disease). Also called the true negative rate.

Standard deviation The square root of the variance. It expresses the spread of a distribution of observations using the same units as the original data.

Standardized effect size An approach that combines the effect size and the measure of variance into a single metric; one way to think of a standardized effect size is the effect size adjusted for standard deviation, such that the effect size is expressed in "standard" units rather than the original measurements units of the dependent variable. Cohen's *d* is an example.

Statistic A characteristic of a sample, usually represented by Latin letters (e.g., the mean of a sample is called a statistic and is represented by $\overline{X}$).

Statistical distribution A type of distribution based on theoretical probability; this describes the way in which a random variable is expected to behave.

Statistical estimation The process by which the population parameters are calculated (or estimated) based on statistics obtained from a sample.

Statistical inference The process of analyzing data from a sample and using the results to infer the related values in the source or target population.

Statistical significance The condition that arises when the null hypothesis is rejected; the determination that the probability of obtaining the given results if there were no factors operating but chance is small.

Statistics The science of learning from data and of measuring, controlling, and communicating uncertainty. It involves summarizing, organizing, presenting, analyzing, and interpreting data.

Stratified random sampling Selection of a random sample of individuals on the basis of the underlying characteristics of the population such as age or gender (strata).

Stratified randomization A randomization process that ensures balance of participants for predefined strata based on prognostic factors such as disease severity among the study groups.

STrengthening the Reporting of OBservational studies in Epidemiology (STROBE) standards A checklist of items for reporting of research based on observational study designs: cross-sectional, case-control, and cohort studies.

Structured (or standardized) interviews Interviews wherein the same set of questions are presented to all the study participants.

Study sample A subset of the target population that participates in the study.

Study validity The degree to which the findings of a study are correct.

Subgroup analysis Analysis of the treatment effect within a category or a subgroup of participants classified based on demographics or other important characteristics.

Surrogate endpoints Indirect or substitute measures of more definitive, clinically meaningful endpoints.

Survey instrument A set of questions aimed at collecting data relevant to the purpose of the study.

Survival analysis A collection of statistical methods commonly employed when the outcome of interest in a study concerns the occurrence and the timing of an event (i.e., a time-to-event outcome); the Kaplan-Meier (KM) method and the Cox proportional hazards regression model are examples.

Survival curve A graphical method for portraying a survival function. In practice, with real data these curves look more like step functions than smooth curves. Sometimes used interchangeably with survival function.

Survival function A function of time that provides the probability of surviving (i.e., not experiencing the event) beyond time *t*; thus, it starts with 100% of the population (probability of survival beyond time 0 is 1) and provides the percentage of the population still surviving at later times.

Systematic review A structured process for identifying and summarizing existing studies that address a specific question; such reviews help patients, healthcare providers, and policy makers understand evidence and formulate best practices.

Target population The group of people with the desired clinical and demographic characteristics who will ultimately benefit from generalization of the study findings.

Temporal ambiguity When it is not clear whether the exposure affects the disease or the disease affects the exposure in observational studies.

Tertiary literature Condensed information from primary sources organized in a format that facilitates efficiency.

Test of difference A type of statistical hypothesis test where the alternate hypothesis is that two quantities are different; the null hypothesis is that the difference between the two quantities is 0 (i.e., the two quantities are the same or equal).

Test of equivalence A type of statistical hypothesis test where the goal is to determine that two quantities are equivalent (e.g., a new generic drug formulation is equivalent to a brand formulation); this requires the selection of some acceptable difference *a priori* (i.e., the margin of equivalence).

Test of noninferiority A type of statistical hypothesis test where the goal is to show that one quantity is no worse than another quantity (e.g., a new treatment is no worse than an existing treatment). It is similar to a test of equivalence but it is directional; the margin of noninferiority must be stated *a priori*.

Test of superiority A type of statistical hypothesis test where the goal is to test whether one quantity is larger than another (e.g., a new treatment is better than an existing treatment); this is similar to a test of difference except that it is directional.

Testing bias Bias that occurs because of changes in outcomes due to repeated (prior) assessments.

Theory A set of ideas that seeks to provide an understanding or explanation of natural phenomenon.

Therapeutic misconception The potential misunderstanding of risks and potential benefits of research participation such that participants in the study have unreasonable expectations about potential individual benefits.

Time series designs Designs that involve multiple observations over time, usually before and after an intervention.

Translational research Scientific research that seeks to apply discoveries generated during research in the laboratory and in preclinical studies to the development of trials and studies in humans. Also refers to research aimed at enhancing the adoption of best practices in the community.

Triple blinding Study design whereby all individuals (patients, investigators, and monitors) are unaware of the intervention assignment.

True negative rate The ability of a diagnostic test to correctly identify individuals without disease; it is the proportion of individuals without the disease who are correctly identified by the test as negative (i.e., do not have the disease). Also called specificity.

True positive rate The ability of a diagnostic test to correctly identify individuals with disease; it is the proportion of individuals with the disease who are correctly identified by the test as positive (i.e., have the disease). Also called sensitivity.

Truncation Use of part of a word to search the secondary literature.

Two-sided test A type of statistical hypothesis test where no direction of effect is specified; for example, the effect in the treatment group is not the same as the effect in the control group. Also referred to as a nondirectional test or a two-tailed test.

Type I error The error of rejecting the null hypothesis when the null hypothesis is actually true. Sometimes referred to as the error

of finding a relationship when none exists. Also known as an alpha (α) error.

Type II error The error of failing to reject the null hypothesis when the null hypothesis is not true. Sometimes referred to as the error of failing to find a relationship when one actually exists. Also known as a beta (β) error.

Unexposed group Subjects who are observed to not have the exposure in a cohort study.

Unobtrusive observation Observation technique whereby the participant is unaware of the observer, who may be either hidden or disguised.

Unstructured interview Interview format that is nonstandardized and flexible; the question and answer categories are not predetermined.

Validity The extent to which an instrument measures what it is intended to measure.

Variable classification schemes Systems used to classify variables according to the values that they can take (e.g., discrete or continuous; nominal, ordinal, interval, or ratio) or their conceptual roles (e.g., independent, dependent, or control variable). Appropriate classification of variables can help determine what types of statistical methods are appropriate for describing data or for making inferences.

Variance A measure of dispersion that shows how far the values of a variable lie from the mean. Can be thought of as the average squared distance of values from their mean.

Washout period The time needed for the outcomes of a previous treatment to dissipate prior to beginning another treatment.

Wilcoxon–Mann–Whitney test A nonparametric statistical method that can be used for testing the differences between two independent groups. It is a nonparametric alternative to the independent groups t-test and can be used to compare two groups when the dependent variable consists of ordinal level data, or with continuous data when the assumption of normality is not tenable.

INDEX

Note: "Page numbers followed by *b*, *f* and *t* indicate material in boxes, figures, tables, respectively."